EDITOR IN CHIEF

NAN BORG, R.N., M.N.

Lieutenant Colonel, Army Nurse Corps
Chief, Clinical Nursing Service
Walter Reed Army Medical Center
Washington, DC

EDITORS

DIANA NIKAS, R.N., M.N., CCRN, CNRN

Clinical Specialist/Neurology-Neurosurgery
LAC-USC Medical Center, Los Angeles, CA

Assistant Professor, Critical Care Specialist Program
California State University, Long Beach, CA

JUNE STARK, R.N.

Critical Care Instructor
Tufts-New England Medical Center Hospital
Boston, MA

SUSAN WILLIAMS, R.N., M.S.N., CCRN

Patient Care Coordinator
VA Medical Center, Shreveport, LA

Formerly:
Director, Critical Care Courses
LDS Hospital, Salt Lake City, UT

SECOND EDITION

CORE CURRICULUM FOR CRITICAL CARE NURSING

American Association of Critical-Care Nurses

W. B. SAUNDERS COMPANY   Philadelphia   London   Toronto   1981

W. B. Saunders Company: West Washington Square
                           Philadelphia, PA 19105

                            1 St. Anne's Road
                           Eastbourne, East Susses BN21 3UN, England

                           1 Goldthorne Avenue
                           Toronto, Ontario M8Z 5T9, Canada

                           9 Waltham Street
                           Artarmon, N.S.W. 2064, Australia

Library of Congress Cataloging in Publication Data

American Association of Critical-Care Nurses.
   Core curriculum for critical care nursing.

    1. Intensive care nursing. I. Title. [DNLM: 1. Critical care–
Nursing texts. 2. Curriculum–Nursing texts. 3. Education,
Nursing–United States.
WY18.3 A508c (P)]
RT120.I5A43 1980a   610.73'6   79-64585
ISBN 0-7216-1215-6

The opinions or assertions contained herein are the private views of the authors and are
not to be construed as official or as reflecting the views of the Department of the Army
or the Department of Defense.

Front and back cover illustrations are modified from illustrations appearing in
Victorian Stained Glass Pattern Book, by Ed Sibbett, Jr.,
published by Dover Publications, Inc., New York, 1979.

Core Curriculum for Critical Care Nursing   ISBN 0-7216-1215-6

Last digit is the print number: 9   8   7   6   5   4   3   2   1

CONTRIBUTORS

KATHLEEN G. ANDREOLI, R.N., D.S.N., F.A.A.N.
Special Assistant to the President for Interdisciplinary Education Office of the President, University of Texas Health Science Center at Houston, Houston, TX.

BETTYE H. BALL, R.N., B.S.N., M.S.N.
Major, Army Nurse Corps
Clinical Coordinator, Medical, Intensive Care Unit, Walter Reed Army Medical Center, Washington, DC.

JOHN L. CARTY, R.N., M.S.N.
Major, Army Nurse Corps
Clinical Specialist, Liaison Psychiatry, Walter Reed Army Medical Center, Washington, DC.

RICHARD DeANGELIS, R.N., B.S., M.S.
Major, Army Nurse Corps
Thoracic–Cardiovascular Clinical Nurse Specialist, Thoracic–Cardiovascular Surgical Unit, Walter Reed Army Medical Center, Washington, DC.

HELEN HOLLMANN, R.N., B.A., CCRN
Adult Critical Care Program, Senior Nursing Instructor, Los Angeles County — University of Southern California Medical Center, Los Angeles, CA.
Head Nurse Emergency Department, Verdugo Hills Hospital, Glendale, CA.

BONNIE MOWINSKI JENNINGS, R.N., M.S.
Major, Army Nurse Corps
Instructor, Department of Nursing, Tripler Army Medical Center, Honolulu, HI.

ROSEANN N. LUTONSKY, R.N., B.S.N., CCRN
Nursing Care Coordinator, Coronary Intensive Care Unit, Audie L. Murphy VA Hospital, San Antonio, TX.

DIANA L. NIKAS, R.N., M.N., CCRN, CNRN

Assistant Professor, Critical Care Clinical Nurse Specialist Program, California State University, Long Beach, CA.

Clinical Nurse Specialist, Neurology/Neurosurgery, Los Angeles County — University of Southern California Medical Center, Los Angeles, CA.

NANCY PIERCE-ERCK, R.N., M.S.N.

Independent Practitioner, Psychiatric-Mental Health Nursing, Bethesda, MD. Formerly Assistant Professor, Catholic University of America.

LINDA SCHAFF, R.N., M.S.N., R.N., C.S.

Formerly Teacher-Practitioner, Rush University College of Nursing, Chicago, IL.

JUNE STARK, R.N.

Critical Care Instructor, Staff Education; Nurse Consultant in Renal Nursing, Tufts-New England Medical Center Hospital, Boston, MA.

SUSAN VAN DeVELDE-COKE, R.N., M.A.

Full-time MBA Student, McGill University, Montreal, Canada. Formerly Teacher-Practitioner, Rush University, Chicago, IL.

SUSAN M. WILLIAMS, R.N., M.S.N., CCRN

Patient Care Coordinator, VA Medical Center, Shreveport. LA.

Formerly Director, Critical Care Courses, LDS Hospital, Salt Lake City, UT.

ACKNOWLEDGEMENTS

The publication of the second edition of *Core Curriculum for Critical Care Nursing* required concerted and dedicated efforts from all individuals involved. It is a distinct pleasure to take this opportunity to express to all participants both our indebtedness and gratitude.

We are especially grateful to the various chapter authors for sharing their expert knowledge based on their professional experience as well as their critical appraisal of pertinent literature in their specialty. We also thank them for their understanding and support throughout this revision process. We also acknowledge Sharon Robert's contribution to the developing phase of the Psychosocial chapter.

A very special note of appreciation for their untiring efforts goes to several physicians and nurses who assisted in an intensive and critical review process required in the development of the manuscripts: Ann Ameigh, R.N., M.S., Michael Apuzzo, M.D., Ronald Bogusky, M.D., Ph.D., Gennaro Carpinito, M.D., Marjorie Cengiz, R.N., M.S., Robert Crapo, M.D., Dan DeVaris, M.D., Walter Flamenbaum, M.D., Ronald George, M.D., Christian Gronbeck, M.D., Robert Hamburger, M.D., Kenneth Herbst, M.D., James Johnson, M.D., Alyce Souden Lanoue, R.N., M.S., Ruth McCormack, M.D., John Michalak, M.D., Pamela Mitchell, R.N., M.S., Georgia Stevens, R.N., M.S., Eileen Watson, R.N., M.S.

To the staff of W.B. Saunders, especially Joan Safko and Katherine Pitcoff, we express our thanks for their advice, concern, and support in this endeavor with AACN.

We are equally pleased to thank the Board of Directors of AACN for allowing us the privilege of being involved in this unique editorial venture. We especially thank JoAnn "Grif" Alspach, R.N., M.S.N., Chairperson, Publications Committee, who shared our constant concern for achieving in this multi-authored text a well integrated and holistic approach to the care of critically ill persons and their families.

NAN BORG
DIANA NIKAS
JUNE STARK
SUSAN WILLIAMS

PREFACE

In 1975 the American Association of Critical Care Nurses (AACN) recognized the need for a core body of knowledge for the critical care nurse practitioner, and published *Core Curriculum for Critical Care Nursing*. Since that time an accumulation of new knowledge and changing technology in critical care is evident throughout the United States. Today's critical care setting offers not only new and exciting challenges for the practicing critical care nurse, but also a greater responsibility in the areas of clinical decision-making.

These ongoing changes require that critical care nurses pursue a more sophisticated level of knowledge, not only to insure better patient care, but also to allow them to relate more meaningfully with others of the health care team. This second edition of the *Core* is designed to expand the knowledge base of the critical care practitioner and may be used as a comprehensive study guide, as a resource document from which a course in critical care nursing can be constructed, and as one resource to prepare for the certification examination in critical care nursing.

In this edition the primary intent was to expand and update the core knowledge required for the critical care nurse practitioner. Each original section has been rewritten and new subject matter has been added. Behavioral objectives have been designed as a means to better assist readers in validating their learning. A systematic approach to assessment of the critically ill individual has been thoroughly addressed in each of these chapters. This should enhance the practitioner's ability to gather data and should insure a more accurate patient assessment.

The first four sections are devoted to the four major body systems — pulmonary, cardiovascular, neurologic, and renal. New material on the "Management of System Conduction Defects With Artificial Pacing" written by Dr. Kathleen Andreoli is included in the Cardiovascular section, as is an expanded discussion on Shock.

The fifth section addresses the critically ill patient with metabolic dysfunction, and two new sections on hematology/oncology and the gastrointestinal system have been added. Hematologic/oncologic patients are

ix

usually seen in the critical care setting for crisis management. A thorough understanding of the physical and psychologic states of these patients will allow the critical care nurse to better meet their total needs. Many critically ill patients with either primary or secondary gastrointestinal problems will be cared for in either a medical or a surgical critical care setting. A more in-depth understanding of the underlying physiologic and psychosocial aspects of these conditions will assist the critical care nurse in the administration of more comprehensive care.

The second edition closes with the Psychosocial section, the purpose of which is to facilitate critical care nurse practitioners' understanding of the foundations of human behavior. They then can more accurately assess needs and appropriately plan and implement nursing interventions that can be evaluated in the process of providing ongoing care to critically ill patients with their family members. This section also addresses an awareness of problems that staff will encounter in the critical care setting.

The success and extensive utilization of the first edition of *Core Curriculum* has indicated the need for its expansion and updating. It must be emphasized that the sophisticated body of knowledge required by critical care nurse practitioners cannot be learned solely from this text. Since the subject of critical care itself necessitates a continuing education process, it is our hope that this edition will serve as a further challenge and stimulus to learning. Correlative clinical practice in the critical care setting is an imperative and vital complement to this learning process.

AACN
SCOPE OF PRACTICE

Critical care nursing practice is a dynamic process the scope of which is defined in terms of the critically ill patient, the critical care nurse and the environment in which critical care nursing is delivered; all three components are essential elements for the practice of critical care nursing.

The critically ill patient

The critically ill patient is characterized by the presence of real or potential life-threatening health problems and by the requirements for continuous observation and intervention to prevent complications and restore health. The concept of the critically ill patient includes the patient's family and/or significant others.

The critical care nurse

The critical care nurse is a registered professional nurse committed to ensuring that all critically ill patients receive optimal care. This nurse's practice is based on the following:

a) individual professional accountability

b) thorough knowledge of the interrelatedness of body systems and the dynamic nature of the life process

c) recognition and appreciation of the individual's wholeness, uniqueness and significant social and environmental relationships

d) appreciation of the collaborative role of all members of the health care team

To continually refine the practice, the critical care nurse participates in ongoing educational activities. In addition to basic preparation, the critical care nurse acquires an advanced knowledge of psychosocial, physiological and therapeutic components specific to the care of the critically ill. Clinical competency and the ability to effectively interact with patients, families and other members of the health care team are developed. Additionally, an awareness of the responsibility for an environment for safe practice is cultivated.

The critical care nurse utilizes the nursing process as a framework for practice. In caring for the critically ill, the nurse will collect data, identify and determine the priority of the patient's problems/needs, formulate an appropriate plan of nursing care, implement the plan of nursing care according to the priority of the identified problems/needs, and evaluate the process and outcome of nursing care.

The critical care environment

A critical care unit is any geographically designated area which is designed to facilitate the care of the critically ill patient by critical care nurses. It is an area where safety, organizational and ethical standards are maintained for patient welfare. Although critical care nursing usually occurs in a critical care unit, it can occur in any setting that meets the environmental and nursing standards such as an area which has a psychologically supportive environment for the patients and families, adequately functioning equipment and supplies, readily available emergency equipment, facilities to meet staff needs, and ready access to support departments.

UTILIZING THE NURSING PROCESS

As stated in the AACN definition of critical care nursing practice, the critical care nurse practitioner utilizes the nursing process as a framework for practice. The format of the second edition of *Core Curriculum* fosters the nursing process in managing the delivery of nursing care in the critical care setting.

The process begins with assessment – the collection of data. Through interview and observation of the patient, the critical care nurse gathers subjective and objective data (for example, a patient on a ventilator with PEEP is comatose; circulatory parameters are decreased, lung compliance reduced, and breath sounds and heart sounds are normal), which is used to arrive at a nursing diagnosis (in the example, decreased venous return related to use of PEEP) and to develop a plan of care.

The second step in the nursing process, care planning, involves coordination of input from nursing and other disciplines that will affect the patient during hospitalization and after discharge. Following the example above, planning for the patient with decreased venous return related to the use of PEEP would include a goal of returning the patient to a stable cardiopulmonary status by increasing cardiac output to previous physiologic levels, and by frequent reassessment of cardiopulmonary status.

Implementation of the plan is the nursing management of the problem. In our example, implementation would include monitoring vital signs and respiratory parameters, reducing PEEP, consideration of Trendelenburg position, administration of short-term vasopressors, and provision of adequate volume intake.

Continuous observation, reinterpretation of data, and the input of new information and knowledge provide the basis for step four, evaluation of the care plan. Determining the response to measures to increase cardiac output and establishment of stable vital signs and respiratory parameters would help to evaluate the example care plan and to change it as required by the patient's condition.

Once you have learned the basic information presented in the *Core Curriculum*, you will be able to use the nursing process effectively in nursing care. This systematic and dynamic method of problem solving has its basis in core knowledge. You must be able to assess a patient's status, use the data from your assessment to plan and implement care, and again use your assessment skills to evaluate and adjust your nursing care. It is an ongoing process requiring integration of all your nursing knowledge and skills.

CONTENTS

THE
PULMONARY
SYSTEM

prepared by
SUSAN M. WILLIAMS, R.N., M.S.N., CCRN

BEHAVIORAL OBJECTIVES

Functional Anatomy

1. Identify the major functions of each given anatomic part of the pulmonary system.

2. Describe the relationship between pulmonary vascular mean pressures and diffusion of gases across the alveolocapillary membrane.

3. Compare the sites and modes of nervous system feedback mechanisms on ventilation.

Physiology

1. List the major functions (in terms of gas transport) performed during each of the four basic steps of respiration.

2. Calculate accurately the values of clinical laboratory tests that measure the first three steps in the gas transport system.

3. Analyze the relationship between the Pa_{O_2} and Sa_{O_2} and between the Pa_{O_2} and O_2 content.

4. Identify the mechanism by which alveolar ventilation is matched to metabolic demand.

5. When given a list of five general physiologic abnormalities that lead to hypoxemia, distinguish between each in terms of etiology, diagnosis, and appropriate oxygen therapy.

6. When given a set of arterial blood gas values, identify the dominant acid-base abnormality involved and the degree of compensation.

7. For each of the four major acid-base abnormalities, list the ways in which the physiologic parameters are altered, the probable causes for the alterations, and the role of compensation and/or correction in normalizing the body's acid-base status.

Assessment

1. Describe a systematic process for assessment of the pulmonary system, utilizing history and physical examination skills.

2. List and justify the diagnostic studies generally used in assessment of the pulmonary system.

3. When given several common pulmonary disease processes, select the characteristic changes in inspection, palpation, percussion, and auscultation that occur with each.

General Patient Care Management

1. Develop a plan for nursing intervention to establish and maintain optimal airway patency in the critically ill patient, while also minimizing the consequences of airway intubation procedures.

2. Describe the physiologic and psychologic consequences of ventilator therapy in terms of etiology, probable complications, and preventive measures.

3. Compare the advantages and disadvantages, and state the therapeutic uses, of pressure-cycled and volume-cycled ventilators.

4. Justify the specific nursing responsibilities required for a patient receiving positive end-expiratory pressure (PEEP).

5. Develop a systematic nursing plan to follow in caring for the patient on continuous ventilatory support, including the weaning phase. Include all essential parameters that must be observed, measured, calculated, and recorded.

6. When presented with a patient who has hypoxemia from a known cause, select the preferred method of oxygen delivery and justify that choice in terms of effectiveness, concentration of oxygen delivered, and possible complications.

Pathologic Conditions and Management

For each of the following: acute respiratory failure, adult respiratory distress syndrome, chronic obstructive pulmonary disease, status asthmaticus, pulmonary embolus, and chest trauma:

1. Describe the specific physiologic derangements that characterize each.

2. Select a systematic approach to the diagnosis of each, based on its clinical presentation, the presence of etiologic or precipitating factors, and the results of diagnostic testing.

3. Outline the essential elements of nursing care that will meet the needs of patients with these diagnoses, and justify the treatment modalities used in the management of each clinical problem or complication.

THE PULMONARY SYSTEM

CONDUCTING AIRWAYS: The entire area from nose to alveoli where gas flows, but is not exchanged, is called "anatomic dead space." The approximate amount is 2 ml per kg body weight.

1. **Nose**
   a. Passageway for movement of air into lung
   b. Preconditions air by action of cilia, mucosal cells, and turbinate bones
      i. Warms air to within 2–3% of body temperature and humidifies it to full saturation before it reaches lower trachea
      ii. Filters by trapping particles greater than 4–6 μm in size
   c. Voice resonance, olfaction, sneeze reflex functions

2. **Pharynx**
   a. Separation of food from air controlled by local nerve reflexes
   b. Opening of eustachian tube regulates middle ear pressure
   c. Lymphatic tissues control infection

3. **Larynx:** incomplete rings of cartilage
   a. Vocal cords — speech function
      i. Narrowest part of conducting airways of adults
      ii. Contraction of muscles of larynx causes vocal cords to change shape
      iii. Vibration of vocal cords produces sound; speech is a joint function of vocal cords, mouth, and respiration, with control by temporal and parietal lobes of cerebral cortex
      iv. Glottis is the opening between vocal cords
   b. Valve action prevents aspiration by epiglottis
   c. Cough reflex — intrathoracic pressure increases to permit coughing or evacuation of colon (Valsalva maneuver)
   d. Cricoid cartilage
      i. Only complete ring
      ii. Narrowest part of child's airway; eliminates need for cuffed endotracheal tube

4. **Trachea:** incomplete rings of cartilage
   a. Conducting air passage
   b. Warms and humidifies air
   c. Mucosal cells trap foreign material
   d. Cilia propel mucus upward through airway

    e. Cough reflex present, especially at bifurcation (carina)

    f. Smooth muscle innervated by parasympathetic branch of autonomic nervous system

5. **Bronchi** (right and left mainstem, lobar, segmental)
   a. Site of division and branching of airways
   b. Right bronchus shorter, wider, and more in line with trachea than left bronchus
   c. Cleansing and humidifying functions
   d. Lined with ciliated mucosal cells

6. **Terminal bronchioles**
   a. Smooth muscle walls (no cartilage); bronchospasm may narrow lumen and increase airway resistance
   b. Ciliated mucosal cells
   c. Sensitive to CO_2 levels — increased levels induce bronchiolar dilation; decreased levels induce bronchiolar constriction

GAS EXCHANGE AIRWAYS: Semi-permeable membrane that permits movement of gases according to pressure gradients.

1. **Respiratory bronchioles, alveolar ducts, alveolar sacs**
   a. Terminal branching of airways
   b. Distribution of inspired air

2. **Alveoli**
   a. Most important structures in gas exchange
   b. Alveolar surface area depends on body size — about $1/m^2/kg$ body weight; less than 1 μm in thickness
   c. Alveolar cells
       i.   Type I — epithelial
       ii. Type II — epithelial, highly active metabolically; thought to be origin of surfactant synthesis
       iii. Alveolar macrophages prevent infection
   d. Pulmonary surfactant
       i.   A phospholipid monolayer at alveolar air-liquid interface that has the property of varying surface tension with alveolar volume
       ii. Enables surface tension to decrease as alveolar volume decreases during expiration
       iii. Decreases work of breathing, permits alveoli to remain inflated at low distending pressures, and reduces net forces causing tissue fluid accumulation
       iv. Reduction of surfactant makes lung expansion more difficult (the greater the surface tension, the greater the pressure needed to overcome it)

e. Alveolocapillary membrane
    i.   Bathed by interstitial fluid; lines respiratory bronchioles, alveolar ducts, alveolar sacs, and alveoli
    ii. About 1 μm in thickness (less than one red blood cell); permits very rapid diffusion of gases; any increases in thickness diminish gas diffusion
    iii. Total surface area of 70 m^2 is in contact with about 60–140 ml of pulmonary capillary blood at any one time
    iv. Endothelium of pulmonary capillaries sensitive to oxygen
f. Gas exchange pathway — alveolar epithelium → alveolar basement membrane → interstitial space → capillary basement membrane → capillary endothelium → plasma → erythrocyte membrane → erythrocyte cytoplasm

PULMONARY CIRCULATION

1. **Oxygen transport:** to pulmonary capillaries where it is absorbed into blood from alveolar air, and CO_2 is excreted by blood into alveoli

2. **Regulation of blood flow through lungs**
    a. Low pressure, low resistance system when compared to systemic circulation
    b. Vessels distend to allow for increases in volume from systemic circulation
    c. Resistance to blood flow decreases as rate of blood flow increases vessel diameter
    d. Pressures in pulmonary vasculature
        i.   Mean pulmonary artery pressure = 13–15 mm Hg
        ii. Mean pulmonary venous pressure = 4–6 mm Hg
        iii. Mean pressure gradient = about 10 mm Hg (far less than systemic gradient)
    e. About 12% of total blood volume is in pulmonary circulation at any given time
    f. Pulmonary hypertension is sometimes caused, and usually aggravated, by hypoxemia that induces pulmonary capillary vasoconstriction

3. **Smooth muscle** surrounding pulmonary vessels is sensitive to oxygen tension; low arterial oxygen pressure (PaO_2) causes vessel constriction, thus shunting blood flow to aerated alveoli

4. **Endothelium:** sensitive to damage by toxic substances — oxygen and endotoxins

LUNG

1. **Anatomic divisions:** right lung (3 lobes), left lung (2 lobes), bronchopulmonary segments (10 on right side, 8 on left), lobules

2. **Lobule:** contains primary functional units of lung (respiratory bronchioles, alveoli, pulmonary circulation); lymphatics surround lobule

3. **Bronchial artery circulation:** supplies nourishment for tracheobronchial tree and lung tissue

THORACIC CAGE: Sternum, spinal column, ribs.

1. **Protection**

2. **Affects ventilation by enlarging and contracting**

PLEURA: Visceral and parietal layers

1. **Pleural fluid:** allows smooth movement of visceral over parietal pleura

2. **Stability:** helps support chest wall

3. **Adherence:** pleural space normally is a potential space or vacuum, and because of a constant "negative" pressure (less than atomospheric by 4–8 mm Hg), any change in volume of thoracic cage is reflected by a similar change in volume of lungs

4. **Nerve supply (pain):** parietal pleura has it, visceral pleura does not

MUSCLES OF RESPIRATION

1. **Act of breathing:** accomplished through muscular actions that alter pressures in intrapleural space, thus changing intrathoracic volumes

2. **Muscles of inspiration:** chest cavity enlarges, an active process brought about by contraction of
    a. Diaphragm
        i. Normal quiet breathing is almost entirely accomplished by this muscle
        ii. Downward contraction lengthens chest cavity
    b. External intercostals
        i. These increase anteroposterior diameter of thorax by elevating ribs
        ii. A-P diameter is about 20% greater during inspiration than during expiration

    c. Small muscles in neck
        i. These pull upward on front of thoracic cage
        ii. Used as accessory muscles for inspiration

3. **Muscles of expiration:** chest cavity decreases in size, a passive act unless forced
    a. Abdominals force abdominal contents upward to elevate diaphragm
    b. Internal intercostals decrease A-P diameter by depressing ribs

NEUROANATOMY

1. **Medullary respiratory center**
    a. Controls rate and depth of ventilation
    b. Adjusts alveolar ventilation to metabolic demands of body
    c. Innervation via phrenic nerve at C4 to diaphragm
    d. Chemoreceptors sensitive to cerebrospinal fluid (CSF) pH levels
    e. Final coordination of respiratory cycle is result of intermingling of actions of inspiratory and expiratory centers, which mutually inhibit each other

2. **Pontine centers:** act upon medullary center to control rhythmic ventilation
    a. Apneustic center stimulates inspiratory medullary center; promotes deep and prolonged inspiration
    b. Pneumotaxic center excites expiratory medullary center

3. **Components of feedback mechanism to respiratory center**
    a. Chemoreceptors in medullary respiratory center
        i. Respond to increased CO_2 tension and decreased pH of CSF, which in turn is affected by $PaCO_2$
        ii. Cause increase in depth (tidal volume) as primary response, and increase in respiratory rate as secondary response; both these responses increase alveolar ventilation to decrease $PaCO_2$
    b. Chemoreceptors in aortic arch and carotid bodies
        i. Sensitive to below-normal oxygen tensions of arterial blood, and to CO_2, pH, and other variables
        ii. Cause increase in tidal volume and respiratory rate
    c. Stretch receptors in alveoli (Hering-Breuer reflex)
        i. Nerve endings that become stimulated via vagus nerve when lungs are distended, causing inhibition of further inspiration
        ii. Prevent overdistention of lungs
    d. Proprioceptors in muscles and tendons of movable joints
        i. Affected by body movements (as with exercise)
        ii. Cause increase in ventilation

    e.   Baroreceptors in aortic arch and carotid bodies
        i.   Respond to increases in arterial blood pressure
        ii.   Cause respiratory inhibition
    f.   Irritant receptors in peripheral airways cause bronchospasm and shallow breathing pattern

3. **Modifying influences**
    a.   Drugs that depress respiratory center
        i.   Depress resting level of alveolar ventilation
        ii.   Blunt normal increase in ventilation in response to increased Pa_{CO_2}
    b.   Chronic hypercapnia — hypoxic drive from aortic and carotid chemoreceptors is primary controlling influence on respiration
    c.   Brain trauma, edema, or increased intracranial pressure

ANATOMIC LANDMARKS: See Assessment of Pulmonary System.

-------------------------- **PHYSIOLOGY** --------------------------

STEPS INVOLVED IN RESPIRATORY (GAS TRANSPORT) SYSTEM:
All processes involved in transfer of respiratory gases (oxygen, carbon dioxide) from room air to mitochondrial chain in cells where oxidative phosphorylation occurs.

1. **Step 1, Ventilation**: process of moving air between atmosphere and alveoli and distributing air within lungs to maintain appropriate concentrations of O_2 and CO_2 in alveoli
    a.   Volumes and capacities (measured by spirometry)
        i.   Volumes — there are four discrete and nonoverlapping pulmonary volumes
            (a)   Tidal volume (V_T) — volume of gas inspired or expired during each respiratory cycle; composed of dead space volume (V_D) and alveolar volume (V_A). Only V_A reaches gas exchange surfaces. $V_T = V_D + V_A$
            (b)   Inspiratory reserve volume (IRV) — maximal amount of gas that can be inspired from end-inspiratory position
            (c)   Expiratory reserve volume (ERV) — maximal volume of gas that can be expired from end-expiratory level
            (d)   Residual volume (RV) — volume of gas remaining in lungs at end of a maximal expiration
        ii.   Capacities — there are four, each of which includes two or more of the primary volumes
            (a)   Total lung capacity (TLC) — amount of gas contained in lung at end of a maximal inspiration

$$TLC = V_T + IRV + ERV + RV$$

(b)   Vital capacity (VC) — maximal volume of gas that can be expelled from lungs by a forceful effort following a maximal inspiration

$$VC = V_T + IRV + ERV$$

(c)   Inspiratory capacity (IC) — maximal volume of gas that can be inspired from resting expiratory level

$$IC = V_T + IRV$$

(d)   Functional residual capacity (FRC) — volume of gas remaining in lungs at resting expiratory level

$$FRC = ERV + RV$$

iii.   Flow Measurements
    (a)   Forced vital capacity (FVC) — vital capacity that is forcibly exhaled
    (b)   Time forced capacity (FEV_t) — FVC over a particular time interval
    (c)   Useful in distinguishing lung conditions
        (1)   Restrictive lung disease — decreased VC without reduction in flow
        (2)   Obstructive lung disease — flow decreased

b.   Alveolar ventilation ($\dot{V}_A$) is that part of total ventilation taking part in gas exchange
  i.   Minute ventilation ($\dot{V}_E$) — amount of air breathed in 1 minute; it equals dead space ventilation plus alveolar ventilation, i.e.:

$$\dot{V}_E = \dot{V}_D \text{ and } \dot{V}_A$$

$$\dot{V} = \text{volume per unit time}$$

  ii. $\dot{V}_A$ cannot be measured directly, however, when a person is in a steady state, CO_2 eliminated per minute from lung is approximately equal to CO_2 production ($\dot{V}_{CO_2}$). Thus, arterial carbon dioxide pressure (Pa_{CO_2}) is inversely related to alveolar ventilation, as shown by this formula:

$$Pa_{CO_2} = \frac{\dot{V}_{CO_2}}{\dot{V}_A} \times P_B$$

Note: P_B (barometric pressure) and $\dot{V}_{CO_2}$ remain the same in a steady state

    iii. Pa_{CO_2} is the only adequate indicator of effective matching of alveolar ventilation to metabolic demand; assessment of ventilation requires measurement of Pa_{CO_2}

    iv. If Pa_{CO_2} is low, alveolar ventilation ($\dot{V}_A$) is high and hyperventilation is present

$$\uparrow \dot{V}_A = \downarrow Pa_{CO_2}$$

    v. If Pa_{CO_2} is within normal limits, $\dot{V}_A$ is adequate

$$\text{normal } \dot{V}_A = \text{normal } Pa_{CO_2}$$

    vi. If Pa_{CO_2} is high, $\dot{V}_A$ is low and hypoventilation is present

$$\downarrow \dot{V}_A = \uparrow Pa_{CO_2}$$

  c. Pressures within chest — pressure changes are due to respiratory muscles alternately decreasing and increasing size of thorax
    i. Air flows into lungs when intrapulmonary air pressure falls below atmospheric pressure
    ii. Air flows out of lungs when intrapulmonary air pressure exceeds atmospheric pressure
    iii. Intrapleural pressure is normally negative with respect to atmospheric pressure, owing to elastic recoil of lungs tending to pull away from chest wall; this "negative" pressure prevents collapse of lung

Approximate changes in pressures throughout ventilatory cycle

Pressures	At Rest (no air flow)	Inspiration	Expiration
1. Atmospheric (P_B)	760 mm Hg	760	760
2. Intrapulmonary	760 mm Hg	757	763
3. Intrapleural	756 mm Hg	750	756

    iv. Increased effort (forced inspiration or expiration) may produce much greater changes in intrapulmonary and intrapleural pressures during inspiration and expiration
  d. Compliance (C) is a measure of expansibility of lungs and/or thorax; it is the reciprocal of elastance
    i. Expressed as volume increases in lungs (liters) for each unit increase in intra-alveolar pressure (cm H_2O)
    ii. Static compliance (C_{st})
      (a) Measured under no flow conditions
      (b) About 100 ml volume per cm H_2O pressure normally
      (c) Measured by dividing tidal volume by plateau pressure (minus PEEP if applicable)
    iii. Dynamic (effective) compliance (C_{dyn})
      (a) Measured during flow conditions

(b) About 50 ml/cm H_2O normally

(c) Measured by dividing tidal volume by peak inspiratory pressure (minus PEEP if applicable)

    iv. Decreased by conditions that make lungs and/or thorax stiffer or reduce expansibility — e.g., atelectasis, pneumonia, pulmonary edema, fibrotic changes, pleural effusion, pneumothorax, kyphoscoliosis, obesity, abdominal distention, flail chest, splinting (pain)

e. Airway resistance

    i. Results from friction between molecules of flowing gas and walls of airways; ratio of alveolar pressure change across airway to rate of air flow

    ii. Increased with bronchospasm, space-occupying lesions, pulmonary emphysema, secretions, artificial airways, laryngeal or tracheal strictures or edema

    iii. Comparison of C_{st} and C_{dyn} gives an indication of airway resistance

2. **Step 2, Diffusion:** alveolar air to pulmonary capillary bed

a. Ability of lung to transfer gases is called diffusing capacity of lung (D_L)

b. CO_2 is 20 times more diffusible across alveolocapillary membrane than is O_2; if membrane is progressively damaged, its decreased capacity for transporting O_2 into blood is almost always more of a problem than its decreased capacity for transporting CO_2 out

c. Diffusion is determined by

    i. Surface area available for gas transfer

    ii. Integrity of alveolocapillary membrane

    iii. Amount of hemoglobin in blood

    iv. Diffusion coefficient of gas

    v. Driving pressure — difference between alveolar gas tension (normal P_{AO_2} = 104 mm Hg, P_{ACO_2} = 40) and gas tension in pulmonary capillary blood (normal $P\bar{v}_{O_2}$ = 40, $P\bar{v}_{CO_2}$ = 45). Po_2 in pulmonary capillaries rises until it is equal or close to P_{AO_2}

        (a) During breathing of 100% O_2, P_{AO_2} becomes so large that difference between P_{AO_2} and $P\bar{v}_{O_2}$ significantly increases, proportionately increasing driving pressure

        (b) Therefore, hypoxemia due solely to diffusion defects is completely obliterated by breathing 100% oxygen

d. A-a gradient $(P_{A-a}O_2$ or A-a $DO_2)$ is difference between alveolar oxygen tension (P_{AO_2}) and arterial oxygen tension (Pa_{O_2}); always a positive figure

    i. Normal gradient in young adult is less than 10 mm Hg (on room air)

      ii.   Provides index of how efficient lung has been in equilibrating pulmonary capillary O_2 with alveolar O_2 ; indicates if gas transfer is normal

     iii. Large A-a gradient generally indicates lung is site of dysfunction (except when true right-to-left shunting is present)

     iv. Formula for calculation (on room air)

$$\text{A-a gradient} = P_{A}O_2 - P_aO_2$$

$$P_{A}O_2 = P_{I}O_2 - (P_aCO_2 \div 0.8)$$

$$P_{I}O_2 = (P_B - 47) \times F_{I}O_2$$

Where: 47 mm Hg is the vapor pressure of water at 37°C;

        $P_{I}O_2$ is pressure of inspired oxygen;

        $F_{I}O_2$ is fraction (concentration) of inspired oxygen

        0.8 is assumed respiratory quotient (ratio of CO_2 produced to O_2 consumed per unit time)

Therefore:

$$F_{I}O_2(P_B - 47) - (P_aCO_2 \div 0.8) - P_aO_2 = \text{A-a gradient}$$

Example:

$$0.21\,(760 - 47) - (40 \div 0.8) - 90 = 10$$

     v.   Normally, values for A-a gradient increase with age and with increased $F_{I}O_2$

     vi. Conditions causing increased A-a gradient
        (a) Ventilation-perfusion ($\dot{V}/\dot{Q}$) mismatching
        (b) Shunting
        (c) Diffusion abnormalities (diffuse pulmonary fibrosis)

3. **Step 3, Transport of gases in blood**
   a. Approximately 97% of oxygen is transported in chemical combination with hemoglobin (Hb) in red blood cell, and only 3% is carried dissolved in plasma; P_aO_2 only measures dissolved O_2

   b. Each gram of Hb can combine maximally with 1.39 ml of oxygen (the value 1.34 is also used).

   c. Amount of oxygen transported per minute in blood is determined by cardiac output and oxygen content of blood (dissolved O_2 is omitted from these formulas in view of its relatively small amounts)

    i.   Oxygen capacity (CaO_2) is maximal amount of oxygen the blood can carry; expressed as ml of O_2 per 100 ml of blood (Vol %)

$$O_2 \text{ capacity} = Hb \times 1.39$$

    ii. Oxygen content is actual amount of oxygen contained in blood; expressed as Vol %

$$O_2 \text{ content} = O_2 \text{ capacity} \times O_2 \text{ saturation}$$

    iii. O_2 saturation (SaO_2) is percentage O_2 capacity actually carried in blood

$$SaO_2 = \frac{O_2 \text{ content}}{O_2 \text{ capacity}} \times 100\%$$

    iv. Oxygen transport is expressed as ml of O_2 per minute.

$$O_2 \text{ transport} = O_2 \text{ content} \times 10 \times \text{cardiac output}$$

The factor 10 converts O_2 content per 100 ml to cardiac output in liters per minute

    v. Focusing only on PaO_2 is unwise — an underestimation of the severity of hypoxemia may result; O_2 content and transport are more reliable measurements because they consider Hb level and cardiac output

  d. Relationship between PaO_2 and O_2 content is expressed in oxyhemoglobin dissociation curve

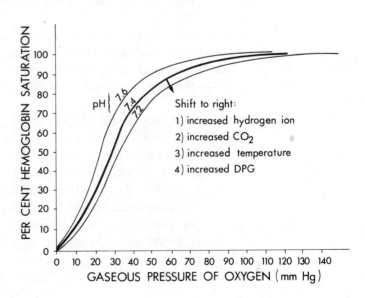

Figure 1-1. Shift of the oxygen-hemoglobin dissociation curve to the right by increases in (1) hydrogen ions, (2) CO_2, (3) temperature, or (4) diphosphoglycerate (DPG). (From Guyton, A.: Textbook of Medical Physiology. W.B. Saunders Co., Philadelphia, 1976.)

Shift to right:
1) increased hydrogen ion
2) increased CO_2
3) increased temperature
4) increased DPG

  i.   Describes oxygen content (and SaO_2) as a function of PaO_2

  ii. "S" shape of curve is very significant — relationship between content and pressure of oxygen in blood is not linear

    (a) Upper flat portion is the arterial-association portion; protects body by enabling Hb to load O_2 despite large decreases in Po_2

    (b) Lower steep portion is the venous-dissociation portion; protects body by enabling tissues to withdraw large amounts of O_2 with small decreases in Po_2

  iii. $Hb - O_2$ binding is sensitive to oxygen tension. Binding is reversible; affinity of Hb for O_2 changes as Po_2 changes

    (a) When Po_2 is increased (as in pulmonary capillaries), O_2 binds readily with Hb

    (b) When Po_2 is decreased (as in tissues), O_2 unloads from Hb

  iv. Increase in rate of O_2 utilization by tissues causes an automatic increase in rate of O_2 release from Hb

  v.   Curve shifts

    (a) to the right (more O_2 unloaded for a given Po_2) caused by

      (1) pH decrease

      (2) Pco_2 increase

      (3) temperature increase

    (b) to the left (O_2 not dissociated from Hb until tissue and capillary O_2 are very low) caused by

      (1) pH increase

      (2) Pco_2 decrease

      (3) temperature decrease

  vi. P50 = partial pressure of O_2 at which Hb is 50% saturated with O_2 at standard temperature and pH (normal P50 = 26 mm Hg)

e. 2,3-diphosphoglycerate (2,3-DPG) is an intermediate metabolite of glucose that facilitates dissociation of O_2 from Hb at tissues; decreased levels of 2,3-DPG impair O_2 release to tissues

f. CO_2 transport — carbon dioxide is carried in blood in three forms

  i.   Physically dissolved CO_2 ($PaCO_2$), which accounts for 7–10% of CO_2 transported in blood

  ii. Chemically combined with hemoglobin as carbaminohemoglobin. Reaction occurs rapidly, and reduced Hb can bind more CO_2 than oxyhemoglobin. Thus, unloading of O_2 facilitates loading of CO_2 (Haldane effect). This accounts for about 30% of CO_2 transport

  iii. As bicarbonate through a conversion reaction:

$$CO_2 + H_2O \overset{CA}{\leftrightarrow} H_2CO_3 \leftrightarrow H + (Hb\ buffer) + HCO_3^{-}$$

(a) This reaction is slow in plasma and fast in red blood cell owing to the enzyme carbonic anhydrase (CA)

(b) When concentration of these ions increases in RBC, bicarbonate (HCO_3^-) diffuses but H^+ remains

(c) In order to maintain electrical neutrality, chloride diffuses from the plasma — "chloride shift"

(d) Accounts for 60–70% of CO_2 in the body

4. **Step 4, Diffusion between systemic capillary bed and body tissues**
   a. Pressure gradients allow for diffusion of O_2 and CO_2 between systemic capillaries and cells

Capillaries		Cells
PaO_2 = 95 mm Hg	diffuses $\rightarrow$	P_{O_2} = 40
$PaCO_2$ = 40 mm Hg	diffuses $\leftarrow$	P_{CO_2} = 45–46 mm Hg

   b. In cells, O_2 reacts with metabolic fuels to form large amounts of CO_2 and produce energy + H_2O

ARTERIAL HYPOXEMIA: Disorders that lead to hypoxemia do so through one or more of the following processes.

1. **Low inspired oxygen tension**
   a. Determined by measuring ambient, i.e., atmospheric, O_2 tension
   b. If lungs are normal, A -a gradient will be normal

2. **Primary alveolar hypoventilation**
   a. "Bellows" of respiratory system function improperly owing to malfunction of
      i. Respiratory center
      ii. Peripheral nerves to muscles of respiration
      iii. Respiratory muscles
      iv. Abnormalities of chest wall
      v. Lungs
   b. If lungs are normal, A -a gradient will be normal, and $PaCO_2$ will be elevated

3. **Mismatching of ventilation ($\dot{V}$) to perfusion ($\dot{Q}$) ($\dot{V}/\dot{Q}$ abnormalities)**
   a. Most common cause of hypoxemia
   b. Ideally, ventilation of each alveolus should be accompanied by comparable amount of perfusion yielding a $\dot{V}/\dot{Q}$ ratio of 1.00; usually, however, there is relatively more perfusion than ventilation, yielding a normal $\dot{V}/\dot{Q}$ ratio of 0.8 (e.g., blood tends to pool in bases of lungs, creating an excess of perfusion to

ventilation). This is termed the respiratory exchange ratio and in a steady state it is equal to the respiratory quotient

c. When $\dot{V}/\dot{Q}$ is decreased (less than 0.8), there is a decrease of ventilation in relation to perfusion, similar to a right-to-left shunt, since more deoxygenated blood is returned to left heart. Hypoxemia and low $\dot{V}/\dot{Q}$ ratios go together as good areas of lung cannot be overventilated to compensate for underventilated areas (Hb cannot be saturated more than 100%). (See also Oxyhemoglobin Dissociation Curve, p. 15.) Example of disease state: atelectasis

d. When $\dot{V}/\dot{Q}$ is increased (greater than 0.8), there is decreased perfusion in relation to ventilation, equivalent to dead space or wasted ventilation. Examples of disease states: pulmonary emboli, shock

e. $\dot{V}/\dot{Q}$ mismatch may be corrected by giving patient 100% O_2 for 10–15 minutes (all nitrogen is washed out, leaving only O_2 and CO_2 in alveoli)

4. True right-to-left shunting

a. Occurs when venous blood goes from right heart to pulmonary artery to pulmonary veins without gas exchange taking place

b. Normal physiologic shunting is 2–5% of cardiac output (this is bronchial, pleural, and thebesian vein blood)

c. True capillary shunting occurs in arteriovenous malformations, adult respiratory distress syndrome, atelectasis, pneumonia, pulmonary edema, pulmonary embolus, vascular lung tumors, intracardiac right-to-left shunts

d. Breathing 100% O_2 will not correct shunting as all blood does not come into contact with open alveoli (Hb cannot super-saturate with O_2 to correct hypoxemia)

e. Shunting does not usually result in elevated Pa_{CO_2} even though shunted blood is rich in CO_2; brain chemoreceptors sense elevated Pa_{CO_2} and respond by increasing alveolar ventilation

f. Shunting is measured by comparing mixed venous O_2 (from pulmonary artery catheter) to arterial O_2; amount of true shunt can be estimated by having patient breathe 100% O_2 for 15 minutes, thereby eliminating effects of abnormal $\dot{V}/\dot{Q}$ and diffusion defects

5. Diffusion defects

a. Seen in patients with thickened alveolar capillary membrane, as in pulmonary fibrosis

b. May be overcome by 100% O_2 breathing

ACID BASE PHYSIOLOGY AND BLOOD GASES

1. **Terminology**
   a. Acid — donator of H^+ ions
   b. Base — acceptor of H^+ ions
   c. pH — negative logarithm of hydrogen ion (H^+) concentration
      i. Increase in (H^+) = lower pH, more acidic
      ii. Decrease in (H^+) = high pH, more alkaline
   d. Acidemia — condition of blood with pH below 7.35
   e. Alkalemia — condition of blood with pH above 7.45
   f. Acidosis — process causing acidemia
   g. Alkalosis — process causing alkalemia

2. **Buffering**: occurs rapidly in response to acid-base disturbances to prevent changes in (H^+) concentration
   a. Bicarbonate buffer system

   $$(H^+) + HCO_3^- \leftrightarrow H_2CO_3 \leftrightarrow CO_2 + H_2O.$$

   This system is very important because HCO_3^- can be regulated by kidneys and CO_2 by lungs.
   b. Phosphate system
   c. Hemoglobin and other proteins

3. **Henderson-Hasselbalch equation**: defines relationship between pH, P_{CO_2}, and bicarbonate
   a.

   $$pH = pK + \log \frac{(HCO_3^-)}{(CO_2)}$$

   $$pK = \text{a constant } (6.1)$$

   b. As long as ratio of HCO_3^- to CO_2 is about 20:1, pH of blood will be normal; it is this ratio that determines blood pH, rather than absolute values of each

4. **Normal adult blood gas values (at sea level)**

	Arterial	Mixed Venous
pH	7.40 (7.35–7.45)	7.36 (7.39–7.41)
P_{O_2}	80–100 mm Hg	35–40 mm Hg
S_{O_2}	95% or more	70–75%

Pco_2	35–45 mm Hg	41–51 mm Hg
HCO_3^-	22–26 mEq/L	22–26 mEq/L
Base Excess	–2 to +2	–2 to +2

Note: Knowledge of blood gas values neither supersedes nor replaces sound clinical judgment.

5. **Effect of altitude on blood gas values**
   a. PO_2 and SaO_2 are lower at high altitudes because of a lower ambient oxygen tension
   b. Normal for 5280 ft (Denver) = PaO_2 of 65–75 mm Hg, SaO_2 of 92–94%

6. **Respiratory parameter:** Pa_{CO_2}
   a. Pa_{CO_2} = tension of CO_2 gas in arterial blood
      i. CO_2 is a by-product of metabolism:

$$Metabolism \rightarrow H_2O + CO_2 + energy$$

      ii. Pa_{CO_2} measures alveolar ventilation
         (a) If elevated — hypoventilation
         (b) If low — hyperventilation
         (c) If normal — adequate ventilation
         (d) Measurements of Pa_{CO_2} should be accompanied by measurements of minute ventilation to assess relationships

   b. Respiratory acidosis (elevated Pa_{CO_2}), caused by hypoventilation of any etiology (may be acute or chronic)
      i. Obstructive lung disease
      ii. Oversedation, head trauma, anesthesia, or reduced function of respiratory center
      iii. Neuromuscular disease
      iv. Inappropriate mechanical ventilation

   c. Respiratory alkalosis (low Pa_{CO_2}) caused by hyperventilation of any etiology
      i. Hypoxia (rare cause)
      ii. Nervousness and anxiety
      iii. Pulmonary embolus
      iv. Pregnancy
      v. Hyperventilation with mechanical ventilator
      vi. Restrictive lung disease

7. **Nonrespiratory (renal) parameters:** HCO_3^- and base excess
   a. Concentration influenced by metabolic processes
      i. When elevated — metabolic alkalosis
         (a) Loss of nonvolatile acid
         (b) HCO_3^- is gained

      ii.   When decreased – metabolic acidosis
         (a) Nonvolatile acid is gained using up HCO_3^-
         (b) HCO_3^- is lost

b. Causes of metabolic alkalosis (elevated HCO_3^-)
      i.   Augmented renal excretion of H^+, K^+, and Cl^-, due to
         (a) Diuretic treatment
         (b) Cushing's syndrome
         (c) Corticosteroids
         (d) Aldosteronism
      ii. Gastric acid loss (nasogastric suction, vomiting)

c. Causes of metabolic acidosis (decreased HCO_3^-)
      i.   Increase in unmeasurable anions (acids that accumulate in certain diseases and poisonings)
         (a) Diabetic ketoacidosis
         (b) Drugs
            (1) Salicylate
            (2) Ethylene glycol
            (3) Methyl alcohol
            (4) Paraldehyde
         (c) Lactic acidosis due to anaerobic metabolism
         (d) Renal failure
      ii. No increase in unmeasurable anions
         (a) Diarrhea
         (b) Drainage of pancreatic juices
         (c) Ureterosigmoidostomy
         (d) Overtreatment with acetazolamide or ammonium chloride
         (e) Renal tubular acidosis

8. **Compensation for acid-base abnormalities:** a physiologic response of body to counteract pH changes
   a. pH is returned to near-normal by changing component not primarily affected
   b. Respiratory acidosis
      i.   Kidneys excrete more acid
      ii. Kidneys increase HCO_3^- reabsorption
      iii. Compensation slow (days)
   c. Respiratory alkalosis
      i.   Kidneys excrete HCO_3^-.
      ii. Compensation slow (days)
   d. Metabolic acidosis
      i.   Compensated by hyperventilation to decrease $PaCO_2$
      ii. Compensation rapid (hours)
   e. Metabolic alkalosis
      i.   Compensation by hypoventilation is limited by fall in PaO_2
      ii. Compensation rapid (hours)
   f. Body never overcompensates; therefore, acidity or alkalinity of pH will identify primary abnormality if there is only one.

Abnormalities may be multiple; each is not a discrete entity; mixed acid-base disturbances occur commonly

9. **Correction of acid-base abnormalities:** effected by a physiologic or therapeutic response
   a. pH returned to normal by altering component primarily affected; blood gas values are returned to normal
   b. For respiratory acidosis — increase ventilation
   c. For respiratory alkalosis — decrease ventilation
   d. For metabolic acidosis
      i. Treat cause
      ii. Give HCO_3^- IV or orally
   e. For metabolic alkalosis
      i. Treat cause
      ii. Give acetazolamide or KCl
      iii. NH_4Cl, arginine monohydrochloride, or hydrochloric acid are used in rare circumstances

_____ ASSESSMENT _____

HISTORY

1. **Pertinent observations:** breathing difficulty, cough, etc.

2. **General:** fatigue, weight loss, fever, sleep patterns, energy level, nervousness, temperature intolerance, general appearance, skin color, appetite, nutritional state

3. **Specific symptoms**
   a. Cough — nature, duration, time of day, length of symptoms, positional, paroxysmal, productive, effort-dependent
   b. Sputum — character, amount, whether bloody, clots, odor, streaks, aggravating factors, alleviating factors, relationship to position
   c. Dyspnea — onset, severity, exercise tolerance, wheeze, tightness, cyanosis, nocturnal, "trouble getting air in?" (often functional), "trouble getting air out?" (more likely organic), positional nature, pursed lip breathing, orthopnea (number of pillows)
   d. Nose — bleeding, discharge, sneezing, occluded
   e. Sinuses — pain, tenderness, discharge
   f. Throat — tenderness, frequent infections
   g. Chest pain — character, relation to respirations (pleuritic), rapidity of onset

4. **Medical history**: current and significant past
   a. Pulmonary diseases
   b. Anemia
   c. Debilitating diseases, chronic diseases
   d. Allergic states
   e. Past operations, injuries, hospitalizations
   f. Cardiac disease
   g. Medication history
   h. Tuberculosis contacts and tests (reason, date, result)
   i. Chest x-ray (date of last examination, reason, result)

5. **Other pertinent history**
   a. Smoking
   b. Hobbies
   c. Exposure to contagions
   d. Occupational history
   e. Environmental pollutants
   f. Family history

PHYSICAL EXAMINATION: A clinical skill that must be learned at the bedside.

1. **Anatomic landmarks**
   a. Midclavicular line
   b. Midsternal line
   c. Anterior axillary line, midaxillary line, posterior axillary line
   d. Vertebral line, spinal processes
   e. Scapular line
   f. Interspaces, ribs
   g. Costal margins, costal angle
   h. Lobes of lung
   i. Bronchopulmonary segments
   j. Point of maximal impulse (PMI)
   k. Suprasternal notch
   l. Manubrium of sternum
   m. Xyphoid process
   n. Inferior angle of scapula
   o. Angle of Louis
   p. Right and left sternal borders

2. **Vital signs/hemodynamic parameters:** CVP, PAP, PAWP

3. **Inspection**
   a. Configuration of thorax
      i. Kyphosis
      ii. Scoliosis

      iii. Kyphoscoliosis
      iv. Barrel chest (increased A-P diameter) indicates prolonged and generalized airway obstruction
      v. Pectus carinatum
      vi. Pectus excavatum

  b. Rate and pattern of breathing
      i. Rate
        (a) Tachypnea
        (b) Hyperpnea or hyperventilation
        (c) Bradypnea
        (d) Eupnea
      ii. Patterns (see Neurologic section)
      iii. Orthopnea
      iv. Labored — use of accessory muscles, flared nares, intercostal retractions
      v. Relation between inspiration and expiration

  c. Movement of chest during ventilation
      i. Abdominal, diaphragmatic, costal, upper thoracic
      ii. Asymmetry — always abnormal
      iii. Intercostal retractions (indicate effort which may be due to decreased dynamic compliance)

  d. Cyanosis
      i. Fundamental mechanism is increase in amount of reduced (deoxygenated) Hb in vessels of skin brought about by
        (a) Decrease in oxygen saturation of capillary blood
        (b) Increase in amount of venous blood in skin as a result of dilation of venules and capillaries
      ii. Visible cyanosis is dependent on presence of at least 5 gm of reduced Hb per 100 ml of blood
        (a) This is an absolute, not a relative, value. It is not percentage of deoxygenated Hb that causes cyanosis, but amount of deoxygenated Hb without regard to amount of oxyhemoglobin. Presence versus absence of cyanosis may be an unreliable clinical sign.
        (b) In anemia, cyanosis may be difficult to detect because absolute amount of Hb is too low
        (c) Conversely, patients with marked polycythemia tend to become cyanotic at higher levels of arterial oxygen saturation than patients with normal hematocrit level
      iii. Cyanosis is also observed when nonfunctioning Hb is in blood (e.g., methemoglobinemia)
      iv. Factors influencing visibility of cyanosis
        (a) Rate of blood flow, perfusion
        (b) Skin thickness
        (c) Skin color
        (d) Hb amount
        (e) Cardiac output
        (f) Perception of examiner

v.   Central versus peripheral cyanosis
  (a) Central cyanosis
    (1) Implies arterial oxygen desaturation or abnormal Hb derivative
    (2) Mucous membrane and skin both affected
  (b) Peripheral cyanosis
    (1) Due to slowing of perfusion to an area such as in cold exposure, shock, obstruction, decreased cardiac output
    (2) SaO_2 may be normal
vi.   In carbon monoxide poisoning, SaO_2 may be dangerously low without cyanosis because carboxyhemoglobin causes a cherry-red color
e. Clubbing — may have nonpulmonary causes
  i.   Pulmonary
    (a) Lung suppuration
    (b) Interstitial fibrosis
  ii. Nonpulmonary
    (a) Right-to-left cardiac shunts
    (b) Liver disease
f. General state of restlessness, pain, disturbed mental status, fright, warmth and moisture of skin, poor posture

4. **Palpation**
  a. Always compare one side with another
  b. Fremitus (vibrations felt through chest wall during phonation)
    i.   Diminished fremitus — any condition that interferes with transference of sound through chest
      (a) Pleural effusions
      (b) Pleural thickening
      (c) Pneumothorax with lung collapse
      (d) Obstruction of bronchus
      (e) Tumors or masses in pleural space
      (f) Emphysema
    ii. Increased fremitus — any condition that favors transmission of sound in chest
      (a) Pneumonia
      (b) Atelectasis, with open bronchus
      (c) Lung tumors
      (d) Pulmonary infarction
      (e) Pulmonary fibrosis
  c. Trachea — midline or deviated
    i.   Deviated toward defect in atelectasis, unilateral pulmonary fibrosis, pneumonectomy, paralysis of hemidiaphragm, inspiratory phase of flail chest
    ii. Deviated to side opposite the lesion in neck tumors, thyroid enlargement, tension pneumothorax, mediastinal mass, pleural effusion, expiratory phase of flail chest

    d. Subcutaneous crepitus — crackling sensation when compressing skin due to air under skin; caused by leak from trachea, mediastinum, abdomen, or pneumothorax

    e. PMI — deviation to left or right

    f. Fractured ribs — pain and tenderness;

5. **Percussion**
   a. May detect organs down to 4–5 cm below surface
   b. Percussion sounds over lung
      i. Normal lung — resonant
      ii. Increased air — tympany or hyperresonance
         (a) Pneumothorax
         (b) Emphysema
      iii. Increased fluid or solid — dull or flat
         (a) Consolidation, as in pneumonia
         (b) Fluid, as in hemothorax
         (c) Mass, as in tumor
   c. Diaphragmatic excursion
      i. Resonance to dullness percussed posteriorly
      ii. Diaphragm level at inspiration and expiration compared
      iii. Decreased excursion with pleurisy, emphysema, overinflation, pain, abdominal disease, sedation, etc.

6. **Auscultation**
   a. Basic points
      i. Terminology often confusing; if in doubt, best to describe sounds rather than label
      ii. Always compare one lung to the other
      iii. Diaphragm of stethoscope best for most lung sounds because they are high-pitched
      iv. Bell of stethoscope is good for localized, low-pitched sounds, such as wheeze from tumor or foreign body obstructing a bronchus, and may be used to listen at apices
      v. Best to have relaxed patient, no forceful exhalation, relaxed inspirations with patient's mouth open, sitting upright, with arms forward
   b. Normal breath sounds
      i. Vesicular
         (a) Heard normally over peripheral lung fields
         (b) Very little expiration heard
         (c) No pause between inspiration and expiration
      ii. Bronchial (tubular)
         (a) Heard over trachea and large bronchi
         (b) More expiration heard
         (c) Short pause between inspiration and expiration
      iii. Bronchovesicular
         (a) Heard in areas of lung near major airways (near sternum, right upper lobe apex, between scapulas)

(b) Sound is combination of vesicular and bronchial
c. Abnormalities of breath sounds
   i. Absent or diminished due to decreased air flow or increased insulation. Examples: obesity, splinting (pain), complete airway obstruction, pleural disease and fluid, muscular weakness, diffuse bronchial obstruction (chronic obstructive pulmonary disease, COPD), pneumothorax
   ii. Bronchial and bronchovesicular sounds heard over lung fields suggest consolidation or an increase of airless tissue. Examples: pneumonia, tumors, infarction, atelectasis
   iii. Adventitious sounds
     (a) Always abnormal
     (b) Superimposed upon normal breath sounds
     (c) Questions to ask: Are they affected by coughing? By position? Are they diffuse or localized?
     (d) Rales (crackles)
       (1) Presence usually means fluid in alveoli and airways
       (2) Sounds may be due to separation of alveoli that are stuck together because of fluid or pus
       (3) Coarse — fluid in large airways; produces continuous bubbling
       (4) Causative conditions: pneumonia, poor mobilization of secretions, pulmonary edema, bronchitis
     (e) Wheeze (rhonchi)
       (1) Indicates obstruction to flow, air passing through narrowed airways, variable or fixed obstructions
       (2) Associated with increased resistance to air flow
       (3) Commonly heard during expiration; may also be heard during inspiration
       (4) Causative conditions: asthma, bronchitis, tumors or foreign bodies, pulmonary edema, pulmonary emboli, mucosal edema (anaphylactic shock), poor mobilization of secretions
     (f) Pleural friction rub
       (1) Due to inflamed pleura, loss of lubricating fluid
       (2) Causative conditions: pleural infections, infarctions, pulmonary emboli, fractured ribs
     (g) Subcutaneous emphysema
       (1) Not a lung sound — no relation to respiratory cycle
       (2) May be mistaken for rales
   iv. Voice sounds on auscultation; spoken or whispered sounds are modified by disease in a fashion similar to breath sounds
     (a) Bronchophony
       (1) Spoken words ("99") heard more distinctly than usual

(2) Heard over lungs in which there are less air-filled spaces than normal

(3) Causative conditions: the same that produce increased tactile fremitus and bronchial breath sounds

(b) Egophony

(1) Patient says "E," sounds like short "A" (nasal "E")

(2) May occasionally occur just above a pleural effusion

(c) Whispered pectoriloquy

(1) Whispered "99" sounds more distinct and audible through stethoscope (normal whispered "99" is barely distinguishable)

(2) Causative conditions: as in bronchophony

DIAGNOSTIC STUDIES

1. **Laboratory**
   a. Sputum
      i. Smear and culture for infectious organisms
      ii. Cytology for malignant cells
   b. Laboratory procedures that provide direct or indirect support for diagnosis
      i. Serum protein (alpha-1 antitrypsin)
      ii. Serology
      iii. Biochemical
      iv. Hematology
      v. Urinalysis
      vi. ECG
   c. Blood gas analysis
      i. Purpose
         (a) Shows end result of what occurs in lung
         (b) Determines presence of respiratory failure and indicates acid-base status
         (c) Absolutely necessary in following patients in acute respiratory failure and patients on ventilators
         (d) Useful in evaluating effects of dyspnea, disability
      ii. Components – PaO_2, $PaCO_2$, pH, base excess, bicarbonate, SaO_2, oxygen content, Hb, FIO_2, body temperature

2. **Radiologic**
   a. Routine – posteroanterior, lateral chest
   b. Special – depends on nature of problem
      i. Decubitus – especially to evaluate effusions
      ii. Apical lordotic – to evaluate apices, look for tuberculosis
      iii. Oblique – for localization of lesions

  iv. Laminography (tomography, planography) — to delineate lesions

  v. Fluoroscopy — diaphragmatic motion

  vi. Bronchography

  vii. Pulmonary angiography

  viii. Lung scans (ventilation and perfusion)

  ix. Bone survey

  x. Extrathoracic studies

 3. **Special**

  a. Skin tests for delayed hypersensitivity (PPD)

  b. Endoscopy

   i. Laryngoscopy — direct and indirect

   ii. Bronchoscopy — rigid or fiberoptic

   iii. Mediastinoscopy

  c. Pleural fluid

   i. Cellular contents

   ii. Chemical constituents

   iii. Character

  d. Biopsy procedure — for histologic diagnosis

   i. Bronchial

   ii. Lymph nodes

   iii. Lung

   iv. Pleural

  e. Pulmonary function testing

   i. Purpose

    (a) Classifies pulmonary function as normal or delineates presence of restrictive or obstructive disease

    (b) Detects minimal disease

    (c) Describes disease in physiologic terms

    (d) Follows patient in quantitative terms for future comparisons

    (e) Permits description of patient to others

    (f) Evaluates risk of surgery

   ii. Components (see also Ventilation section)

  f. Diffusion studies, using carbon monoxide, measure amount of functioning gas exchange surface

GENERAL PATIENT CARE MANAGEMENT

AIRWAY OBSTRUCTION

 1. **Common causes**

  a. Upper airway (mouth to larynx)

   i. Relaxation of tongue against hypopharynx

   ii. Foreign body aspiration, vomitus, dentures

        iii.   Laryngeal spasm (adduction of vocal cords due to irritation), laryngeal edema
    b. Lower airway (larynx to terminal alveoli); cough reflex important here
        i.   Foreign bodies, secretions, hemorrhage
        ii. Pneumonia
        iii. Space-occupying lesions, tumors
        iv. COPD
        v. Bronchospasm

2. **Diagnosis**
    a. Partial or complete
        i.   Partial — air movement present, producing
           (a) Snoring
           (b) Retractions
           (c) Stridor
           (d) Wheeze, rhonchi
           (e) Altered speech
           (f) Coughing
        ii. Complete — no air movement; symptoms include
           (a) Deep retractions (sternal, intercostal, paraclavicular)
           (b) "Rocking boat" chest movement
           (c) Extreme anxiety
           (d) Tracheal tug
    b. Inspiratory or expiratory
        i.   Inspiratory phase
           (a) Obstruction usually at or above larynx (extrathoracic)
           (b) Causes: mucus, secretions, paralyzed vocal cords, tracheal tumor
        ii. Expiratory phase
           (a) Obstruction in airway (intrathoracic)
           (b) Causes: foreign body, asthma, hay fever, obstructive pulmonary disease, tumors, secretions, mucus, hemorrhage in airways
    c. Upper or lower airway
        i.   Upper — symptoms often more obvious, onset more rapid
        ii. Lower — symptoms may be less evident; auscultation and chest x-ray examination often required to confirm diagnosis

3. **Contributory drugs**
    a. Sedatives — barbiturates, narcotics, anesthetic agents
    b. Muscle relaxants
        i.   Depolarizing (succinylcholine)
        ii. Nondepolarizing (curare preparations)
    c. Alcohol

ESTABLISHMENT AND MAINTENANCE OF A PATENT AIRWAY:

Principle of care is always to use the simplest technique for which one is qualified; progress to more complex maneuvers and equipment only as the patient's condition warrants. Necessary skills include the following.

1. **Head tilt and forward displacement of mandible:** this simple maneuver will correct most airway patency problems and should always be attempted first

2. **Foreign body removal:** manual or by use of suction apparatus

3. **Suctioning of tracheobronchial tree:** nasotracheal, endotracheal, tracheostomy
   a. Signs and symptoms that may indicate need for suctioning
      i. Increase in respiratory rate and pulse, BP decrease
      ii. Dyspnea, noisy or shallow respirations
      iii. Development of low grade fever
      iv. Restlessness, anxiety
      v. Obvious visible secretions
      vi. Ventilator findings
         (a) Change in sound of positive pressure machine
         (b) Excessive coughing during ventilator inspiratory phase
         (c) Increased pressure on a volume ventilator; sounding of pressure alarm
         (d) Decreased volume on a pressure ventilator
      vii. Auscultatory findings — rales, rhonchi
   b. Complications from suctioning respiratory tract
      i. Hypoxemia from prolonged suctioning or failure to oxygenate patient
      ii. Dysrhythmias from hypoxemia and from sympathetic discharge (e.g., premature ventricular contractions [PVCs], bradycardia)
      iii. Cardiovascular collapse, cardiac arrest
      iv. Trauma to trachea and bronchi from excessive negative pressure or rough use of catheter
      v. Infection from unsterile technique
   c. Prevention of complications
      i. Oxygenation required before, during, and after suctioning (several deep inflations of 100% oxygen using sigh volume on ventilator or self-inflating bag)
      ii. Use two-person technique (one to suction, one to ventilate patient in between suctioning)
      iii. Monitor ECG for dysrhythmias during and after suctioning
      iv. Never use more than 10 seconds' total time for tracheal suctioning

    v.   Full suctioning of both bronchi necessary. To achieve this, use curved catheter for left mainstem bronchus; also, patient's head may be turned to opposite side, and opposite shoulder elevated, or patient may be turned on his side

    vi. Entire procedure for suctioning must be sterile

    vii. Adequate humidification required at all times

4. **Oropharyngeal airways**
   a. Purpose: to maintain airway by holding tongue anteriorly
   b. Complications
      i. Vomiting and aspiration
      ii. Malposition due to improper length

5. **Nasopharyngeal airways**
   a. Purpose: useful in facial and jaw fractures when oral airway cannot be used; patients tolerate it more readily than oropharyngeal airway
   b. Complications: nosebleed
   c. Adequate humidification essential to insure patency of narrow lumen

6. **Ventilation by "mouth-to-mouth" methods**
   a. Mouth-to-mouth
      i. Can deliver good volumes (1–2 liters) of approximately 17–18% oxygen
      ii. Difficult to achieve a good seal in some patients. Use of mask from Ambu-type bag facilitates this maneuver; keep dentures in place
   b. Mouth-to-nose: used in oral injuries or any condition that prevents use of mouth; patient's mouth must be closed
   c. Mouth-to-stoma: used in laryngectomies and tracheostomies

7. **Ventilation by self-inflating bag-valve-mask apparatus**
   a. Useful device in hands of experienced persons
   b. Good tidal volumes attained if bag squeezed properly
   c. Should have oral airway in; also head should be tilted and chin elevated
   d. Watch chest excursion
   e. Allow bag to release completely during expiration, or patient may be unable to empty lungs
   f. Oxygen enrichment
      i. An advantage of using this technique; 40–100% O_2 depending on device
      ii. Maintain good O_2 concentrations by
         (a) Adjusting flow rate for maximal delivery
         (b) Slow release of bag to decrease air entrainment
         (c) Avoidance of hyperventilation
         (d) Use of reservoir tube attachment

    g. Complications
        i. Inadequate ventilation if operator inexperienced
           (a) Tendency of operator to hyperventilate patient
           (b) Poor seal with mask
           (c) Inexpert manual dexterity of operator
        ii. Jamming of exhalation valve on bag
        iii. Gastric dilatation

8. **Ventilation by demand positive pressure devices:** "Elder" valve, "Handy" valve
    a. Of some use in experienced hands (as during CPR) but potentially dangerous
    b. Must be run off high flow pressure outlet, never through flow meter
    c. Patient can trigger device to cycle on
    d. Difficult to attain good seal around mask

9. **Cricothyroidotomy:** restricted to extreme emergencies when other methods fail or are unavailable — use is seldom indicated; involves making incision through cricothyroid membrane

10. **Esophageal obturator airway**
    a. Temporary emergency use only
    b. Usually easier to insert than endotracheal tube, requiring less training and skill; reduces risk of aspiration while tube is in place
    c. Disadvantages
        i. Suctioning is difficult
        ii. Stimulates vomiting; do not use if patient is conscious
        iii. If patient vomits during or before passage of tube, device can be flooded
        iv. Vomiting usually follows removal of tube; place patient on his side before removing and be ready to suction
        v. Esophagus may be perforated
        vi. May inadvertently intubate trachea

11. **Endotracheal intubation**
    a. Thorough training and retraining in this procedure is an absolute necessity for competency
    b. Key points
        i. Preoxygenate with 100% oxygen for at least 2 minutes if possible
        ii. Check for correct placement of tube after insertion
           (a) Air movement through tube opening
           (b) Chest excursion during inspiration
           (c) Auscultate both sides of chest peripherally
           (d) Chest x-ray — end of tube should be about 3 cm above carina

   c. Nasotracheal intubation — used when oral route not available, also for long-term intubation; allows patient to eat and drink

   d. Nursing care considerations
     i. Frequent mouth care essential
     ii. Placement of tube should be checked often
     iii. Adequate humidity mandatory
     iv. Obstruction from kinking may develop
     v. Oral tubes should be moved from one side of mouth to the other every 8 hours, or daily at least
     vi. Infection due to contaminated equipment or unsterile procedures may develop
     vii. Suction as indicated
     viii. Prolonged intubation procedure — Xylocaine may be used down tube or injected into vocal cords to help increase patient tolerance

   e. Nursing measures regarding cuffs
     i. Qualities of a good cuff
       (a) Low sealing pressure; intracuff pressure should not exceed capillary filling pressure of trachea (25 cm water pressure, 20 mm Hg pressure) to avoid tracheal necrosis
       (b) Cuff pressure distributed over large contact area
       (c) Large volumes of air accepted with minor increases in balloon tension
       (d) Maintains enough pressure to keep a good seal during exhalation — necessary to prevent aspiration
       (e) Does not distort tracheal wall
     ii. Low pressure soft cuffs offer best solution for meeting above qualities
       (a) Soft cuffs — conform to tracheal wall, fewer complications
       (b) Rigid hard cuffs — tracheal wall conforms to them, associated with more complications
     iii. Inflation-deflation of cuffs — methods vary from institution to institution, and are controversial
       (a) Inflation of low pressure cuffs: inflate with sufficient air to ensure no leak, or only minimal leak during peak inspiration. If increasing amounts of air needed to obtain a seal, this may be due to tracheal dilation or to leak in cuff; condition should be corrected
       (b) Inflation of high pressure cuffs: inflate with only enough air to allow for small leak around cuff during peak inspiration
       (c) Deflation of cuffs
         (1) Periodic deflation not absolutely necessary if low pressure cuffs used; routine deflation during tracheal suctioning may be useful so that patient can breathe around tube during suctioning, but aspiration is a possible consequence

(2)   Periodic deflation not necessary if minimal leak technique used

(3)   If using rigid cuff, periodic deflation necessary, although usefulness questionable

(4)   If patient is on continuous controlled ventilation, tidal volume must be adjusted when cuff is deflated in order to maintain desired tidal volume to compensate for leak around deflated cuff

    iv.   Regardless of cuff design or pressure characteristics, all cuff pressures should be routinely measured at least every 4–8 hours, and must be readjusted as patient's peak inspiratory pressure changes

f.   Extubation

    i.   Criteria — depend on purposes for which tube originally inserted

(a)   Vital signs stable

(b)   Patient awake and oriented or able to keep airway open

(c)   Blood gases within acceptable limits, after a trial of 30 minutes on nebulizer T tube at 40% O_2

(d)   Ventilatory measurement within acceptable limits

    ii.   Key points

(a)   Suction trachea, then pharynx

(b)   Deflate cuff and remove tube at peak lung inflation (use self-inflating bag)

(c)   Repeat blood gases 20 minutes after extubation, and periodically thereafter

(d)   Observe for laryngospasm (stridor, breathing difficulties). Treatment may consist of high humidity, steroids to reduce laryngeal edema, positive pressure breathing with O_2

(e)   Monitor patient's tolerance to extubation by clinical observation, ventilatory measurements, blood gas studies

12.   Tracheostomy

a.   Reasons

    i.   To remove secretions from tracheobronchial tree

    ii.   To decrease dead space ventilation

    iii.   To bypass upper airway obstruction

    iv.   To prevent aspiration of oral or gastric secretions

    v.   To deliver assisted or controlled ventilation over an extended period

b.   Uncuffed tracheostomy tubes

    i.   Used in children and in patients with laryngectomies

    ii.   Never used in adults who may require ventilatory support

c.   Cuffed tracheostomy tubes: used when patient is receiving artificial ventilation, also to prevent aspiration

    d. Nursing care considerations (see also section on Endotracheal Tube Care) — stoma must be kept clean and dry

    e. Tracheostomy tube changing

        i. Change only as necessary, especially in unstable patients (some clinicians advise more frequent changes; opinions vary widely)

        ii. Use precautions to maintain open airway

            (a) Be prepared to intubate or otherwise support ventilation

            (b) Have self-inflating bag and mask, adequate suction, oxygen, intubation materials, tracheal spreader all ready

    f. Weaning from tracheostomy tube

        i. Criteria for extubation (see section on Extubation from Endotracheal Tube)

        ii. Several variations in technique may be used; patient must first demonstrate physiologic and psychologic independence of artificial airway and of ventilator

            (a) T tube

            (b) Tracheostomy button

            (c) Fenestrated tubes

            (d) Progression from original-size tube to smaller one of same make

            (e) Breathing with cuff deflated or through fenestration

        iii. Patient monitored carefully to see how weaning is tolerated; blood gases and clinical observations utilized

        iv. Complete sealing of tracheostomy incision may occur in 72 hours; remember patient cannot produce adequate coughing pressure until this is accomplished

COMPLICATIONS OF AIRWAY INTUBATION PROCEDURES

1. **Physiologic alterations created by airway diversion**

    a. Inspired air is inadequately conditioned and is irritating to delicate pulmonary membranes

    b. Plastic or metal tubes are foreign bodies, causing body to respond by increasing production of mucus

    c. Accumulated secretions are good medium for bacterial growth

    d. Bypassing larynx produces aphonia

    e. Eliminating glottis from air route prevents patient from developing back pressures in airways below epiglottis, thereby making effective coughing difficult

2. **Complications during placement of airway**

    a. Endotracheal tube

        i. Mucous membrane disruption and tooth damage or dislodgment

    ii. With nasotracheal route, one may see
      (a) Nosebleed
      (b) Submucosal dissection
      (c) Introduction of polyp or plug from nose into lungs, resulting in infection or obstruction
  b. Tracheostomy (problems are fewer and less severe if this is an elective procedure done in operating room)
    i. Cardiac arrest
    ii. Hemorrhage
    iii. Pneumothorax
    iv. Damage to adjacent structures in neck
    v. Mediastinal emphysema

3. **Complications occurring while tube is in place**
  a. Obstruction due to
    i. Plugging with secretions that have become dried and inspissated; entirely preventable by use of humidification and suctioning
    ii. Herniation of cuff over end of tube
    iii. Kinking of tube
    iv. Cuff overinflation that collapses tube
  b. Displacement or dislodgment out of trachea
    i. Especially hazardous during first 48 hours of tracheostomy; avoid by using tube of proper length and fixing it securely to patient
    ii. Dislodgment out of trachea into tissue causes mediastinal emphysema, subcutaneous emphysema, pneumothorax. Diagnosis by: poor blood gas values, poor chest excursion, inability to introduce suction catheter properly, poor air movement
    iii. Low tube placement into one bronchus or at level of carina; leads to obstruction or atelectasis of nonventilated lung. Check placement with auscultation, then x-ray or fiberoptic scope
      (a) Displacement into one bronchus. Signs and symptoms are
        (1) Decreased or delayed motion of one side of chest
        (2) Unilateral diminished breath sounds
        (3) Excessive coughing
        (4) Localized expiratory wheeze
      (b) Placement at level of carina. Signs and symptoms are
        (1) Excessive coughing
        (2) Localized expiratory wheeze
        (3) Difficulty in introducing suction catheter
        (4) Bilateral diminished breath sounds
  c. Poor mouth hygiene; oral care absolutely essential

    d. Local infection of tracheostomy wound, tracheal tissue, or lungs; tracheostomy should be treated as a surgical wound, cultures obtained routinely

    e. Massive hemorrhage resulting from erosion of tracheostomy tube into innominate vessels; may be fatal; occurs most often with low placement of tube, excessive "riding" of tube within trachea, or pulling torsion on tube

    f. Disconnection between tracheal tube and ventilator
      i. Most likely to occur when patient is being turned
      ii. Adequate alarms on all ventilators are a necessity
      iii. Frequent checking of all connections should be routine

    g. Leaks due to broken cuff balloon
      i. Diagnosis by: ability of previously aphonic patient to talk, air movement felt at nose and mouth, pressure changes on ventilator, decreased exhaled volumes as measured with Wright respirometer or ventilator spirometer
      ii. Necessary to remove and replace tube. Always check cuff for leaks before inserting; note amount of air required to fill cuff

    h. Tracheal ischemia, necrosis, dilation
      i. Owing to oval shape of trachea and round shape of tube, there is a tendency for erosion in anterior and posterior trachea
      ii. Diagnosis by necessity to use larger and larger amounts of air to inflate balloon
      iii. May progress to tracheoesophageal fistula; this is indicated if food is aspirated through trachea, air is in stomach, or a methylene blue dye test is made
      iv. Prevent through use of low pressure cuffs, frequent monitoring of cuff pressures

4. **Early postextubation complications**

    a. Acute laryngeal edema
      i. Most frequently seen in children
      ii. In adults, commonly associated with use of oversized tube or with pre-existing inflammation of upper airway
      iii. Prevention
        (a) Close observation for several hours after extubation
        (b) Patient should receive well humidified air or oxygen after prolonged intubation
      iv. Treatment
        (a) Humidified O_2 and steroids
        (b) Smaller endotracheal tube introduced or tracheostomy performed
        (c) 2% racemic epinephrine administered to larynx with intermittent positive pressure breathing (IPPB)

    b. Hoarseness
      i. Almost universal after long endotracheal intubation
      ii. Usually disappears during first week

    c. Aspiration of food, saliva, gastric contents
        i.   Presence of tube over long period results in loss of usual protective reflexes of larynx
       ii.   Monitor patient carefully during feedings: watch for excessive coughing; start with soft food, then liquids
    d. Difficulties with decannulation of a tracheostomy
        i.   More frequently seen in infants
       ii.   Related to narrow lumen of trachea, which is further narrowed by swelling

5. Late postextubation complications
    a. Fibrotic stenosis of trachea
        i.   Cause: prolonged use of any tube with rigid inflatable cuff
       ii.   Follows earlier ulceration and necrosis of site
      iii.   Lesions may become advanced before clinical evidence appears (dyspnea, stridor); tracheoesophageal fistula may form
      iv.   Prevention: use of low pressure cuffs, frequent monitoring of cuff pressure
    b. Stenosis of larynx
        i.   Cause: discrepancy between anatomy of larynx and size and shape of tube
       ii.   Treatment
          (a)   Dilation or surgical intervention
          (b)   Permanent tracheostomy

MAINTENANCE OF ADEQUATE VENTILATION THROUGH USE OF CONTINUOUS VENTILATORY SUPPORT

1. Negative external pressure ventilators (iron lung, cuirass)
    a. Subambient pressure applied to thorax
    b. Permit long-term ventilator support without an artificial airway
    c. Use restricted to patients with nonpulmonary problems, e.g., neuromuscular disorders
    d. Make patient care difficult

2. Positive pressure ventilators: all apply positive pressure to airway during inspiration; the most important types used in critical care area
    a. Classified according to preset factors responsible for cessation of inspiratory cycle
        i.   Volume-cycled
       ii.   Pressure-cycled
      iii.   Time-cycled
      iv.   Flow-cycled
    b. Classified according to initiation of inspiratory cycle
        i.   Assisted — triggered by patient's inspiratory effort
       ii.   Controlled — not affected by patient's inspiratory effort; mechanically controlled

      iii. Combination — may be set so that if patient does not trigger ventilator, it will automatically start inspiratory cycle

3. **Comparison of pressure-cycled and volume-cycled ventilators**
   (*Note:* Models and their capabilities are continually changing. Refer to instructions supplied by manufacturer.)
   a. Pressure-cycled
      i. Advantages
         (a) Relatively inexpensive
         (b) Mobility
         (c) Run on compressed air or O_2
         (d) Can usually be repaired on site
      ii. Disadvantages
         (a) Varying resistance interferes with flow (since flow is a function of pressure and resistance), so delivered volume varies as resistance varies
         (b) Relatively low pressure capability
         (c) Inspired O_2 concentrations may be variable and unreliable
            (1) Air mix-O_2 dilutions must be verified with O_2 analyzer
            (2) Mixes are available, or O_2 and/or compressed air may be "bled in"
         (d) All settings can change with change in patient's rate, compliance, and airway resistance, so they must be checked frequently
         (e) Lack of adequate alarm systems
         (f) Cannot compensate for leak in system or around tube, so will have continuous inspiratory phase if pressure limit not reached
   b. Volume-cycled
      i. Advantages
         (a) More reliable in delivering volume of air wanted; deliver a measured amount of air at whatever pressure is required, up to peak pressure capabilities of machine
         (b) Better delivery of accurate O_2 concentrations
         (c) Built-in monitoring alarms
         (d) Allows modification of pressure delivered to chest
         (e) Equipped with or modified to have PEEP, intermittent mandatory ventilation (IMV)
      ii. Disadvantages
         (a) Expensive, large, difficult to transport
         (b) May deliver excessive pressures

4. **Guidelines for setting up ventilator**
   a. Minute ventilation (usually 6–10 liters/minute)
      i. Governed by estimated tidal volume of 7–10 ml/kg body weight and respiratory rate

      ii. Respiratory rate variable according to flow rate, inspiratory-expiratory time ratio (usually 1:2) and whether ventilator is on control or assist mode

  b. Oxygen concentration is variable

      i. Adjust inspired partial pressure of oxygen so that arterial PO_2 is at least 60 mm Hg

      ii. Excessive high levels may cause oxygen toxicity

  c. Continuous humidification necessary, warmed to appropriate temperature

  d. Establish parameters concerning sighing or bagging of patient (frequency and volume)

      i. Rate is usually average of 6 deep sighs per hour, with volume approximately twice the ordered tidal volume

      ii. If sigh not possible, can be done manually by changing machine settings, or preferably by bagging patient every hour

  e. Establish parameters concerning sensitivity settings, i.e., when patient can trigger machine for "assistance." This is adjusted so that minimal patient effort is required

  f. Flow rate should usually be 40-60 liters/minute or more

      i. Adjusted so that inspiratory volume can be completed in time allowed based on respiratory rate, inspiratory-expiratory ratio, etc.

      ii. Must be adjusted to patient's comfort

  g. Adjust amount of PEEP, expiratory resistance or retard

  h. Pressure limits to be used during continuous ventilation

      i. Should be based on cardiovascular response of patient and ventilator needs

      ii. Are usually set 10–20 cm above current required settings

  i. Check that alarms are working and set

  j. Orders for ventilators

      i. Require considerable technical knowledge of machines, combined with awareness of pathophysiology of each patient

      ii. Necessitate consultation of technical manual that accompanies each machine

5. Complications associated with use of positive pressure ventilators

  a. Cardiac effects

      i. Decreased cardiac output

          (a) Pulse changes, urine output decrease, BP decrease, decreased venous return

          (b) Treatment: Trendelenburg position, fluids, adjustment of volumes delivered by ventilator

      ii. Dysrhythmias very common

          (a) Causes

              (1) Hypoxemia

              (2) Acidosis or alkalosis

          (b) Patients on ventilators should have cardiac monitoring

b. Pneumothorax
   i. Positive pressure ventilation, especially PEEP, subjects patient to pulmonary barotrauma
   ii. Treatment: chest tube
c. Atelectasis
   i. Cause: obstruction, also lack of periodic deep inflations (this is controversial)
   ii. Diagnosis
      (a) Rales, diminished breath sounds
      (b) Chest x-ray
      (c) A-a gradient increases
      (d) Compliance decreases
   iii. Prevention
      (a) Use of sighing (this is controversial) or large tidal volumes
      (b) Humidity
      (c) Chest physical therapy, repositioning
d. Positive water balance — may be overhydrated with humidifiers, nebulizers, physiologic changes; interstitial pulmonary edema may develop. Symptoms include
   i. Increased A-a gradient
   ii. Decreased vital capacity
   iii. Weight gain
   iv. Intake greater than output
   v. Decreased compliance
   vi. Increased V_D/V_T (dead space/tidal volume) ratios
   vii. Hemodilution (decreased hematocrit and decreased Na)
   viii. Increased bronchial secretions
e. Decreased urinary output
   i. Decreased renal blood flow
   ii. Increased antidiuretic hormone (ADH) controlled by vagal stimulation and influence of left atrial pressor receptors on ADH levels
f. Infection
   i. Debilitated and aged have lower resistance to infection
   ii. Intubation bypasses normal upper airway defense mechanisms
   iii. Ventilatory equipment may be carrier
   iv. Improper suctioning technique may be employed
g. Subcutaneous emphysema
   i. Tracheal or bronchial tear, puncture of pleural lining by chest tube or broken rib, air leak or pneumothorax
   ii. Crepitus felt under skin — may extend to upper face, around eyes, down arms and trunk, even into feet
   iii. Treated by controlling cause; pressure may be relieved by making small skin incisions and milking air out

   h.   Tracheal damage, tracheoesophageal fistula, vessel rupture

   i.   Oxygen toxicity

      i.   Impaired surfactant activity, progressive capillary congestion, fibrosis, edema, and thickening of interstitial space

      ii.   Caused by prolonged administration of high oxygen concentrations

      iii.   Prevented by frequent monitoring of blood gases and administration of oxygen in lowest possible concentration to maintain adequate PaO_2 and oxygen saturation

   j.   Inability to wean

      i.   Occurs in patients with COPD, cystic fibrosis, debilitation

      ii.   Mechanical ventilator eases work of breathing for these patients, making weaning difficult

   k.   Hypercapnia — respiratory acidosis

      i.   Due to inadequate ventilation leading to retention of CO_2 and decreased pH

      ii.   Treated by increasing alveolar ventilation

   l.   Hypocapnia — respiratory alkalosis

      i.   Due to hyperventilation, causing increased diffusion, decreased CO_2 and increased pH

      ii.   If lowering of CO_2 is too rapid, may cause shock or seizures (particularly in children)

      iii.   Treated by slowing rate, decreasing V_T if inappropriately high, or adding mechanical V_D

   m.   Gastrointestinal effects

      i.   Causes

         (a)   Stress ulcer and bleeding

         (b)   Adynamic ileus

         (c)   Gastric dilatation due to loss of adequate nervous supply; may lead to shock from fluid shifts

      ii.   Prevention

         (a)   Listening for bowel sounds

         (b)   Stool charting

         (c)   Antacids

         (d)   Hematest and pH of stomach aspirate and stools for blood

6. **Positive end-expiratory pressure (PEEP):** a pressure above atmospheric is maintained at airway opening at end-expiration. Its purpose is to prevent alveolar collapse at end-expiration

   a.   At end of quiet expiration lung volume is increased; therefore, functional residual capacity (FRC) is increased. Increase in FRC is dependent on both amount of PEEP used and functional state of lungs

   b.   Major goal is enhanced oxygen transport. PEEP serves to reduce shunt effect of collapsed alveoli, and may increase PaO_2 dramatically

    c. Clinical use

        i. Adult respiratory distress syndrome and pulmonary infiltrates (characterized by closure of airways or collapse of alveoli at end-expiration, resulting in hypoxemia and need for increased F_{IO_2})

        ii. Acute respiratory failure that has caused persistent hypoxemia even though F_{IO_2} of 0.5 or greater has been maintained via IPPB

        iii. Pulmonary edema from heart failure

        iv. Avoidance of pulmonary oxygen toxicity from high F_{IO_2}'s

    d. Amount of PEEP is tailored to patient's need — there is no arbitrary upper limit; determination of optimal level requires accurate assessment of cardiopulmonary function, including lung compliance and cardiac output studies

    e. Side effects

        i. Hemodynamic consequences of positive pressure breathing are accentuated by PEEP

           (a) Venous return may be impaired not only during inspiration, but also during expiration, resulting in decreased cardiac output

           (b) Venous return, cardiac output, and oxygen delivery may be decreased even though Pa_{O_2} is increased

           (c) Goal of increased oxygen transport cannot be met if cardiac output decrease is disproportionate to gain in arterial oxygenation (because oxygen transport is a product of oxygen content and blood flow)

        ii. Barotrauma — rupture of lung tissue

    e. Nursing responsibilities: PEEP is safe only if monitored by qualified personnel

        i. Essential to monitor those parameters that indicate status of cardiac output; these include blood pressure, urine output, pulse (central and peripheral), intake-output, mental status, skin color and temperature, arterial blood gases (specifically Pa_{O_2}), mixed venous O_2 ($P\bar{v}_{O_2}$)

        ii. Ideally patient should have arterial pressure monitoring catheter and pulmonary artery pressure catheter in place

        iii. If significant drop in cardiac output occurs, PEEP may be reduced, or Trendelenburg position may be indicated

        iv. Hypovolemia must be corrected if this is a contributing factor in decreased cardiac output

        v. Short-term vasopressor therapy may sometimes be employed to correct decreased cardiac output in normovolemic patient

MEASURES FOR WEANING PATIENTS FROM CONTINUOUS VENTILATORY SUPPORT

1. **Indications for weaning**
   a. Signs that disease process is manageable
   b. Patient's strength and vigor adequate
   c. Patient does not require PEEP or more than 40% O_2
   d. Measurements of arterial blood gases, V_T, vital capacity, minute ventilation, inspiratory and expiratory pressure, A-a gradient, compliance, V_D/V_T ratio are within normal limits
   e. Level of consciousness
   f. Patient is psychologically prepared

2. **Key points of weaning procedures**
   a. Explain to patient what will take place
   b. Perform ventilatory measurements frequently while patient is off ventilator to assess ability to ventilate adequately without mechanical assistance. Measurements include $\dot{V}_E$, V_T, P_{insp} (peak inspiratory pressure), P_{exp} (peak expiratory pressure), VC, V_D/V_T ratio
   c. Stay with patient throughout weaning period; be prepared to give periodic manual ventilation as needed
   d. Consider putting patient back on ventilator if signs of tiring occur, such as
      i. Decreased V_T, increased respiratory rate
      ii. Increased $P_{A CO_2}$
      iii. Diaphoresis
      iv. Cardiac dysrhythmias
   e. If patient tolerates being off for 20 to 30 minutes, determine blood gas values
   f. Progress slowly with increasing lengths of time off ventilator; monitor respiratory and hemodynamic parameters frequently
   g. Schedules for weaning vary with patient response; there should be no rigid timetables

3. **Intermittent mandatory ventilation (IMV)**
   a. Used in support and weaning of patients from continuous mechanical ventilation. Delivers preset mechanical ventilation between spontaneous ventilations of patient. Intermittent demand ventilation (IDV) is similar, but augmentation through respirator breath is on demand rather than mandatory. Both IMV and IDV may be used as initial mode of ventilatory support rather than only as weaning mode

   b. Indications (variable)
- i. Patients who fail to meet previously established criteria for attempting a trial of spontaneous ventilation (e.g., those placed on ventilator because of respiratory failure due to COPD)
- ii. Patients who have been on a ventilator for extended periods
- iii. Abnormal ventilatory measurements

   c. Advantages
- i. Can start early in phase of controlled ventilation, as soon as respiratory parameters have stabilized
- ii. More physiologic $PaCO_2$ may be achieved with IMV than with assisted or controlled breathing; this may reduce weaning time
- iii. Safer than trial-and-error method of complete removal from ventilator because it prevents precipitous fall in PaO_2 or rise in $PaCO_2$
- iv. Good acceptance by patients when procedure is carefully explained, as in any weaning process
- v. Can effect rapid changeover from spontaneous ventilation to ventilatory support if patient's condition warrants it
- vi. Decreased risk of contamination from switching machine and equipment
- vii. Good control of FIO_2 and reliable humidification
- viii. Same PEEP valve on ventilator serves for both machine and spontaneous breaths
- ix. System of IMV adaptable to almost any pressure- or volume-cycled ventilator; newer models have system built in

   d. Disadvantages
- i. Ventilator checks and measurements sometimes more difficult owing to continuous flow system
- ii. Apnea or low pressure alarms are a necessity
- iii. Uses more water; cascade empties faster with continuous flow
- iv. Mechanical problems (air lines, connections, bag hookups)
- v. CO_2 buildup in circuitry is potential problem

   e. Nursing responsibilities
- i. Assess patient's response to weaning, make adjustments in IMV rate as indicated; monitor by serial arterial blood gases
- ii. Check oxygen concentration delivered frequently
- iii. Check water level often
- iv. Monitor spontaneous V_T, inspiratory rate, minute ventilation

PHYSIOLOGIC MONITORING AND ASSESSMENT OF PATIENT'S CONDITION AND OF VENTILATOR FUNCTION

1. **General measures**
   a. Do not leave patient unattended or unobserved
   b. When medications are to be used, specific orders must be written. A bronchodilator cannot be administered continuously by aerosol
   c. All ventilator alarms should be on unless patient is being suctioned or weaned from ventilator
   d. Most patients will have an arterial line, pulmonary artery catheter, cardiac monitor

2. **Daily monitoring**
   a. Pressure monitoring (arterial and venous, pulmonary artery and wedge)
   b. Cardiac monitoring, ECG, heart sounds, pulses, pulse pressures
   c. Pulmonary function studies
   d. Biochemical, hematologic and electrolyte studies
   e. Cardiac output, blood volume status
   f. Intake/output, hydration, body weight
   g. Respiratory patterns, breath sounds, vital signs
   h. Dressings and drainages, tubes and suction apparatus
   i. Neurologic state, level of consciousness, pain
   j. Response to treatments, medications

3. **Complete ventilatory monitoring:** performed for any patient on continuous ventilation
   a. Ventilation checks should be done
      i. When blood gases are drawn
      ii. When changes are made in ventilator settings
      iii. Frequently on any unstable patient
      iv. Routinely at least twice a shift
   b. Components of ventilation check (to be recorded on flow sheet)
      i. Blood gas values — record source (arterial, mixed venous, etc.) along with ventilator settings and measurements so that decisions about changes may be made
      ii. Ventilator settings (read off machine)
         (a) Ventilatory mode (control/assist)
         (b) Tidal volume, rate, flow rates
         (c) Sigh volume, frequency
         (d) Temperature of humidification device, temperature of inspired gas

        (e)   Oxygen concentration

        (f)   Inflation hold, expiratory time (only on some machines)

        (g)   Inspiratory pressure

   iii. Ventilation measurements (taken on patients)

        (a)   Peak, plateau, and end-expiratory pressures

        (b)   Partial pressure of inspired oxygen, fraction of inspired oxygen

        (c)   Minute ventilation, respiratory rate, tidal volume

        (d)   Compliance, static and dynamic

        (e)   Inspiratory/expiratory ratio, V_D/V_T ratio

PHYSICAL THERAPY, INTERMITTENT OR CONTINUOUS POSITIVE PRESSURE BREATHING AND HUMIDIFICATION

1. **Chest physical therapy (PT)**

   a. Breathing exercises to increase aeration to underventilated areas of lung

   b. Percussion to loosen bronchial secretions and improve aeration

      i.   Performed with patient in postural drainage position

      ii. Done at slow rhythmic rate over area containing secretions

     iii. Contraindicated if patient has pain, acute pulmonary inflammatory process, acute cardiac condition, or hemorrhage

     iv. Follow with suctioning

   c. Manual or mechanical vibrations (artificial cough) — increase velocity of expired tidal volume, loosening secretions and propelling them to larger airways

      i.   Applied over chest wall during prolonged expiration

      ii. Follow with suctioning

   d. Postural drainage — promotes more efficient clearing of bronchial tree with less time and less energy expenditure for patient

      i.   Physical means of forcing secretions from lung toward trachea

      ii. Enlists aid of gravity in draining local areas of lung

     iii. Positions used are modified as necessary for patients with traction and cardiac and neurosurgical patients

2. **Intermittent positive pressure breathing (IPPB):** application of moderate pressure above ambient air pressure during patient's inspiratory phase

   a. Purpose

      i.   To provide greater expansion of lungs and even distribution of gases and aerosol throughout lungs

      ii. To prevent or correct atelectasis by deep lung inflations

     iii. To deliver medications and humidity in order to provide bronchodilation and aid in loosening bronchial secretions

     iv. To decrease work of breathing

    b. Possible indications (controversial)
        i. Hypoventilation
            (a) In acute or chronic obstructive lung diseases
            (b) Postoperatively, caused by anesthetic gases, pain, and depressant drugs
        ii. Retention of secretions
        iii. Respiratory acidosis
        iv. Pulmonary congestion or edema
        v. Carbon dioxide narcosis
        vi. Preoperative training
    c. Contraindications
        i. Absolute
            (a) Massive pulmonary hemorrhage
            (b) Massive subcutaneous emphysema of unknown etiology
        ii. Relative (use IPPB with caution)
            (a) Hypovolemia
            (b) Severe cardiac diseases
            (c) Active tuberculosis
            (d) Hemoptysis
            (e) Sensitivities to various drugs that may be used
            (f) Pneumothorax
    d. Hazards and side effects
        i. Causes increased intrathoracic pressure, thereby reducing venous return to heart and reducing total cardiac output
        ii. Hyperventilation (excessive removal of CO_2)
        iii. Reaction to drugs used
        iv. Infection, transmitted by equipment
        v. Potential hazard when administered by untrained personnel or when there is inadequate supervision of therapy sessions
        vi. Rupture of alveoli resulting in mediastinal and subcutaneous emphysema and pneumothorax, caused by distention of alveoli
    e. Use and benefits: controversial and insufficiently studied at present; alternatives include nebulizers, voluntary deep breathing, chest PT

3. **Continuous positive airway pressure (CPAP)**
    a. A nonventilator technique – a means of maintaining positive pressure during breathing (similar to PEEP but without a ventilator)
    b. Net result is improved arterial O_2 tensions, and technique allows for a reduction in inspired O_2 concentration
    c. Used in weaning, pediatrics

4. **Humidification therapy**
    a. Oxygen from tanks and wall outlets is completely dry; even when mixed with room air, drying effect is detrimental and irritating to mucous membrane

    b. IPPB must never be given without humidification; all ventilators should be supplied with heated humidification devices for long-term use

    c. Humidifying devices increase water vapor content of air (not associated with bacterial contamination of airways)

        i. Cold bubble humidifiers

        ii. Heated cascade humidifiers

        iii. Humidification tents and chambers

    d. Nebulizer therapy delivers water in particle form for deposition along airway; droplets may contain living bacteria

        i. Brief, intermittent therapy

           (a) Small hand nebulizers

           (b) IPPB devices

           (c) Ultrasonic nebulizers

        ii. Continuous aerosol therapy

OXYGEN THERAPY: Used to prevent or treat hypoxia.

  1. **Hypoxia-hypoxemia relationships**

    a. Definition of hypoxia: decrease in tissue oxygen; oxygen supply inadequate to meet tissue needs. Must be immediately corrected

    b. Definition of hypoxemia: decrease in arterial blood oxygen tension. A good PaO_2 does not guarantee adequate tissue oxygenation; conversely, a low PaO_2 may not mean tissue hypoxia and may be clinically acceptable

    c. Organs most susceptible to lack of oxygen — brain, adrenals, heart, kidneys, liver

    d. Factors governing effective oxygenation of blood and tissues in body

        i. Sufficient oxygen supply in inspired air

        ii. Ventilation must be sufficient to provide exchange between atmosphere and alveoli of lungs

        iii. Exchange of gases must readily occur across alveolocapillary membrane

        iv. Circulation of blood from lungs to tissues, volume of blood, and Hb levels must be adequate. A decreasing cardiac output will cause a compensatory rise in O_2 extraction at tissue level

        v. Oxygen brought to tissues must be readily released from Hb molecule, and readily diffused into and taken up by various tissues

    e. Examples of disease states

        i. Hypoxemia without hypoxia: severe COPD with increased Hb

        ii. Hypoxia without hypoxemia: carbon monoxide and cyanide poisoning

2. **Diagnosis of hypoxia**
   a. Clinical signs and symptoms
      i. Restlessness, anxiety, apprehension
      ii. Headache, angina
      iii. Confusion, disorientation, impaired judgment
      iv. Hypotension, tachycardia
      v. Shallow respirations, hypoventilation, dyspnea, yawning
      vi. Cyanosis
   b. Arterial blood gas analysis, specifically Pa_{O_2}, $P\bar{v}_{O_2}$ O_2 content, Hb, arteriovenous oxygen content difference

3. **Areas in nursing care where periodic administration of oxygen may benefit patient**
   a. Before tracheal suctioning
   b. When patient is ambulatory (use self-inflating bag and oxygen if patient's tidal volume is inadequate)
   c. Before any activity or nursing care given to cardiac patient
   d. When transferring an unstable patient

4. **Rationale for use of low flow oxygen in patient with chronic carbon dioxide retention** (as in severe COPD)
   a. Because of decreased sensitivity to blood CO_2 levels, carbon dioxide no longer serves as a respiratory stimulus; only remaining stimulus is hypoxemia. Therefore, high flow concentrations of oxygen depress hypoxic drive, leading to depression of respiration and apnea. Figure 1–2 illustrates a clinical application
   b. Nursing implications
      i. Administer oxygen only enough to raise patient's Pa_{O_2} to what are adequate levels for him (usually above 50–60mm Hg)
      ii. Safety lies in controlled low flow rates, frequent monitoring of blood gases, and nursing observation

5. **Hazards of oxygen therapy**
   a. Oxygen-induced hypoventilation
      i. Prevent by use of controlled low flow rates of 1–2 liters/minute; may be given continuously
      ii. Greatest risk is when Pa_{CO_2} is greater than 50 mm Hg
      iii. Oxygen therapy should be used with special caution in
         (a) Obstructed patient with hypoxia
         (b) Respiratory center depression due to sedatives or narcotics
   b. Atelectasis, caused by elimination of nitrogen and effect of oxygen on pulmonary surfactant
   c. Retrolental fibroplasia in neonates
      i. Fibrotic process behind lens due to retinal vasoconstriction caused from high Pa_{O_2}

Figure 1–2.

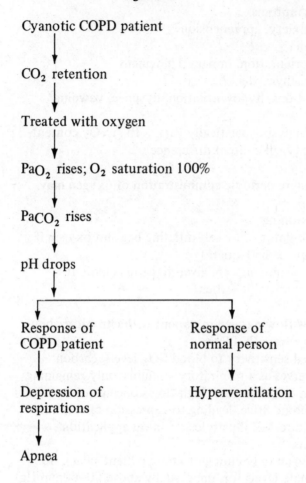

Cyanotic COPD patient

$\downarrow$

CO_2 retention

$\downarrow$

Treated with oxygen

$\downarrow$

PaO_2 rises; O_2 saturation 100%

$\downarrow$

$PaCO_2$ rises

$\downarrow$

pH drops

$\downarrow$

Response of COPD patient	Response of normal person
$\downarrow$	$\downarrow$
Depression of respirations	Hyperventilation
$\downarrow$	
Apnea	

    ii.   Keep oxygen concentration as low as necessary to
           maintain adequate PaO_2
   d. Oxygen toxicity
      i.   Related to FIO_2 and PIO_2 (not PaO_2)
     ii.   Caused by too-high a concentration over too long a time
           (from 6–30 hours)
    iii. May be mild or fatal
    iv. Early signs and symptoms
        (a) Substernal distress
        (b) Paresthesias in extremities
        (c) Nausea, vomiting
        (d) Fatigue, lethargy, malaise
        (e) Dyspnea
        (f) Anorexia
        (g) Restlessness

v.   Late signs and symptoms
(a)   Progressive respiratory difficulty
(b)   Cyanosis
(c)   Dyspnea
(d)   Asphyxia
vi. Pathologic process is not fully understood
(a)   Local pulmonary toxicity to pulmonary capillaries
(b)   Possibly a change in surfactant
(c)   Hyaline membrane production may be a factor
(d)   Absorption atelectasis and nitrogen washout
vii. Both oxygen concentration and duration of therapy are critical (40% oxygen or greater over several days is potentially dangerous)
viii. Changes seen in oxygen toxicity
(a)   Decreased compliance
(b)   Increasing A -a O_2 gradient

6. **Summary of oxygen use**
   a. Oxygen is a potent drug that should be used with reason and according to indications
   b. If high concentrations are necessary, duration of administration should be kept to a minimum and reduced as soon as possible
   c. Objective is to maintain Pa_{O_2} of at least 50–60 mm Hg to produce acceptable Sa_{O_2} of 85–90%, without damaging lungs or causing CO_2 retention
   d. Frequent arterial blood gas monitoring is a mandatory safety measure when concentrations above 40% are used
   e. Exact concentration of inspired O_2 should be measured with an O_2 analyzer, especially when gas is used in mechanical ventilators, as settings may not be accurate

7. **Means of oxygen administration**
   a. Important preliminary points
       i.   Remember airway – no oxygen treatment is of any use without an adequate airway
       ii. Pathology of disease under treatment is major determinant of effectiveness of oxygen therapy
       iii. Delivered concentration of gas from any appliance is subject to
            (a)   Condition of equipment
            (b)   Technique of application
            (c)   Cooperation of patient
            (d)   Ventilatory pattern of patient
       iv. Low flow oxygen systems do not provide the total inspired atmosphere, and therefore are adequate only if V_T is adequate, respiratory rates are not excessive, and ventilator pattern is stable

     v.   High flow oxygen systems provide the entire inspired atmosphere, and are adequate only if flow rates exceed patient's $\dot{V}_E$, and reservoirs meet peak flow rates

b.   Appliances capable of delivering oxygen
- i.   Masks
  - (a) General points
    - (1) Useful if O_2 needed quickly and for short periods
    - (2) Concentrations of 24–100% oxygen are delivered, depending on device
  - (b) Disadvantages
    - (1) Uncomfortable and hot
    - (2) Necrosis of skin caused by tight fit
    - (3) Difficult to control F_{IO_2} precisely
  - (c) Dangers to watch
    - (1) Patients who are prone to vomit may aspirate
    - (2) Obstruction by flaccid tongue may occur in comatose patient. Use oral airway and stay with patient
    - (3) May cause CO_2 retention and hyperventilation if flow is too low and exhalation ports are too small
  - (d) Types of masks
    - (1) Simple – 35–55% O_2 at 6–10-liter flows
    - (2) Rebreathing – used only for administration of anesthesia
    - (3) Partial rebreathing
      - (a) Deliver 35–60% at 6–10-liter flows
      - (b) Flow must be adjusted so that reservoir bag does not collapse during inspiration, otherwise CO_2 retention may occur
    - (4) Non-rebreathing
      - (a) Delivers 90–100% concentration of gases provided there are no leaks in system
      - (b) Is most precise method of delivering a specific gas concentration for short-term purposes
    - (5) Venturi (dilution)
      - (a) Adjustments allow for delivery of precise O_2 concentrations of 24%, 28%, 35%, 40%, and 50%
      - (b) Total air flow must be adequate for ventilatory needs of patient
- ii.   Cannula (nasal)
  - (a) Low O_2 concentrations delivered (below 40%, but depends on patient's tidal volume)
  - (b) Cooperative patient necessary
  - (c) Advantages: easy to apply, light, economical, disposable, allows patient mobility

      (d)   Disadvantages: easily dislodged, excessive flow rates uncomfortable

   iii. Nasal catheter

      (a)   Disadvantages: technique of insertion, gastric distention, nasopharyngeal injury

      (b)   Low O_2 concentrations delivered (below 40%)

      (c)   Better for less dependable and restless patient

      Note: Data show that eventual delivery of oxygen to blood is not significantly different when either cannula or catheter is used, and whether mouth is open or closed (Egan, 1977).

   iv. IPPB

      (a)   21–100% O_2

      (b)   Errors in O_2 air dilution; check with O_2 analyzer

   v. Heated nebulizer

      (a) O_2 settings are not adequate

      (b)   Flow rates important

   vi. Tracheal masks

      (a)   6–12 liters/minute, 35–70% O_2

      (b)   Use with heated nebulizer, large bore tubing

   vii. T-piece

      (a)   6–12 liters/minute, 25–70% O_2

      (b)   Use with heated nebulizer, large bore tubing

   viii. Hyperbaric oxygenation

      (a)   Administration of oxygen under greatly increased pressure: e.g., F_{IO_2} of 100% at sea level produces Pa_{O_2} of 650 mm Hg; at 3 atmospheres pressure, Pa_{O_2} is 2000 mm Hg

      (b)   Used in CO poisoning, radiation therapy, gas gangrene, burns, decubiti

COMPLICATIONS ARISING FROM PATIENT'S MEDICAL CONDITION OR HOSPITAL CARE

1. **Infection**

   a. Primary sources

      i.   Respiratory therapy equipment – a major source

      ii.   Cross-contamination between patients

      iii.   Indwelling catheters of all kinds

      iv.   Suction catheters

   b. Preventive measures

      i.   Rigorous hand washing by staff

      ii.   Isolation techniques as needed

      iii.   Routine cultures of patient and machines

      iv.   Antibiotics as indicated

      v.   Bronchial hygiene, chest physical therapy

      vi. Basic bedside nursing activities

      vii. Restriction of numbers of patient contacts (staff and visitors)

2. **Machine and equipment problems**
   a. Loose connections
   b. Leaks
   c. Asynchronization with patient
   d. Inadequate water levels in respiratory therapy equipment
   e. Oxygen source failures
   f. Failure of temperature regulation
   g. Mechanical failure

3. **Electrical hazards**
   a. Electrically susceptible patients
   b. Physiologic effects of electrical current
   c. Inadequate equipment preparation and precautions
   d. Faulty hospital wiring and inadequate safety precautions
   e. Dangerous electrical devices and equipment

4. **Hazards of immobility on respiratory system:** decreased respiratory movements lead to stasis and pooling of secretions, $\dot{V}/\dot{Q}$ mismatches
   a. Nursing measures for patient
      i. Sitting-up rather than supine position, if possible
      ii. Deep breathing and coughing
      iii. Force fluids unless contraindicated
      iv. Blow bottles and other measures to increase ventilation; incentive spirometry

EMOTIONAL AND PSYCHOLOGIC SUPPORT FOR PATIENT AND FAMILY

1. **Communication skills**
   a. Intubated patients
      i. Talk to patient and encourage him to try to talk, lip-read
      ii. If patient able, provide pencil and paper, magic slate, letter board
      iii. Explain all procedures and equipment
      iv. Identify yourself to patient
      v. Ask questions answerable by "yes" or "no" so that patient can express needs
   b. Paralyzed patients
      i. Explain all procedures fully
      ii. Do not touch or move patient abruptly
      iii. Talk to patient as you care for him
      iv. Orient patient to time, place, and person

    v.   Remember that an apparently asleep patient may be mentally alert

2. **Anxiety factors for patient**
    a. Patient's main fears center around his body and the machinery supporting it
        i. New unidentifiable sounds without explanation, enhancing fantasies
        ii. Medications causing confusion, disorientation
        iii. Inability to talk
        iv. Machinery seen as taking over bodily functions — e.g., ECG machine makes heart beat
        v. Fears of mechanical and human failure
    b. Conversation around patient regarded as all pertaining to himself
        i. If patient cannot understand all of conversation, he will fill in the blanks
        ii. Hospital jargon can cause strange fantasies
    c. Frustration and fright caused by inability to communicate
        i. Patient may express frustrations behaviorally, becoming uncooperative or disoriented
        ii. He may withdraw to extremely passive behavior

──────── PATHOLOGIC CONDITIONS AND MANAGEMENT ────────

ACUTE RESPIRATORY FAILURE: Acute inability of the lungs to maintain adequate oxygenation of the blood with or without impairment of ventilation.

1. **Pathophysiology**
    a. Hypoxemia leads to hypoxia which stimulates sympathetic nervous system, producing selective tissue vasoconstriction, increased peripheral resistance, and tachycardia
    b. When hypoxia is caused by hypoventilation or circulatory deficiences, hypercapnia may occur. Hypercapnia has a local depressant effect on cellular and tissue function, resulting in cerebral depression, hypotension, and circulatory failure
    c. Excess of carbon dioxide stimulates sympathetic nervous system, increasing heart rate and cardiac output. High levels of carbon dioxide in blood may also lead to acidosis
    d. Process may be acute or chronic
        i. Chronic — renal compensation for hypercapnia occurs, and arterial pH remains close to normal owing to increases in serum bicarbonate
        ii. Acute — renal compensation does not have time to develop, and pH falls

    e. Disease may be hypoxic or hypoxic/hypercapnic
- i. Hypoxic – decreased PaO_2 (e.g., ARDS)
- ii. Hypoxic/hypercapnic – decreased PaO_2 with increased $PaCO_2$ and decreased pH (e.g. narcotic overdose)

2. **Etiology or precipitating factors**
   a. Impaired ventilation
      - i. Chronic airway obstruction – emphysema, chronic bronchitis, asthma, bronchiectasis
      - ii. Restrictive defects
         - (a) Decreased lung expansion – pleural effusion, pneumothorax
         - (b) Limited thorax expansion – kyphoscoliosis, multiple rib fractures, thoracic surgery
         - (c) Decreased diaphragmatic movement – abdominal surgery, peritonitis
      - iii. Neuromuscular defects – polio, Guillain-Barré syndrome, multiple sclerosis, myasthenia gravis, brain or spinal injuries, drugs or toxic agents (e.g., acetylcholinesterase inhibitors, colistin, curare)
      - iv. Respiratory center damage or depression – narcotics, barbiturates, tranquilizers, anesthetics; cerebral infarction or trauma; high dose, uncontrolled oxygen therapy
   b. Impaired gas exchange and diffusion
      - i. Adult respiratory distress syndrome, atelectasis, diffuse viral pneumonia, fat emboli, postperfusion syndromes, aspiration
      - ii. Pulmonary edema
      - iii. Pulmonary fibrosis
      - iv. Anatomic loss of functioning lung tissue
      - v. Pneumonectomy or tumor
   c. Ventilation-perfusion abnormalities
      - i. Chronic airway obstruction
      - ii. Thomboembolism

3. **Clinical presentation**
   a. Manifestations of the primary disease plus manifestations of hypoxia (see diagnosis of hypoxia)
   b. Manifestations of hypercapnia with acidemia
      - i. Headache
      - ii. Confusion
      - iii. Unconsciousness, somnolence
      - iv. Dizziness
      - v. Muscle twitching, asterixis
      - vi. Miosis, papilledema, engorged fundal veins
      - vii. Diaphoresis
      - viii. Hypertension

4. **Diagnostic findings**
   a. History
      i. Presence of one or more precipitating factors
      ii. History of clinical manifestations
   b. Physical examination (see Clinical presentation)
   c. Diagnostic studies
      i. Laboratory
         (a) Respiratory failure is defined by arterial blood gas measurements.
         (b) Criteria – PaO_2 below 50 mm Hg, $PaCO_2$ above 50 mm Hg, or both
            (1) Acute – acidosis, normal or mildly increasing blood buffers (HCO_3^-)
            (2) Chronic – relatively normal pH, elevated blood buffers
      ii. Radiologic findings depend on primary disease

5. **Complications**
   a. Cardiac dysthythmias associated with hypoxia, alkalosis
   b. Infection, pneumonia, O_2 toxicity, atelectasis, pulmonary edema
   c. Psychosis, depression
   d. Renal failure, acid-base imbalance, electrolyte disturbances, hypokalemia
   e. Hypotension
   f. Abdominal distention, ileus, GI hemorrhage (especially with steroid treatment)
   g. Thromboembolism
   h. Alkalosis – when $PaCO_2$ normalized rather than pH; clinical manifestations include tachypnea, confusion, tremors, asterixis, dysrhythmias, seizures, death

6. **Specific patient care**
   a. Improve ventilation and $\dot{V}/\dot{Q}$ ratio (open airways, bronchial hygiene, intubation, ventilators, PEEP)
   b. Decrease shunting, decrease A-a gradient (O_2 administration; maintain adequate Hb)
   c. Follow arterial blood gases closely to achieve
      i. PaO_2 above 50 mm Hg (with normal Hb, which will insure adequate tissue oxygenation)
      ii. pH in range of 7.40 ± 0.04 (regulates vascular resistance and Hb binding of O_2)
      iii. $PaCO_2$ is less important by itself. Regulates blood flow and influences O_2 binding by Hb. Better to regulate pH rather than $PaCO_2$

ADULT RESPIRATORY DISTRESS SYNDROME (ARDS): Also called congestive or hemorrhagic atelectasis, adult hyaline membrane disease, postperfusion lung, pump lung, post-traumatic pulmonary insufficiency, progressive pulmonary consolidation, wet lung, and shock lung.

1. **Pathophysiology:** may represent final common pathway of response of lung to many different kinds of injuries (stressors)
   a. Altered capillary permeability permits protein and H_2O to leak out into interstitial and alveolar spaces, producing interstitial edema and decreased FRC
   b. Vascular reactivity in pulmonary circulation, pre- and post-capillary constriction or obstruction
   c. Alteration of surfactant, creating rise in surface tension (this role is not as clear in ARDS as it is in infants with hyaline membrane disease)
   d. Decreased compliance

2. **Etiology or precipitating factors:** any condition or event producing stress, such as
   a. Trauma — thoracic or extrathoracic
   b. Shock
   c. Multiple transfusions
   d. Amniotic fluid embolism
   e. Infections — pneumonia
   f. Fat embolism
   g. Smoke inhalation
   h. Drug ingestion
   i. Aspiration
   j. Disseminated intravascular coagulation
   k. Fluid overload

3. **Clinical presentation**
   a. Dyspnea
   b. Tachypnea
   c. Cyanosis
   d. Other manifestations of hypoxia
   e. Hypotension

4. **Diagnostic findings**
   a. History: presence of precipitating factors as listed, along with sudden, marked respiratory distress
   b. Physical examination: findings of primary disease (see Clinical presentation)
   c. Diagnostic studies
      i. Laboratory: arterial blood gases
         (a) Hypoxemia is hallmark of the disease
         (b) Hypercapnia usually is not initially present

    ii.   Radiologic: x-ray examination demonstrates bilateral alveolar infiltrates

    iii.   Special
        (a) Pulmonary compliance reduced
        (b) Spirometry — lung volumes reduced, functional residual capacity low
        (c) Shunt studies demonstrate large right-to-left shunt (usually greater than 20% of cardiac output) measured during 100% oxygen breathing
        (d) Increased A -a gradient

5. **Complications**: ultimate outcome depends on nature and degree of original pulmonary injury, ability to support oxygenation, and success in avoiding further pulmonary injury

6. **Specific patient care**
   a. Support alveolar ventilation and oxygen transport, and prevent further fluid sequestration in lungs
     i.   Tracheostomy for long-term ventilatory support and suctioning
     ii.   Appropriate ventilator with high pressure and flow capabilities
     iii.   Use of PEEP — a major treatment modality, increases FRC
     iv.   Diuretics, restriction of fluids, to minimize sequestration of fluid within lung
     v.   Corticosteroids (controversial)
     vi.   Antibiotics — reserved for specific infections
     vii.   Careful respiratory monitoring — especially mixed venous PO_2 (pulmonary artery blood), which is a measure of O_2 delivery to the tissues in relation to their need
     viii.   Extracorporeal membrane oxygenation (ECMO) — an experimental therapy now being evaluated
   b. Psychologic support — preparation of family for high mortality rate of ARDS

CHRONIC OBSTRUCTIVE PULMONARY DISEASE (COPD): A functional category of respiratory disorders; comprises those conditions characterized by obstruction to air flow within the lung — principally, chronic bronchitis, asthma, and emphysema.

1. **Pathophysiology**
   a. Chronic bronchitis — commonly precedes and accompanies pulmonary emphysema
     i.   Pathologic changes
        (a) Inflammatory, mononuclear infiltrate in bronchial wall
        (b) Hypertrophy and hyperplasia of mucus-secreting bronchial glands and mucosal goblet cells

          (c)   Metaplasia of bronchial and bronchiolar epithelium
          (d)   Loss of cilia
          (e)   Eventual distortion and scarring of bronchial wall
          (f)   Often accompanied by cor pulmonale
      ii.   Excessive mucous secretions in bronchi
      iii.   Chronic or recurrent productive cough
  b. Asthma (technically is often not included in COPD since it is reversible)
      i.   Recurrent, generalized airway obstruction
      ii.   Increased responsiveness of trachea and bronchi to various stimuli
      iii.   Manifested by difficulty in breathing caused by generalized narrowing of airways
      iv.   Increased contraction of smooth muscles and hypersecretion of bronchial mucus
      v.   Mucus abnormally tenacious
      vi.   Also may be associated with cor pulmonale and emphysema
      vii.   Paroxysmal and recurrent in early stages
      viii. Allergic response to specific allergens in some patients
  c. Emphysema — an anatomic disorder characterized by
      i.   Enlargement of air spaces distal to terminal nonrespiratory bronchiole, with destruction of alveolar wall
      ii.   Lungs are large, pale, and relatively bloodless; do not collapse readily; contain many superficial blebs or bullae

2. **Etiology or precipitating factors**
  a. Smoking
      i.   Most important cause of COPD in United States
      ii.   Increases frequency and severity of asthma attacks
  b. Air pollution and occupation
      i.   Pollution related to chronic bronchitis
      ii.   Smog worsens dyspnea by increasing bronchospasm
      iii.   Irritating fumes and certain vegetable dust aggravate COPD
      iv.   Occupational exposures less important than cigarette smoking
  c. Repeated respiratory infections
      i.   No specific viral or bacterial agent causes COPD
      ii.   Greater susceptibility to bronchopulmonary infections
  d. Heredity
      i.   Familial emphysema — deficiency of serum $alpha_1$ globulin (alpha$_1$-antitrypsin)
      ii.   Cystic fibrosis patients fit category of COPD
      iii.   Possible tissue defect involved
  e. Aging
      i.   High prevalence of COPD among older smokers
      ii.   Not primary cause of COPD
  f. Allergy — role in asthma

3. **Clinical presentation**
    a. Chronic cough and expectoration
    b. Wheezing
    c. Dyspnea
    d. Pursed lip breathing
    e. Use of accessory muscles of respiration
    f. Disease may not show progression until aggravated by respiratory infection or debilitating states

4. **Diagnostic findings**
    a. History
        i. Shortness of breath, exercise intolerance
        ii. Production of sputum; amount and characteristics may vary
        iii. Smoking, lower respiratory tract infections, fever, tuberculosis, wheezing (identify precipitating events)
        iv. Occupational or residential hazards, allergy to pets, hobbies
        v. Family history positive for asthma, other lung disease, cardiac symptoms
        vi. Anorexia and weight loss, general debilitation
        vii. Medications and previous therapy
    b. Physical examination
        i. Increased A-P diameter
        ii. Use of accessory muscles of respiration
        iii. Restriction of lateral motion of rib cage during respiration
        iv. Decreased diaphragmatic excursion (by percussion)
        v. Hyperresonance (not an accurate sign, varies with chest wall thickness)
        vi. Breath sounds quiet, expiration and forced expiratory time prolonged
        vii. Wheezes and rhonchi on inspiration and expiration
        viii. Rales (early inspiratory)
        ix. Liver may be enlarged if cor pulmonale is present
        x. Increased development of abdominal musculature
        xi. Cyanosis, plethora, edema
        xii. Neck vein distention
    c. Diagnostic studies
        i. Laboratory
            (a) Hematologic
                (1) Polycythemia
                (2) Eosinophilia
            (b) Chemistries (nonspecific)
            (c) Sputum examination
                (1) Wet mount demonstrates whether prevalence is due to eosinophils or neutrophils
                (2) Gram stain: secondary bacterial infections in pooled secretions may exist with either gram-

positive or gram-negative organisms. *Streptococcus pneumoniae* and *Haemophilus influenzae* are often found

   ii. Radiologic: PA, lateral chest

     (a) Signs of overinflation

       (1) Low, flat diaphragms

       (2) Retrosternal space greater than 2.5 cm

       (3) Sternodiaphragmatic angle on lateral film of over 90°

     (b) May be evidence of emphysema

     (c) Heart may be enlarged

   iii. Special

     (a) Spirometry – frequently identifies airway obstruction not obvious on physical examination

       (1) Screening spirometry – decreased vital capacity, response to bronchodilators

       (2) Maximal midexpiratory flow rate: sensitive for early involvement

       (3) FEV_1 decreased

       (4) TLC may be increased as a result of air trapping

     (b) Arterial blood gases – evaluates degree of hypoxemia, hypercapnia, acidosis, renal compensation

5. **Complications**

   a. Cor pulmonale

   b. Respiratory failure

   c. Pneumonia

   d. Pulmonary thromboembolism

   e. Perforation or hemorrhage from peptic ulcer

   f. Spontaneous pneumothorax

6. **Specific patient care**

   a. Physiologic defects that have been identified should be corrected, and factors believed to be of pathogenic significance eliminated

     i. Patient education – self-care classes, texts

     ii. Removal of bronchial irritants (smoking, etc.)

     iii. Postural drainage

     iv. Breathing education and exercise

     v. Abdominal support

     vi. Acute situations – e.g., tracheal aspiration, controlled or assisted ventilation

     vii. Drug therapy (antibiotics, bronchodilators)

     viii. Hydration

     ix. Oxygen

   b. Assist patient to adjust to psychosocial effects of living with chronic disease

PULMONARY EMBOLISM: The most common pulmonary complication in hospitalized patients. A massive pulmonary embolism is a sudden, mechanical obstruction of 50% or more of the pulmonary arterial bed.

1. **Pathophysiology**
   a. Conditions predisposing to thrombus formation — Virchow's triad
      i. Hypercoagulability of blood, which exists during pregnancy, in postoperative period, after abrupt discontinuation of anticoagulants, during fever, with use of oral contraceptives, in certain malignancies, in sickle cell anemia, and with abnormal "stickiness" of platelets
      ii. Alterations in integrity of blood vessel walls due to local trauma or venous disease
      iii. Venous stasis — causes clots and their extension. Most thrombi causing pulmonary embolism originate in the peripheral venous system, primarily the legs
   b. Mechanisms causing thrombi to dislodge or fragment
      i. Intravascular pressure changes due to direct trauma, muscle action, changes in rate of blood flow
      ii. Natural mechanisms of clot dissolution
   c. Emboli may cause increased pulmonary circulatory resistance and right heart failure

2. **Etiology or precipitating factors**
   a. Immobility
   b. Oral contraceptives
   c. Previous congestive heart failure
   d. Thrombus formation in heart from cardioversion, bacterial endocarditis, atrial fibrillation, or myocardial infarction
   e. Age increase
   f. Obesity
   g. Recent surgery
   h. Pregnancy
   i. Trauma to vessel wall due to venipuncture
   j. Vasculitis

3. **Clinical presentation:** varies from mild to severe
   a. Massive pulmonary embolism
      i. Sudden shock — frequently profound
      ii. Cyanosis
      iii. Tachypnea and respiratory distress
      iv. Mental clouding, anxiety
      v. Feeling of impending doom
   b. Pulmonary embolism — symptoms may be vague and nonspecific
      i. Tachypnea, tachycardia
      ii. Pleuritic chest pain (late), diffuse chest discomfort
      iii. Hemoptysis

          iv.   Anxiety, restlessness

          v.   Dyspnea, cough

4. Diagnostic findings

   a. History

        i.   Positive for one or more precipitating factors

        ii.   Palpitations, apprehension

        iii.   Dyspnea – sudden, unexplained

   b. Physical examination – may be entirely normal or nonspecific (see also Clinical presentation)

        i.   Rales, although lower lungs may sound clear

        ii. S_3 or S_4 gallop with associated heart failure

        iii.   Accentuated pulmonic closure sound due to pulmonary hypertension

        iv.   Pleural friction rub

        v.   Cyanosis

        vi.   Elevated temperature

   c. Diagnostic studies

        i.   Laboratory – not specific

           (a)   Decreased WBC unless infection present

           (b)   Increased LDH, increased SGOT (possibly)

           (c)   Increased bilirubin – correlated with right heart failure

           (d)   Arterial blood gases – usually will show hypoxemia; if Pa_{O_2} is above 80 mm Hg on room air, pulmonary embolism is not a likely diagnosis

        ii.   Radiologic

           (a)   Chest x-ray is nonspecific. Frequently normal, it may show patterns of infarction, parenchymal abnormalities.

        iii.   Special

           (a)   Lung scan

               (1)   Useful in diagnosis. May show nonspecific uptake of radiopaque material

              (2)   Ventilation–perfusion scans are preferred, demonstrating ventilation in excess of perfusion

           (b)   Pulmonary angiography

               (1)   If clots are actually demonstrated, positive diagnosis may be made

              (2)   May show significant obstruction in pulmonary arterial tree

           (c)   ECG – nonspecific, usually no changes, but may show tachycardia or patterns of right ventricular strain

5. Complications

   a. Pulmonary infarction

   b. Extension of emboli, blocking additional vessels

   c. Cerebrovascular occlusion

   d. Acute myocardial infarction

    e. Intractable cardiac dysrhythmias
    f. Hepatic congestion and necrosis
    g. Bronchopneumonia
    h. Pulmonary abscess
    i. Shock, ARDS

6. **Specific patient care**: varies with severity
    a. Arrest thrombosis
        i. Heparin – anticoagulant of choice
            (a) Loading dose, followed by continued dosages sufficient to prolong clotting time as desired
            (b) May be given as continuous IV or intermittent injection
            (c) Dosage is reduced with graded ambulation and administration of oral anticoagulants
       ii. Thrombolytic therapy
            (a) An experimental therapy using streptokinase or urokinase
            (b) Appears to lyse pulmonary emboli, increase pulmonary capillary perfusion, decrease hemodynamic abnormalities
      iii. Surgical interruption of inferior vena cava
            (a) Used in cases in which anticoagulant therapy has been a failure or is contraindicated, and for recurrent cases
            (b) Procedures – ligation, clipping, plication, filter
            (c) Intracaval umbrella – avoids major surgery
      iv. Pulmonary embolectomy
            (a) Rarely indicated
            (b) Reserved for select cases of massive pulmonary embolism with profound cardiovascular collapse or cardiac arrest who fail to stabilize with therapy
       v. Oral anticoagulants – long-term maintenance
    b. Use nursing measures to prevent development of pulmonary embolism in susceptible hospitalized patients
        i. Encourage ambulation
       ii. Schedule exercise (active and passive) for nonambulatory patients
      iii. Elastic stockings
      iv. Elevation of legs
       v. Avoid strain, avoid Valsalva maneuver
      vi. Adequate fluid intake, steady IV flow rates
     vii. Deep breathing exercises
    viii. Medical orders may include heparin, low molecular weight dextran
    c. Maintain adequate oxygenation, ventilation, and circulation
    d. Reduce apprehension, fear, anxiety
        i. Sedation

   ii. Quiet, nonstimulating environment
   iii. Calm reassurance
   iv. Patient and family education

STATUS ASTHMATICUS: A severe unabated attack of asthma that does not respond to sympathomimetic drugs. A self-perpetuating complex.

1. **Pathophysiology**
  a. Bronchi constrict in response to antigen/histamine mechanism, producing increased airway resistance
  b. Airway secretions become tenacious due to water loss as a result of tachypnea
  c. Blood vessels dilate
  d. Bronchial vessel walls hypertrophy
  e. Bronchiolar obstruction reduces alveolar ventilation
  f. Severe atelectasis occurs

2. **Etiology or precipitating factors**
  a. Respiratory infection
  b. Inappropriate use of asthmatic medications
  c. Exposure to allergens
  d. Emotional factors
  e. Unusually hot, cold, or dusty environment

3. **Clinical presentation**
  a. Extreme dyspnea
  b. Hyperpnea
  c. Cyanosis (not always present)
  d. Physical exhaustion
  e. Dehydration

4. **Diagnostic findings**
  a. History
   i. Symptoms of infection
   ii. Medication history that suggests errors in taking drugs (too many or too few)
   iii. Antecedent asthma
   iv. Dyspnea, cough, wheezing
   v. Inability to sleep
  b. Physical examination (see also Clinical presentation)
   i. Tachypnea
   ii. Tachycardia
   iii. Breath sounds — wheezing and rhonchi may be absent (ominous sign) or present
   iv. Use of accessory muscles of respiration
   v. Labored breathing
   vi. Hyperresonance
   vii. Pallor — cyanosis

    c. Diagnostic studies
      i. Laboratory
        (a) Arterial blood gases — low PaO_2, normal or decreased $PaCO_2$, increased $PaCO_2$ with respiratory failure
        (b) Sputum — evidence of infection, allergy
      ii. Radiologic — chest x-ray normal or hyperlucent

5. Complications
    a. Respiratory failure
    b. Pneumothorax

6. Specific patient care
    a. Clear airway obstruction and reduce bronchospasm
      i. Bronchodilators (aminophylline and others)
      ii. IV corticosteroids if attack does not subside promptly
    b. Provide adequate oxygenation (guided by arterial blood gases)
    c. Support ventilation
      i. Used if hypoxemia not controlled or if CO_2 retention occurs
      ii. Endotracheal tube, volume ventilator
    d. Reduce anxiety, provide reassurance
    e. Maintain fluid balance, correct dehydration
      i. IV fluids
      ii. Oral fluids as tolerated
      iii. Humidification
    f. Prevent infection, exposure to irritants
      i. Antibiotics if current infection
      ii. Quiet, air-conditioned room
      iii. Allergen-proof pillows, blankets
    g. Monitor carefully for complications, response to therapy
      i. Cardiac monitoring for dysrhythmias
      ii. Arterial blood gases
      iii. Vital signs
      iv. Airway patency
      v. Serial monitoring of FEV_1, other expiratory flow studies

CHEST TRAUMA

1. Pathophysiology
    a. Chest injuries are usually a part of multisystem trauma (head, abdomen, etc.)
    b. Chest injuries are particularly serious in patients with impaired physiologic reserves such as
      i. Advanced age
      ii. Obesity
      iii. Cardiac disease
      iv. Chronic respiratory ailments
    c. Pressure dynamics of thoracic cage must be understood to enable intelligent decisions about treatment to be made

    d. Classification of injury
       i. Blunt (nonpenetrating)
          (a) Chest wall involved; no communication with pleural cavity
          (b) Severe blunt trauma is often associated with serious intracranial and intra-abdominal injury
      ii. Penetrating
          (a) Pleural cavity as well as chest wall has been entered
          (b) Generally able to predict organs likely to be injured by course of wound
     iii. Perforating
          (a) Through and through (wound of entrance and wound of exit)
          (b) In a gunshot wound, wound of exit is usually larger and more ragged because bullet has tumbled or become deformed during passage (exception: shotgun blast)
     iv. Open/closed
          (a) Open — Constant exchange of air between atmosphere and pleural cavity
          (b) Closed — no communication between underlying pleura and atmosphere

2. **Etiology or precipitating factors**
    a. Blunt trauma — automobile accidents, falls, assaults, explosives
    b. Penetrating/perforating trauma — knives, pistol fire, free-flying objects, industrial accidents

3. **Clinical presentation** (see discussion of specific injury to follow)

4. **Diagnostic findings:** vary with specific injury
    a. History of traumatic epidsode
    b. Physical examination — specific to injury; complete examination of all apparently noninvolved systems is necessary to rule out additional covert injuries
    c. Diagnostic studies — as indicated by specific injury

5. **Complications** (see specific injury): patients with pre-existing borderline pulmonary function are prone to ventilatory insufficiency progressing to respiratory failure

6. **Specific patient care**
    a. Restore adequate cardiopulmonary function
    b. Correct damage to chest and other structures

7. **Major types of chest trauma**
    a. Rib fractures
       i. Clinical presentation
          (a) Pain

          (b) Splinting on movement

          (c) Dyspnea

          (d) Ecchymosis

    ii. Complications specific to rib fractures

          (a) Fracture of first rib — takes hard blow to produce; look for neck injuries, brachial plexus injury, pneumothorax, aortic rupture/tears

          (b) Ribs 9–12 — injuries to spleen, liver

    iii. Specific patient care

          (a) Intercostal nerve block (pain relief without impairment of cough)

          (b) Analgesics

          (c) Binders or taping should rarely be used, as these tend to limit respiratory excursion

          (d) Bronchial hygiene, physical therapy

b. Flail chest

    i. Clinical presentation

          (a) Rapid, shallow respirations

          (b) Cyanosis

          (c) Severe chest wall pain

          (d) Shock

          (e) Paradoxical chest motion

          (f) Bony crepitation at sites of fracture (rib is fractured in more than one location)

    ii. Specific patient care

          (a) Emergency use — stabilizing pressure over chest wall segment (adhesive, sandbags, hands)

          (b) Hospital care usually includes intubation, early tracheostomy, positive pressure ventilation; there may be pulmonary contusion

c. Pneumothorax

    i. Clinical presentation (varies with degree of collapse and patient's previous clinical state)

          (a) Increased chest pain

          (b) Dyspnea

          (c) Diminished or absent breath sounds on affected side

          (d) Increased resonance

          (e) Spontaneous emphysema

          (f) Shock

    ii. Specific patient care

          (a) Apply occlusive dressing, vaseline gauze if there is an open wound

          (b) Chest tubes — in appropriate position to drain air

d. Tension pneumothorax

    i. Clinical presentation

          (a) Respiratory distress

          (b) Progressive cyanosis

          (c) Mediastinal shift (away from affected side)

        (d) Tracheal displacement (away from affected side)

        (e) Hyperresonant percussion note (affected side)

        (f) PMI shift (away from affected side)

        (g) Distant or absent breath sounds (affected side)

        (h) Widening intercostal spaces (affected side)

    ii. Specific patient care

        (a) Emergency decompression of air under tension in pleural cavity. Use large (14 G) needle in 2nd–3rd interspace, midclavicular line, directly between ribs; aim posteriorly toward shoulder

        (b) Chest tube drainage, water seal

e. Hemothorax

    i. Clinical presentation

        (a) Respiratory embarrassment

        (b) Dullness to percussion (affected side)

        (c) Absent or distant breath sounds (affected side)

        (d) Shock if hemorrhage is extensive

    ii. Specific patient care

        (a) Thoracocentesis or tube drainage. Use large-size tube in dependent position

        (b) Have blood available for replacement

        (c) Direct repair of bleeding vessels

f. Cardiac tamponade

    i. Clinical presentation

        (a) Distended neck veins

        (b) Falling systolic blood pressure

        (c) Elevated central venous pressure

        (d) Muffled or distant heart sounds

        (e) Various degrees of shock

        (f) Narrow pulse pressure

        (g) Pulsus paradoxus

    ii. Specific patient care

        (a) Aspiration of pericardial fluid (pericardiocentesis)

        (b) Thoracotomy, pericardiotomy, direct repair of wound

g. Diaphragmatic injuries (rupture, herniation)

    i. Clinical presentation

        (a) Respiratory distress

        (b) Shoulder pain on same side as tear

        (c) Inability to pass nasogastric tube

        (d) Signs/symptoms of cardiorespiratory collapse

    ii. Additional diagnostic studies and findings

        (a) Elevated hemidiaphragm on x-ray examination

        (b) Contrast studies demonstrate elevation or depression of diaphragm

       iii. Specific patient care
- (a) Surgical repair of tear, to prevent movement of abdominal contents into thoracic cavity, or replace if herniated
- (b) Ventilatory support

h. Esophageal tear
      i. Clinical presentation
- (a) Severe substernal chest pain, localized to midline (gastric contents extremely irritating)
- (b) Back pain
- (c) Vomiting of blood
- (d) Dyspnea
- (e) Cyanosis
- (f) Pain on swallowing
- (g) Change of voice
- (h) Severe thirst
- (i) Subcutaneous emphysema

      ii. Specific patient care
- (a) Intubation
- (b) Bedrest
- (c) Antibiotics
- (d) Chest tube
- (e) Surgical repair

i. Fracture of trachea, bronchus — often associated with severe chest trauma and fracture of upper ribs
      i. Clinical presentation
- (a) Cough
- (b) Bloody sputum
- (c) Respiratory distress
- (d) Subcutaneous emphysema

      ii. Additional diagnostic studies — bronchoscopy shows internal trauma of trachea

      iii. Specific patient care
- (a) Intubation
- (b) Assisted ventilation
- (c) Operative repair

REFERENCES

Alspach, J.: Critical care nursing of the patient with chest injuries. Crit. Care Update 6:18–26, 1979.

Ayers, S., and Lagenson, J.: Pulmonary physiology at the bedside: O_2 and CO_2 abnormalities. Cardiovasc. Nurs. 9:1–6, 1973.

Baier, H., Begin, R., and Sackner, M.: Effect of airway diameter, suction catheters, and the bronchofiberscope on airflow in endotracheal and tracheostomy tubes. Heart Lung 5:235–238, 1976.

Bates, B.: A Guide to Physical Examination, 2nd ed. J. B. Lippincott Co., Philadelphia, 1979.

Bates, D. V., Macklem, P. T., and Christie, R. V.: Respiratory Function in Disease. In Respiratory Failure, 2nd ed. W. B. Saunders Co., Philadelphia, 1971, Chap. 22.

Baum, G. L.: Textbook of Pulmonary Medicine, 2nd ed. Little, Brown & Co., Boston, 1974.

Beall, C. E., Braun, H. A., and Cheney, F. W.: Physiologic Bases for Respiratory Care. Mountain Press Publishing Co., Missouli, Montana, 1974.

Bergofsky, E. H.: Pulmonary insufficiency after nonthoracic trauma: shock lung. Am. J. Med. Sci. 264:92–101, 1972.

Blaisdel, F. W., and Schlobohm, R. M.: The respiratory distress syndrome: a review. Surgery 74:251–262, 1973.

Bloomfield, D. A.: The recognition and management of massive pulmonary embolism. Heart Lung 3:241–246, 1974.

Brammell, H. L.: Arrhythmias in acute respiratory failure associated with chronic airway obstruction. Heart Lung 2:888–892, 1973.

Brannin, P. K.: Oxygen therapy and measures of bronchial hygiene. Nurs. Clin. North Am. 9:111–121, 1974.

Broughton, J. O.: Chest physical diagnosis for nurses and respiratory therapists. Heart Lung 1:200–206, 1972.

Bryant, L., Trinkle, J., and Dubilier, L.: Reappraisal of tracheal injury from cuffed tracheostomy tubes. J.A.M.A. 215:625–628, 1971.

Bryson, T. K., Benumof, J. L., and Ward, C. F.: The esophageal obturator airway: a clinical comparison to ventilation with a mask and oropharyngeal airway. Chest 74:537–539, 1978.

Butler, E. K.: Dyspnea in the patient with cardiopulmonary disease. Heart Lung 4:599–614, 1975.

Carden, B., and Bernstein, M.: Investigation of the nine most commonly used resuscitation bags. J.A.M.A. 212:589–592, 1970.

Carroll, R.: Evaluation of tracheal tube cuff designs. Crit. Care Med. 1:45–46, 1973.

Cherniack, R. M., Cherniack, L., and Naimark, A.: Respiration in Health and Disease. 2nd ed. W. B. Saunders Co., Philadelphia, 1972.

Christensson, P., et al.: Early and late results of controlled ventilation in flail chest. Chest 75:456–460, 1979.

Comroe, J. H., et al.: The Lung: Clinical Physiology and Pulmonary Function Tests, 2nd ed. Year Book Medical Publishers, Inc., Chicago, 1962.

Comroe, J. H.: Physiology of Respiration, 2nd ed. Year Book Medical Publishers, Inc., Chicago, 1974.

Cook, W. A.: Shock lung: etiology, prevention, and treatment. Heart Lung 3:933–938, 1974.

Cooper, J. D., and Grillo, H.: Analysis of problems related to cuffs on intratracheal tubes. Chest 62 (Suppl.): 21S–27S, 1972.

Crosby, L. J., and Parsons, L. C.: Measurements of lateral wall pressures exerted by tracheostomy and endotracheal tube cuffs, Heart Lung 3:797–803, 1974.

Davenport, H. W.: The ABC of Acid-Base Chemistry, 6th ed. University of Chicago Press, Chicago, 1974.

DeLaney, M.: Examination of the chest, Part I: The lungs. Nursing 75 5:12–14, 1975.

Desautels, D.: Methods of administering intermittent mandatory ventilation. Resp. Care 19:187–190, 1974.

Downs, J.B.: Intermittent mandatory ventilation: a new approach to weaning patients from mechanical ventilators. Chest 64:331–334, 1973.

Egan, D. P.: Fundamentals of Respiratory Therapy, 3rd ed. C. V. Mosby Co., St. Louis, 1977.

Fishman, A. P.: Shock lung: a distinctive nonentity. Circulation XLVII:921–923, 1973.

Fitzgerald, L.: Mechanical ventilation. Heart Lung 5:939–949, 1976.

Fitzgerald, L., and Huber, G.: Weaning the patient from mechanical ventilation. Heart Lung 5:228–234, 1976.

Fitzmaurice, J. B., and Sasahara, A.: Current concepts of pulmonary embolism: implications for nursing practice. Heart Lung 3:209–218, 1974.

Forgacs, P.: The functional basis of pulmonary sounds. Chest 73:399–405, 1978.

Franklin, W.: Treatment of severe asthma. N. Eng. J. Med. 290:1469–1472, 1974.

Frownfelter, D. L.: Chest Physical Therapy and Pulmonary Rehabilitation. Year Book Medical Publishers, Inc., Chicago, 1978.

Gracey, D. R.: Acute respiratory distress syndrome. Heart Lung 4:280–283, 1975.

Greenbaum, D. M.: Decannulation of the tracheostomized patient. Heart Lung 5:119–123, 1976.

Greenbaum, D. M., et al.: Continuous positive airway pressure without tracheal intubation in spontaneously breathing patients. Chest 69:615–620, 1976.

Guenter, C. A., and Welch, M. H.: Pulmonary Medicine. J. B. Lippincott Co., Philadelphia, 1977.

Guyton, A. C.: Textbook of Medical Physiology, 5th ed. W. B. Saunders Co., Philadelphia 1976, pp. 516–583.

Hudson, L. D.: The acute management of the chronic airway obstruction patient. Heart Lung 3:93–96, 1974.

Keyes, J. L.: Basic mechanisms involved in acid-base homeostasis. Heart Lung 5:239–246, 1976.

Keyes, J. L.: Blood-gas analysis and the assessment of acid-base status. Heart Lung 5:247–255, 1976.

Keyes, J. L. Blood-gases and blood-gas transport. Heart Lung 3:945–954, 1974.

Kirby, R. R., et al.: High level positive end expiratory pressure (PEEP) in acute respiratory insufficiency. Chest 67: 156–163, 1975.

Lake, K. B., and Van Dyke, J. J.: Prolonged nasotracheal intubation. Heart Lung 9:93–97, 1980.

Levy, M. M., and Stubbs, J. A.: Nursing implications in the care of patients treated with assisted mechanical ventilation modified with positive end-expiratory pressure. Heart Lung 7: 299–305, 1978.

Magovern, G. J., et al.: The clinical and experimental evaluation of a controlled-pressure intratracheal cuff. J. Thorac. Cardiovasc. Surg. 64:747–756, 1972.

Mittman, C.: Chronic obstructive lung disease: The result of the interaction of genetic and environmental factors. Heart Lung 2:222–226, 1973.

Murray, J. F.: The Normal Lung. W. B. Saunders Co., Philadelphia, 1976.

Naclerio, E. A.: Chest Injuries. Grune & Stratton, New York, 1971.

Naclerio, E. A.: Chest Trauma–Clinical Symposia. Ciba Found. Symp. 22, No. 3, 1970.

Naigow, D., and Powaser, M. M.: The effect of different endotracheal suction procedures on arterial blood gases in a controlled experimental model. Heart Lung 6:808–816, 1977.

Nett, L.: The use of mechanical ventilators. Nurs. Clin. North Am. 9:123–136, 1974.

Nett, L., and Petty, T.: Oxygen Toxicity. Am. J. Nurs. 73: 1156–1158, 1973.

Oaks, A., and Morrow, H.: Understanding blood gases. Nursing 73 3:15–21, 1973.

Pace, W. R.: Pulmonary Physiology in Clinical Practice, 2nd ed. F. A. Davis Co., Philadelphia, 1970.

Patient Assessment: Examination of the Chest and Lungs (Programed Instruction). Am. J. Nurs. 76:1–22, 1976.

Petty, T. A.: A chest physician's perspective on asthma. Heart Lung 1:611–620, 1972.

Petty, T. A.: Complications occurring during mechanical ventilation. Heart Lung 5:112–118, 1976.

Petty, T. A.: Intensive and Rehabilative Respiratory Care, 2nd ed. Lea & Febiger, Philadelphia, 1974.

Petty, T. A.: Respiratory failure and the heart. Heart Lung *1*:84–89, 1972.

Powaser, M., et al.: The effectiveness of hourly cuff deflation in minimizing tracheal damage. Heart Lung *5*: 734–741, 1976.

Prior, J. A., and Silberstein, J. S.: Physical Diagnosis: The History and Examination of the Patient, 5th ed. C. V. Mosby Co., St. Louis, 1977.

Risser, N. L.: Preoperative and postoperative care to prevent pulmonary complications. Heart Lung *9*:57–67, 1980.

Safar, P.: Recognition and management of airway obstruction. J.A.M.A. *208*: 112–115, 1969.

Selecky, P.: Tracheal damage and prolonged intubation with a cuffed endotracheal or tracheostomy tube. Heart Lung *5*:733, 1976.

Selecky, P.: Tracheostomy—a review of present day indications, complications, and care. Heart Lung *3*:272–283, 1974.

Shapiro, B., Harrison, R. A., and Trout, C. A.: Clinical Application of Respiratory Care. Year Book Medical Publishers, Chicago, 1975.

Shapiro, B. A., Harrison, R. A., and Walton, J. R.: Clinical Application of Blood Gases 2nd ed. Year Book Medical Publishers, Inc., Chicago, 1977.

Shimada, Y., et al.: Evaluation of the progress and prognosis of adult respiratory distress syndrome. Chest *76*: 180–186, 1979.

Slonim, N. B., and Hamilton, L. H.: Respiratory Physiology, 3rd ed. C. V. Mosby, St. Louis, 1976.

Stone, E. W., and Zuckerman, S.: The esophageal obturator airway. Am. J. Nurs. *75*:1148–1149, 1975.

Supplement on cardiorespiratory intensive care. Chest *62*:1S–125S, 1972.

Suter, P. M., Fairley, H. B., and Isenberg, M. D.: Optimum end-expiratory pressure in patients with acute pulmonary failure. N. Eng. J. Med. *292*:284–289, 1975.

Suter, P. M., Fairley, H. B., and Isenberg, M. D.: Effect of tidal volume and end-expiratory pressure on compliance during mechanical ventilation. Chest *73*:158–162, 1978.

The asphyxiating patient: what you can do to save him. Nurs. Update *3*:2–13, 1972.

Thorn, G. W., et al.: Harrison's Principles of Internal Medicine, 8th ed. McGraw-Hill Book Co., New York, 1977, pp. 1330–1419.

Traner, G.: Assessment of the thorax and lungs. Am. J. Nurs. *73*:466–471, 1973.

Turner, H. G.: The anatomy and physiology of normal respiration. Nurs. Clin. North Am. *3*:383–401, 1968.

Tyler, M.: Artificial airways. Nursing 73 *3*:22–36, 1973.

Venus, B., Jacobs, H. K., and Lim, L.: Treatment of the adult respiratory distress syndrome with continuous positive airway pressure. Chest *76*: 257–261, 1979.

Votteri, B. A.: Hand-operated emergency ventilation devices. Heart Lung *1*: 277–282, 1972.

Wade, J.: Respiratory Nursing Care, 2nd ed. C. V. Mosby Co., St. Louis, 1977.

Wenger, N. K., Stein, P. D., and Willis, P.W.: Massive acute pulmonary embolism: the deceivingly nonspecific manifestations. J.A.M.A. *220*:834–844, 1972.

Wen-Hsi en, et al.: Pressure dynamics of endotracheal and tracheostomy cuffs. Crit. Care Med. *1*:197–202, 1973.

Winslow, E. H.: Visual inspection of the patient with cardiopulmonary disease. Heart Lung *5*:421–429, 1975.

Wyper, M.: Pulmonary embolism: fighting the silent killer. Nursing 75 *5*:31–38, 1975.

THE CARDIOVASCULAR SYSTEM

prepared by

RICHARD DeANGELIS, R.N., B.S., M.S.

KATHLEEN G. ANDREOLI, R.N., D.S.N., F.A.A.N.

LINDA SCHAFF, R.N., M.S.N., C.S. and

BETTYE H. BALL, R.N., B.S.N., M.S.N.

BEHAVIORAL OBJECTIVES

Functional Anatomy

1. Describe the normal anatomy of the cardiovascular system and its respective function(s).

2. Describe the conduction system of the heart.

Physiology

1. Delineate the electromechanics of the heart muscle.

2. Explain the neural innervation of the cardiovascular system.

3. Compare the relationship of pressures in the heart to the mechanical events of the cardiac cycle.

4. Describe the effects of the relationship between stroke volume and end-diastolic volume (Starling's law of the heart) on cardiac output.

5. Describe the physiologic events that create and maintain arterial pressure.

6. List the factors that determine venous pressure.

7. Discuss the cardiac conduction system: its inherent characteristics, its normal sequence of activation in the heart, and its relationship to pump action.

Assessment

1. Describe a systematic approach for assessment of the cardiovascular system, including history-taking and physical examination components.

2. Explain the diagnostic studies generally used in the assessment of the cardiovascular system.

3. Identify basic cardiac dysrhythmias and describe a systematic approach to accurate interpretation.

4. When given several common cardiovascular disease processes, select the characteristic changes in inspection, palpation, percussion, and auscultation that occur with each.

General Patient Care Management

1. Develop a plan for nursing intervention to assist in the maintenance of optimal cardiovascular functioning.

2. Identify the underlying physiologic concepts of hemodynamic monitoring techniques utilized in the care of the critically ill cardiovascular patient.

Pathologic Conditions and Management

For each of the following: arteriosclerosis, angina pectoris, acute coronary insufficiency, myocardial infarction, congestive heart failure, pericarditis, and hypertensive crisis:

1. Describe the specific physiologic alterations that characterize each condition.

2. Utilize a systematic approach to the identification of each condition based on clinical presentation, presence of etiologic or precipitating factors, and diagnostic findings.

3. Describe the treatment modalities used in the management of the acutely ill cardiovascular patient.

4. Identify the specific patient care management designed to meet the needs of the critically ill cardiovascular patient.

5. Describe the therapeutic indications for temporary and permanent cardiac pacing, including nursing management, and emphasizing the prevention of potential complications.

In the case of shock:

6. Describe the pathophysiology of shock, including both total body and individual organ response.

7. Discuss the compensatory mechanisms seen in the shock syndrome.

8. Delineate the syndromes of hypovolemic, neurogenic, septic, and cardiogenic shock, and the treatment modalities pertinent to each.

9. Develop a nursing management model that depicts an orderly and systematic manner of determining the nursing care of the patient in shock.

With regard to cardiovascular surgery:

10. Describe the treatment modality of cardiovascular surgery, including indications for the specific procedures, types of procedures, and potential complications.

11. Outline the essential elements of nursing care that meet the needs of the post-operative cardiovascular surgical patient.

THE CARDIOVASCULAR SYSTEM

_____ FUNCTIONAL ANATOMY _____

SKELETAL MUSCLE

1. **Central nucleus**

2. **Sarcoplasma**: intracellular proteinaceous fluid

3. **Sarcolemma**: the membrane that surrounds the muscle fiber (a single cell)

4. **Fiber**: composed of many fibrils, each surrounded by a sarcotubular system

5. **Sarcotubular system**: a membranous continuation of sarcolemma
   a. T tubules function to transmit action potential (AP) rapidly from sarcolemma to all fibrils in muscle
   b. Sarcoplasmic reticulum houses calcium ions. Action potential in T tubules causes release of calcium from reticulum, resulting in a contraction

6. **Contractile unit**: sarcomere
   a. Muscle fiber composed of fibrils
      i. Each fibril is divisible into filaments
      ii. Each filament is made up of contractile proteins
      iii. Contractile proteins consist of actin, myosin, troponin, tropomyosin
         (a) Myosin forms the thick filaments
         (b) Actin, troponin, and tropomyosin form the thin filaments
         (c) Thick and thin filaments interdigitate with onset of ionic movement across membrane (depolarization – for further definition, see Electrophysiology section) and produce a contraction

CARDIAC MUSCLE: Differs from skeletal muscle. It has more mitochondria, and can provide more adenosine triphosphate (ATP) and energy required for repetitive action.

1. **Fibers**: connected to each other by intercalated discs forming a lattice arrangement called a functional syncytium

81

2. **Syncytium:** when one fiber is depolarized, AP spreads along syncytium to all other fibers, stimulating them also. Thus, whole syncytium contracts, not just one fiber (an all or none response)

STRUCTURE OF THE CARDIAC WALL

1. **Pericardium:** a fibroserous membranous sac that encloses heart and roots of great vessels. Functions to protect heart from friction. Composed of two layers
   a. Fibrous pericardium – outermost layer
   b. Serous pericardium – has two layers
      i. Parietal layer
      ii. Visceral layer – this is outer surface of heart itself (epicardium)

2. **Epicardium:** equivalent to visceral layer of serous pericardium

3. **Myocardium:** muscular portion of heart

4. **Endocardium:** inner membranous surface of heart lining chambers of heart

5. **Papillary muscles:** arise from endocardial surface of ventricles, and attach to chordae tendineae

6. **Chordae tendineae:** attach to tricuspid and mitral valves. Papillary muscles and chordae tendineae work together to permit opening and closing of valves during relaxation and contraction of ventricles. Chordae tendineae also serve to prevent eversion of valves during systole

CHAMBERS

1. **Atria:** thin-walled, low pressure chambers
   a. Both right and left atria act as reservoirs of blood for their respective ventricles
   b. 70% of blood flows passively from atria into ventricles during early ventricular diastole (protodiastole)
   c. Right atrium receives systemic venous blood via superior vena cava, inferior vena cava, and coronary sinus
   d. Left atrium receives oxygenated blood returning to heart from lungs via the four pulmonary veins

2. **Ventricles:** the major "pumps" of the heart
   a. Right ventricle
      i. Contracts (ventricular systole) and propels deoxygenated blood into pulmonary circulation via pulmonary artery (PA) (the only artery in body that carries deoxygenated blood)

      ii.   Functions in a low pressure system.
  b. Left ventricle — main "pump"
      i.   Ejects blood into systemic circulation during ventricular systole via aorta
      ii.   Functions in a high pressure system

3. **Factors influencing atrial function**
  a. Fiber length
  b. Sympathetic and parasympathetic (vagal) innervation

4. **Factors influencing ventricular function**
  a. Atrial function
  b. Neuronal control
  c. Drugs, electrolytes, pH
  d. Electrical stimulation
  e. Preload
      i.   Resting force of myocardium determined by volume in ventricles at end of diastole (left ventricular end-diastolic pressure — LVEDP)
      ii.   Preload can be related to a number of variables, e.g., fiber length, stretch
      iii.   Increase in preload stretches myocardial muscle fibers, which increases force of ventricular contraction, increasing stroke volume and thus cardiac output
      iv.   Increase in preload is accomplished by increasing the volume returning to ventricles
      v.   Muscle fibers reach a point of stretch beyond which contraction is no longer enhanced; stroke volume decreases, leading to heart failure
      vi.   Above concepts are known as the Frank-Starling Law of the Heart
  f. Afterload
      i.   Since initial resistance that must be overcome for ejection is opening of aortic valve, afterload is more or less equivalent to aortic pressure
      ii.   In systemic arterial circulation, resistance is primarily a function of arteriolar diameter
      iii.   As afterload increases, amount of tension against which ventricles must pump increases
      iv.   Thus, increase in systemic arterial pressure, e.g., increases afterload and causes more resistance for left ventricle to overcome in order to propel blood
      v.   Intra-aortic balloon pump works on this concept — it decreases resistance (decreases afterload) that left ventricle must pump against; consequently, ventricle requires less oxygen in order to function

VALVES OF THE HEART: Two types.

1. **Atrioventricular valves**
   a. Opening and closing are controlled by papillary muscles and chordae tendineae
   b. Consist of tricuspid and mitral valves
      i. Allow unidirectional blood flow from each respective atrium to each respective ventricle during ventricular diastole, and prevent retrograde flow during ventricular systole
         (a) With ventricular diastole, papillary muscles relax and valve leaflets open
         (b) With increased ventricular pressure and systole, valve leaflets approximate completely
         (c) Closing of valves produces a sound that constitutes first heart sound, S_1. This consists of a mitral and a tricuspid component ($M_1 T_1$). M_1 is initial and major component of S_1
      ii. Tricuspid valve is situated between right atrium and right ventricle; mitral valve between left atrium and left ventricle

2. **Semilunar valves**
   a. Consist of pulmonary and aortic valves
      i. Allow unidirectional blood flow from respective ventricle to arterial outflow tract during ventricular systole, and prevent retrograde blood flow during ventricular diastole
         (a) Opening occurs when respective ventricle contracts — pressure is greater than in arterial outflow tract, and valve opens
         (b) After ventricular systole, pressure in arterial outflow tract exceeds that in respective ventricle, and retrograde blood flow causes valve to close.
         (c) Closing of valves produces a sound that constitutes initial and major component of second heart sound, S_2. This consists of an aortic and pulmonary component ($A_2 P_2$). A_2 is the initial major component of S_2
      ii. Pulmonary valve is situated between right ventricle and pulmonary artery; aortic valve between left ventricle and aorta

VASCULATURE

1. **Major functions:** are to supply tissues with blood and nutrients, and remove metabolic wastes

2. **Resistance to flow:** depends on viscosity of blood and diameter of vessels, in particular the arterioles

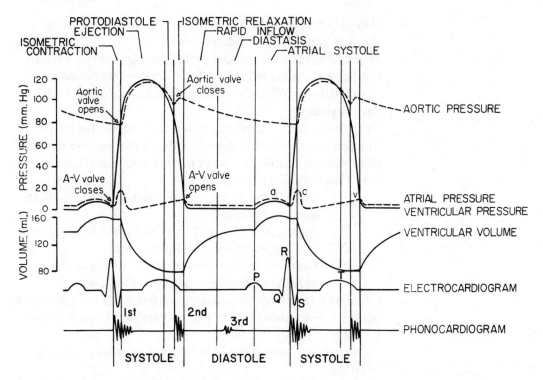

Figure 2-1. The events of the cardiac cycle, showing changes in left atrial pressure, left ventricular pressure, aortic pressure, ventricular volume, the electrocardiogram, and the phonocardiogram. (From Guyton, A.C.: Textbook of Medical Physiology, 5th ed. W.B. Saunders Co., Philadelphia, 1976, p. 164.)

3. **Blood flow to tissues:** controlled via local chemical reactions and nerves which dilate or constrict blood vessels

4. **Major components of vasculature system**
    a. Arteries
        i.   Strong, compliant, elastic-walled vessels that carry blood away from heart and distribute it to capillary beds throughout body
        ii. This is a high pressure system
        iii. Owing to elastic fibers located within arterial wall, arteries are able to stretch during systole and recoil during diastole
    b. Arterioles
        i.   Contain smooth muscle innervated by adrenergic sympathetic nerves, the stimulation of which causes constriction of vessels. Decreased adrenergic discharge dilates vessels, thus controlling blood distribution to various capillary beds
        ii. Controlled by autonomic nervous system (ANS) and by autoregulation
        iii. The major vessels controlling total peripheral resistance, and thus arterial blood pressure

    iv.   May give rise directly to capillaries — regulation of flow is through constriction or dilatation

    v.   May first give rise to metarterioles (precapillaries), which then give rise to capillaries. They serve as thoroughfare channels to venules or conduits to supply capillary beds

c. Capillary system

    i.   Nutritional flow — capillary blood flow allows for exchange of gases and solutes between blood and tissues, and permits fluid volume transfer between plasma and interstitium

        (a) Capillary filtration

            (1) Due to sum of hydrostatic and osmotic pressures across membrane

            (2) Increased hydrostatic pressure leads to movement of fluid from vessel to interstitium

            (3) Greater capillary osmotic pressure leads to fluid movement from interstitium into vessels

    ii. Capillaries lack smooth muscle. Control of their diameter is passive owing to changes in precapillary and postcapillary resistance

    iii. Capillaries can withstand high internal pressures without bursting

    iv. Diffusion — the process most important in moving substrates and wastes between blood and tissues via capillary system

d. Venous system

    i.   Stores approximately 65% of total volume of blood in circulatory system

    ii. Venules

        (a) Receive blood from capillaries

        (b) Serve as collecting channels and capacitance (storage) vessels

    iii. Veins

        (a) Also capacitance vessels

        (b) Conduct blood back to heart within a low pressure system

        (c) Venous pump — skeletal muscle pump; veins are surrounded by skeletal muscles. When these contract, they compress veins moving blood toward heart. Valves in veins prevent retrograde blood flow

            (1) Under normal conditions, venous pump keeps venous pressure in lower extremities at 25 mm Hg or less

            (2) Gravity has profound effects on the erect, immobile individual. Pressures can rise to 90 mm Hg in the lower extremities, which results in swelling and a decrease in blood volume due to leakage of fluid from circulatory system into interstitium

CONDUCTION SYSTEM

1. **Sinoatrial (S-A) node**
    a. Normal pacemaker of heart, since it possesses fastest inherent rate of depolarization
    b. Initiates a rhythmic, self-excitatory impulse

2. **Internodal atrial pathways** (Goldman, 1976, pp. 36–37)
    a. Composed of three internodal tracts
        i. Bachmann's – anterior
        ii. Wenckebach's – middle
        iii. Thorel's – posterior
    b. Pathways conduct impulse generated in S-A node through atria, causing depolarization, followed by atrial contraction and ejection of blood into ventricles

3. **Atrioventricular junction (A-V node)**
    a. Delays impulse from atria before it goes to ventricles
    b. Allows time for both ventricles to fill prior to ventricular systole

4. **Bundle of His:** arises from A-V node and conducts impulse from it to bundle branch system

5. **Bundle branch system:** pathways that arise from bundle of His, and composed of three parts
    a. Right bundle branch (RBB)
        i. Transmits impulse down right side of interventricular septum toward right ventricular myocardium
        ii. Divides into three parts – anterior, lateral, posterior – that then further divide, becoming parts of Purkinje system (see below)
    b. Left bundle branch (LBB)
        i. Left posterior fascicle arises from LBB and transmits impulse over posterior and inferior endocardial surface of left ventricle
        ii. Left anterior fascicle arises from LBB and transmits impulse to anterior and superior endocardial surfaces of left ventricle

6. **Purkinje system**
    a. Arises from distal portion of bundle branches
    b. Transmits impulse into subendocardial layers of both ventricles, and provides for depolarization (from endocardium to epicardium), followed by ventricular contraction and ejection of blood out of ventricles

_____ PHYSIOLOGY _____

CARDIAC MUSCLE MECHANICS*

1. **Electromechanics**
   a. Ionic exchange during depolarization-repolarization process (sodium and potassium ions primarily involved)
   b. AP produced during depolarization is transmitted to interior of cell via T tubules, which transmit AP to all myofibrils of muscle
   c. Calcium is stored in lateral sacs of sarcoplasmic reticulum, and is released when AP reaches sarcoplasmic reticulum from T tubules
   d. Calcium enters interior of cell, and through a complex interaction with enzymes, causes interaction between actin and myosin filaments, which ultimately ends in a contraction of muscle fibers

2. **Contractile process**
   a. Actin filaments move progressively inward on myosin filaments as successive electrochemical interactions take place (interdigitation: the sliding filament hypothesis)
   b. This results in shortening of sarcomeres, causing shortening of muscle fibers, and thus myocardial contraction
   c. Free calcium is then absorbed back into sarcoplasmic reticulum, resulting in relaxation

3. **Principle of cardiac muscle function:** Frank-Starling Law
   a. The more cardiac muscle fiber is stretched in diastole (i.e., augmented venous return, increased preload, increased LVEDP) to a point, the stronger the contraction is in the next systole
   b. Increase in myocardial contractility results in increase in stroke volume, and thus in cardiac output
   c. There is an optimal level of muscle fiber stretch beyond which contraction of myocardium weakens, causing decreased stroke volume and cardiac output (varies with each individual)

4. **Variables affecting contractility**
   a. Inotropy — affects strength of cardiac contraction
      i. Positive inotropy — increase in myocardial contractility (which may increase cardiac output)
      ii. Negative inotropy — decrease in myocardial contractility
   b. Cardiac drugs
      i. Positive inotropic drugs — digitalis, isoproterenol, calcium, catecholamines (norepinephrine, dopamine, epinephrine, dobutamine)
      ii. Negative inotropic drugs — quinidine, barbiturates, propranolol

_____

*See also electrophysiology section on pp. 93–95.

    c. Changes in cardiac rate and rhythm (force-frequency ratio, increase rate → increase in myocardial contractility)

    d. Available oxygen — hypoxia (O_2 saturation $< 50\%$) depresses myocardial contractility

    e. Hypercapnia — increased CO_2 directly depresses myocardium

    f. Pharmacologic depressants such as barbiturates depress myocardial contractility

    g. Intrinsic depression — heart failure depresses myocardial contractility owing to overstretch of myofibrils (Frank-Starling Law)

    h. Muscle condition — loss of functional myocardial tissue decreases myocardial contractility (e.g., scar secondary to myocardial infarction)

    i. Excessive afterload/preload increases depress myocardial tissue (when they increase above optimal functional level)

    j. Neural control
        i. Sympathetic stimulation increases myocardial contractility (mechanism not fully understood)
        ii. Parasympathetic stimulation (via vagus nerve) has depressive effects on S-A node, atrial myocardium, and A-V junctional tissue that decrease myocardial contractility (mechanism not fully understood and remains hypothetical)

    k. Concentration of cations in plasma
        i. Hyponatremia and hyperkalemia diminish myocardial contractility
        ii. Hypercalcemia increases myocardial contractility

CONTROL OF PERIPHERAL BLOOD VESSELS

1. **Local control mechanisms:** autoregulation (three hypotheses exist)
    a. Myogenic response — as pressure rises, vessels stretch, stimulating contraction of smooth muscles (feedback mechanism). As tension decreases, smooth muscles relax
    b. Metabolic hypothesis — metabolic activity of tissue is thought to cause a decrease in O_2 saturation, an increase in CO_2, acidosis, hyperkalemia, prostaglandins, and phosphatemia. This gives rise to formation of metabolites, which cause vasodilation that increases blood flow to area; thus, waste products of metabolic activity are diluted and removed from the area. There may be a delicate balance between these two mechanisms: myogenic response → vasoconstriction → decreases blood supply → local increase in metabolites → vasodilation → wastes removed
    c. Tissue pressure hypothesis — not described since very few data support this mechanism

2. **Autonomic regulation of vessels**
    a. Sympathetic nervous system secretes norepinephrine at nerve endings (adrenergic effect) → producing vasoconstriction

       i.   In arterioles, this mechanism helps regulate blood flow and arterial pressure

      ii.   In veins, this mechanism helps vary amount of blood stored; i.e., venoconstriction → an increase in venous return to heart

  b. Parasympathetic nervous stimulation secretes acetylcholine at nerve endings (cholinergic effect), producing vasodilation

3. **Baroreceptors (pressoreceptors):** stretch receptors

  a. Receptor sites located in aortic arch, carotid sinus, vena cava, pulmonary arteries, and atria

  b. Sensitive to arterial pressures above 60 mm Hg

  c. Action with elevated blood pressure

      i.   Response to stretching of arterial walls

      ii.   Impulse transmitted from aortic arch via vagus nerve to medulla, and from carotid sinus via Hering's nerve to glossopharyngeal nerve to medulla

      iii. Sympathetic action inhibited

      iv. Vagal reflex dominates

      v.   Result — decreased heart rate and contractility, dilation of peripheral vessels, BP back to normal

  d. Action with decreased blood pressure

      i.   Vagal tone decreased

      ii.   Sympathetic system becomes dominant

      iii. Result — increased heart rate and contractility, arterial and venous constriction and thus BP elevated to near normal

4. **Vasomotor center in medulla:** also called cardioaccelerator center or cardiac center. Consists of two areas, vasoconstrictor and vasodepressor

  a. Stimulation of vasoconstrictor area causes

      i.   Increased heart rate, stroke volume, and cardiac output, and ultimately increased arterial BP

      ii.   Venoconstriction, which decreases stores of blood in venous system

  b. Inhibition of vasoconstrictor area stimulates vasodepressor area, which causes vasodilation — there is an increase in storage of blood in venous system, thereby decreasing stroke volume and cardiac output, and thus arterial BP

  c. Vasomotor center works with baroreceptors and chemoreceptors located in carotid sinus and aortic arch

      i.   Rise in BP stimulates carotid sinus, which in turn inhibits vasoconstrictor area. This induces vasodilation via stimulation of vasodepressor area, and sequence of events follows as listed above; the converse also occurs

      ii.   Fall in O_2 saturation, rise in CO_2, or fall in pH stimulates chemoreceptors, which then stimulate vasoconstrictor center and cause a rise in arterial BP.

CONTROL OF THE HEART

1. **Stimulation of sympathetic nervous system:** causes release of nor-epinephrine, a neurotransmitter, eliciting two types of effects
   a. Alpha-adrenergic — produces arteriolar vasoconstriction
   b. Beta-adrenergic
      i.   Increases S-A node discharge, and thus increase in heart rate
      ii. Has positive inotropic effects

2. **Stimulation of parasympathetic nervous system:** occurs through action of right vagus (affecting S-A node) and left vagus (affecting A-V conduction tissue). Releases acetylcholine — also a neurotransmitter (cholinergic effect)
   a. Decreases rate of discharge from S-A node to produce brady-cardia, or even sinus arrest
   b. May slow A-V conduction tissue, producing various degrees of A-V block
   c. Both "a" and "b" above lead to decreased heart rate

3. **Chemoreceptors (carotid and aortic bodies):** sensitive to fall in O_2 and rise in CO_2, causing increase in heart rate via stimulation of vasomotor center in medulla

4. **Baroreceptors (pressoreceptors):** respond to pressure changes (see page 90)
   a. Increase in arterial pressure stimulates vasodepressor area of vasomotor center, which then increases vagal tone and slows heart rate, tending to decrease BP
   b. Decrease in arterial pressure inhibits vasomotor center, which decreases vagal tone and accelerates heart rate, tending to increase BP

5. **Other reflexes that affect heart rate**
   a. Atrial (Bainbridge) reflex, via stretch receptors in atria — increase in atrial pressure causes increase in heart rate
   b. Respiratory-heart reflexes — inspiration stimulates stretch receptors in lungs and thorax, which then cause increased heart rate
   c. Hormonal reflexes that increase pacemaker activity

ARTERIAL PRESSURE

1. **Definition:** cardiac output times total peripheral resistance

2. **Regulation**
   a. Arterial pressure is controlled by various mechanisms outlined in section on Control of peripheral blood vessels (pages 89–90)

    b. Arterial pressure controlled by hormonal mechanisms
       i. Renin-angiotensin system
          (a) Renin, a protease secreted by kidney, converts angiotensin I to angiotensin II
          (b) Release of renin from kidney is stimulated by
              (1) Baroreceptors in juxtaglomerular cells that are sensitive to changes in BP
                  (a) Decreased BP → increased renin secretion
                  (b) Increased BP → decreased renin secretion
              (2) Increased sympathetic output causes increased renin secretion
              (3) Fall in sodium concentration causes increased renin secretion
       ii. Angiotensin II is most potent vasoconstrictor known; produces arteriolar constriction and rise in systolic and diastolic pressures
    c. Capillary fluid shift mechanisms
    d. Local control mechanisms (see section on Control of peripheral blood vessels)
    e. Renal — fluid volume process
       i. With rise in arterial pressure, kidneys excrete more fluid, causing reduction in extracellular fluid and blood volumes that reduces circulating blood volume and cardiac output, leading to normalization of arterial pressure
       ii. With fall in arterial pressure, kidneys retain fluid, causing increased blood volume and cardiac output that results in normalization of arterial pressure

3. **Factors affecting arterial blood pressure**
    a. Cardiac output
    b. Peripheral resistance
    c. Arterial elasticity
    d. Blood volume
    e. Blood viscosity
    f. Age
    g. Weight
    h. Exercise
    i. Emotions

4. **Mean arterial BP** (Berne and Levy, 1977, 103): "The average pressure during a given cardiac cycle that exists in the aorta and its major branches . . . It is dependent on the mean volume of blood in the arterial system and the elastic properties of the arterial walls."
    a. Equivalent to diastolic pressure plus pulse pressure (difference between systolic and diastolic pressures) multiplied by 0.3 to 0.4 D + (PP × 0.4) (Wilson, 1977, p. 33)

b. Example: BP of 120/70 has a pulse pressure of 50 mm Hg

$$(D + PP \times 0.4) = 70 + (50 \times 0.4) = 70 + 20 = 90$$

PULSE PRESSURE

1. **Definition**: numerical difference between systolic and diastolic pressures

2. **A function of stroke volume and arterial capacitance**

CARDIAC OUTPUT

1. **Determined by stroke volume** (amount of blood ejected by left ventricle at each beat — about 60 ml) times heart rate

$$CO = SV \times HR$$

2. **Regulation**
   a. Changes in heart rate
   b. Changes in stroke volume
      i. Increased sympathetic activity causes increased myocardial contractility (positive inotropy), and thus more blood is ejected (increased stroke volume); this increases cardiac output
      ii. Preload — when muscle fibers are stretched owing to increased preload, force of contraction increases; thus, stroke volume and cardiac output increase
      iii. Afterload — high afterloads decrease stroke volume and cardiac output
   c. Changes in venous return to heart
      i. Reduction in total blood volume decreases venous return. This causes a fall in cardiac filling, stroke volume, and cardiac output
      ii. Venous constriction decreases venous pooling and promotes venous return to heart. This increases cardiac filling, stroke volume, and cardiac output
   d. Myocardial contractility (see section on factors affecting myocardial contractility, pp. 88–89)

ELECTROPHYSIOLOGY

1. **Resting membrane potential (RMP)**
   a. Sodium ion concentration higher outside of cell
   b. Potassium ion and anion (proteins) concentration higher inside of cell

    c. More sodium outside of cell than inside, and so outside is more positively charged than inside (therefore, inside is "negative" with respect to outside)

    d. RMP = -80 to -90 mV for myocardial muscle fibers

    e. To control concentrations of sodium and potassium there is a "pump" ("sodium pump") that regulates concentration of these cations in resting membrane and during depolarization-repolarization process. It continuously extrudes sodium out of cell and pumps potassium into cell

2. **Cell membrane:** passively permeable to sodium and potassium

    a. This permeability is variable in time

    b. Resting cell membrane is more permeable to potassium and less to sodium

3. **Stimulation of resting membrane**

    a. Must be of certain strength in order to produce change in RMP; this change is recorded in the form of an AP

        i. Threshold intensity — minimal intensity of stimulus needed to generate change in RMP sufficient to produce an AP

    b. Causes reversal in membrane potential (sodium diffuses into cell and potassium diffuses out) that results in an AP (see Figure 2–2)

        i. Membrane is now more positive inside cell (+ 40 mv)

        ii. This process is called depolarization — AP spreads in a wave-like form throughout cells. Depolarization lasts for only milliseconds before membrane potential returns to RMP level

        iii. Repolarization — return of membrane potential RMP level (See Figure 2–2)

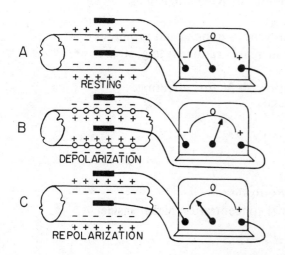

Figure 2-2. Sequential events during the action potential, showing: (A) the normal resting potential, (B) development of a reversal potential during depolarization, and (C) re-establishment of the normal resting potential during repolarization. (From Guyton, A.C.: Textbook of Medical Physiology, 5th ed. W.B. Saunders Co., Philadelphia, 1976, p. 117).

c. Two forces that move potassium across membrane during depolarization are
    i.   Chemical force — based on a concentration gradient, potassium diffuses out to where it is less concentrated
    ii. Electrostatic counterforce —
         (a) Anions (proteins that are negatively charged) remain inside cell when potassium moves out
         (b) Positively charged potassium ions, when out of cell, are attracted to anions inside cell
d. Same forces, chemical and electrostatic, also act to pull extracellular sodium into cell

_____ ASSESSMENT*_____

HISTORY

1. **Chief complaint**: consists of patient's own words as to why he is seeking help — one sentence is sufficient

2. **History of present illness**: determine
    a. Date of onset
    b. Description of complaint
    c. Mode of onset, course, duration
    d. Location
    e. Exacerbations, remissions of all signs and symptoms
        i.   Pain — character, location, radiation, quality, duration, factors that aggravate or produce, factors that alleviate
        ii.   Fatigue — with or without activity
        iii. Edema — location, degree
        iv.   Syncope — with or without dizziness, and time of occurrence
        v.   Dyspnea, orthopnea, paroxysmal nocturnal dyspnea, dyspnea on exertion
        vi.   Palpitations or dysrhythmias
        vii. Hemoptysis
        viii. Cyanosis (circumoral, extremities)
        ix.   Intermittent claudication
        x.   Clubbing

3. **Past medical history**: includes all previous illness, injuries, surgical procedures

_____

*In the section on ECGs, heart sounds, heart valves, and other physiologic aspects, refer to the diagrams for additional graphic information.

4. **Family history**: determine
    a. State of health or cause of death of immediate family members
    b. Hereditary familial diseases pertaining to cardiovascular system
        i.   Diabetes
        ii. Hypertension
        iii. Cardiovascular disease (stroke, transient ischemic attacks)
        iv. Gout
        v.   Obesity
        vi. Allergies

5. **Social history**: determine
    a. Present and past work experiences
    b. Smoking patterns
    c. Drinking habits
    d. Daily living patterns
    e. Types of foods eaten
    f. Relationship with significant others
    g. Recreational habits
    h. Sex life

6. **Medication history**: note all medications prescribed or bought over counter, and dosages being taken by patient

PHYSICAL EXAMINATION

1. **Inspection**
    a. Note general overall appearance
    b. Check skin and mucous membranes
        i.   Color
        ii. Turgor
        iii. Edema – usually found in extremities, sacrum, behind scapula, or in periorbital area
        iv. Nailbeds – color, clubbing
        v.   Angiomas
        vi. Petechiae
    c. Observe neck veins – internal rather than external jugular veins are more reliable. They reflect pressure and volume changes in right atrium
        i.   Check for distention and pulsation
             (a) Place patient in 45-degree angle position
             (b) Shine a bright light tangentially to illuminate vessels
        ii. Determine CVP (roughly) – norm = 4–15 cm H_2O
             (a) Place patient in position above
             (b) Manubrial joint is roughly 4 cm above atrium
             (c) Measure distance from manubrium to top of distended neck vein
             (d) Value obtained plus the 4 cm provides a rough estimate of CVP

    d. Check for a hepatojugular reflex (HJR)
       i.   Place patient in 45-degree angle position
      ii.   Compress upper abdomen for 30–45 seconds
     iii.   If HJR is present, jugular pulses will become more
           pronouced and level of filling of the neck veins will rise
    e. Extremities – note and compare both sides for
       i.   Edema
      ii.   Color/temperature changes
     iii.   Hair distribution
     iv.   Clubbing of nail beds
      v.   Ulcerations
     vi.   Peripheral pulses
    f. Precordium
       i.   Observe for heaves
      ii.   Shape and contour of chest
     iii.   Symmetry
     iv.   Breathing pattern
      v.   Pulses
     vi.   Visible point of maximal intensity (PMI)

2. **Palpation:** bilateral, simultaneous (except for carotids)
    a. Arteries
       i.   Check rate, rhythm, contour, and volume
      ii.   Rated on scale of 0 to 4
          (a)   0 = absent pulses
          (b)   1+ = palpable
          (c)   2+ = normal
          (d)   3+ = full
          (e)   4+ = full and bounding
     iii.   Most common sites for palpation
          (a)   Carotid
          (b)   Brachial
          (c)   Radial
          (d)   Femoral
          (e)   Popliteal
          (f)   Dorsalis pedis
          (g)   Posterior tibialis
     iv.   Note following types of pulses
          (a)   Pulsus magnus – strong, bounding pulse with a rapid
              upstroke and downstroke. Found in
             (1)   Essential hypertension
             (2)   Thyrotoxicosis
             (3)   Aortic insufficiency (AI)
             (4)   Patent ductus arteriosus (PDA)
             (5)   Arteriovenous fistula
          (b)   Pulsus parvus – small, weak pulse with a delayed
              upstroke and a prolonged downstroke. Found in

        (1)   Aortic stenosis (AS)
        (2)   Mitral stenosis (MS)
        (3)   Constrictive pericarditis
        (4)   Cardiac tamponade

   (c) Pulsus alternans — owing to weakened myocardium, pulse waves alternate, every other beat being weaker than preceding beat. Found in
        (1)   Severe arterial hypertension
        (2)   Left ventricular failure

   (d) Pulsus paradoxus — an exaggeration of normal physiologic response to inspiration. Normally, upon inspiration, there is a fall of less than 10 mm Hg in arterial systolic pressure. With pulsus paradoxus, arterial pressure drop upon inspiration exceeds 10 mm Hg. To be significant, fall must occur during normal inspiratory effort. Found in
        (1)   Pericardial effusion
        (2)   Constrictive pericarditis
        (3)   Severe pulmonary emphysema

   (e) Pulsus bisferiens ("double beating" pulse) — characterized by two impulses palpated during systole. Found in
        (1)   AI
        (2)   AS

b. Precordium
   i.   Palpate in order to note
      (a) Pulsations (like PMI)
      (b) Thrills (palpable murmurs, analogous to sensation felt on throat of purring cat)
      (c) Friction rubs (analogous to sensation felt when rubbing two pieces of leather together)

   ii. Palpate following seven areas and note pulsations or thrills, and their location in cardiac cycle
      (a) Sternoclavicular area — suprasternal notch
      (b) Aortic area — second right intercostal space (2RICS) near sternum
      (c) Pulmonic area — second left intercostal space (2LICS) near sternum
      (d) Anterior precordium — lower half of sternum and ICS both to left and right, adjacent to sternum
      (e) Apical area — area of PMI. Note location, size, and character of impulse — normally found in 5 LICS, midclavicular line, and is approximately 2 cm in size
      (f) Epigastric area — inferior to xiphoid process
      (g) Ectopic area — left cardiac border midway between pulmonary and apical areas

3. **Percussion**
   a. Limited use in this system owing to extracardiac factors interfering with the technique
   b. Used to determine outer limits of cardiac dullness, i.e., heart size

4. **Auscultation** (Lehmann, 1972, pp. 1242–1246)
   a. Sound – an object is set in motion (vibration), initiating a sound wave cycle
   b. Characteristics of sound
       i. Frequency/pitch – frequency (number of wave cycles per second) determines pitch of sound
           (a) High frequency (high number of wave cycles per second) vibrations produce high-pitched sounds.
           (b) Low frequency vibrations produce low-pitched sounds.
       ii. Intensity/loudness (will be considered synonymous) determined by amplitude of sound wave. This depends on the energy producing the vibration – more energy produces high amplitude of sound wave, and thus louder sound
       iii. Quality – sounds of same loudness and pitch coming from a different source are distinguished by their quality
       iv. Duration – pertains to number of continuous vibrations set in motion: the more vibrations, the longer the sound lasts
   c. Origin of heart sounds – opening and closing of valves and muscular contraction can cause turbulent blood flow, or rapid acceleration or deceleration of blood, producing either low or high frequency sounds
       i. High frequency, high intensity sounds are called heart sounds
       ii. Low frequency, low intensity sounds are called heart murmurs
   d. Auscultation recording instruments
       i. Stethoscope
           (a) Bell used to hear low-pitched sounds (heart sounds S_3, S_4 and ventricular filling murmurs)
           (b) Diaphragm used to hear high-pitched sounds (heart sounds S_1 and S_2, ejection clicks, opening snaps, and murmurs due to stenosis of values)
       ii. Phonocardiogram – used to demonstrate cardiac sounds graphically
   e. Normal heart sounds (refer to Figure 2–1)
       i. First heart sound (S_1) is produced when mitral and tricuspid valves close
           (a) Ventricles contract asynchronously – left before right
           (b) Component parts of S_1 may be heard, (M_1 and T_1)

(c) Occurs at onset of ventricular systole

ii. Second heart sound (S_2) is produced when aortic and pulmonary valves close

(a) Due to asynchronous ventricular contraction.

(b) Component parts of S_2 may be heard (A_2 and P_2)

(c) Occurs at end of ventricular systole

iii. Third heart sound (S_3) may normally be heard in diastole

(a) Usually heard in young adults and children (physiologic S_3)

(b) If heard in older age-groups or in association with disease entities, probably abnormal

iv. Variant splitting of heart sounds

(a) Physiologic (normal) split of S_2 ($A_2 P_2$)

(1) P_2 is delayed on inspiration owing to increased venous return to heart on inspiration, and since right ventricle is slower to contract than left ventricle

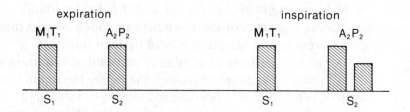

(2) Aortic component (A_2) precedes pulmonary (P_2) and is generally louder

(3) Heard best over aortic and pulmonary areas

(4) May be heard best in recumbent position and in young adults

f. Abnormal heart sounds

i. Fixed splitting of S_2

(a) Persistent splitting of A_2 and P_2 in both inspiration and expiration

(b) Seen in atrial septal defect (ASD)

ii. Expiratory splitting of S_2 — second sound is split on expiration in addition to inspiration seen in

(a) ASD

(b) RBBB

(c) Pulmonary stenosis

(d) Severe mitral insufficiency

(e) Pulmonary hypertension

iii. Paradoxical splits (reversed splitting of S_2)

(a) When split widens on expiration and narrows on inspiration, implication is that P_2 came first, i.e.:

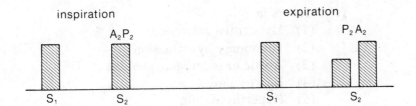

       (b)   Second component of split will be louder and is A_2

       (c)   Occurs when left ventricular ejection time is prolonged, delaying aortic closure

          (1)   LBBB

          (2)   AS

          (3)   PDA

       (e)   Having patient sit or stand may help detect a para- doxical split

  iv.   Ventricular (diastolic or S_3) gallop

       (a)   Is pathologic counterpart of normal S_3

       (b)   Occurs during rapid phase of ventricular filling and is due to resistance to ventricular filling, resulting from increased volume load or decreased compliance

       (c)   Sound is low-pitched (best heard with bell)

       (d)   When originating in left ventricle, best heard at apex with patient in left lateral decubitus position

       (e)   When originating in right ventricle, best heard along 3–4 LSB*

       (f)   Heard transiently in mitral insufficiency (MI), advanced congestive heart failure (CHF), tricuspid insufficiency (TI), left-to-right shunts

       (g)   Sounds like Ken-tuc-ky

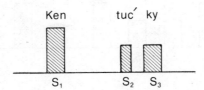

  v.   Atrial (presystolic or S_4) gallop

       (a)   Occurs after atrial contraction and just before S_1, during late phase of ventricular filling

       (b)   Occurs when there is an overload of either ventricle, and diastolic pressure in increased

---

*3rd to 4th intercostal space, left sternal border. This standard abbreviation should be interpreted thus throughout this Section on the Cardiovascular System.

    (c) Occurs in
      (1) Myocardial infarction
      (2) Pulmonary hypertension
      (3) Aortic or pulmonary stenosis
      (4) Heart failure
      (5) Hyperthyroidism
    (d) If heard over apex, probably left ventricular in origin
    (e) If heard over left lower sternal border, probably right ventricular in origin
    (f) A right-sided S_4 is usually louder on inspiration
    (g) A left-sided S_4 is usually louder on expiration
    (h) Sounds like Ten-nes-see

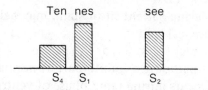

  vi. Summation gallop
    (a) Occurrence of an atrial and ventricular gallop simultaneously
    (b) Heard with tachycardias or any situation causing shortening of diastole
    (c) Summation sound is louder than S_1 or S_2
    (d) Usually mid-diastolic, and commonly found in advanced heart failure

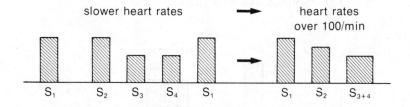

  vii. Extracardiac sounds
    (a) Clicks
    (b) Pericardial rubs
    (c) Mediastinal crunch
    (d) Systolic snap
    (e) Venous hum
  viii. Murmurs
    (a) Sounds produced by turbulent blood flow. Examiner should note
      (1) If murmur is in systole or diastole

      (a)   First, listen in systole and examine all areas
           of precordium

      (b)   Second, listen in diastole, examining all
           seven areas

      (c)   Listen with both bell and diaphragm

(2)   Site of maximal intensity

(3)   Radiation of sound

(4)   Its duration and location in systole

      (a)   Pansystolic (holosystolic) — heard
           throughout systole

S_1 S_2

      (b)   Ejection murmur — starts after S_1 and ends
           before S_2

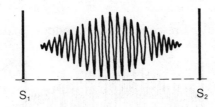

S_1 S_2

(5)   Its duration and location in diastole

      (a)   Protodiastole — a diastolic murmur in early
           diastole

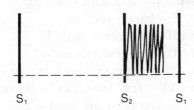

S_1 S_2 S_1

      (b)   Presystolic — a diastolic murmur in late
           diastole

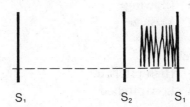

S_1 S_2 S_1

(6) Effect of ventilation on murmur — does it increase or decrease with either inspiration or expiration?

(7) Characteristic pattern of murmurs

    (a) Crescendo — builds up in intensity

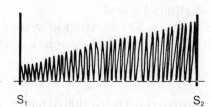

    (b) Decrescendo — decreases in intensity

    (c) Crescendo-decrescendo — peaks in intensity

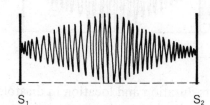

(8) Intensity — based on grade of I to VI
    (a) I — barely audible
    (b) II — just easily audible
    (c) III–IV — intermediate
    (d) V — loudest but requiring a stethoscope
    (e) VI — very loud, can be heard with stethoscope off chest
    (f) Recorded with grade over VI to show scale being used, i.e., II/VI

(9) Quality
    (a) Blowing
    (b) Musical
    (c) Rough

(10) Pitch
    (a) High-pitched
    (b) Low-pitched

   (b)   Innocent murmurs (benign — physiologic, functional)
      (1)   Definition — murmurs that are not associated with cardiovascular disease
      (2)   Common in children and pregnant women
      (3)   Found in hyperthyroidism
      (4)   Found in anemia
      (5)   Example: physiologic S_3 ("functional murmur")
   (c)   Abnormal murmurs
      (1)   Systolic
          (a)   Mitral insufficiency (regurgitation)
              (i)   Pansystolic
              (ii)   Loudest at apex
              (iii)   Referred to left axilla
              (iv)   Intensity will vary, grades I–V
              (v)   May be associated with a thrill at apex and axilla
              (vi)   Harsh and low-pitched
          (b)   Tricuspid insufficiency (regurgitation)
              (i)   Pansystolic
              (ii)   Loudest at lower LSB
              (iii)   Constant in intensity
              (iv)   Usually *not* associated with a thrill
              (v)   Harsh in quality
              (vi)   Increases on inspiration
              (vii) Radiates to RSB
          (c)   Aortic stenosis (AS) — obstruction may be supravalvular or subvalvular, or may involve aortic valve itself
              (i)   Valvular stenosis
                  a)   Systolic ejection murmur
                  b)   Crescendo-decrescendo
                  c)   Intensity varies — no relation to severity of murmur
                  d)   Thrill usually found at 2RSB, i.e., aortic area
                  e)   Radiates to neck, upper back, apex of heart
                  f)   Harsh in quality
                  g)   Maximal intensity at base of heart, usually 2RSB
              (ii)   Subvalvular AS (idiopathic hypertropic subaortic stenosis — IHSS) — occurs when septal wall just below aortic valve is hypertrophied
                  a)   Maximal intensity 2, 3, 4RSB
                  b)   May radiate to apex
                  c)   Thrill may be found at lower LSB

          d) Ejection murmur
          e) Crescendo-decrescendo
          f) Increases during expiration and valsalva maneuver

    (iii)   Supravalvular AS
          a) Ejection murmur
          b) Maximal intensity 2RSB or in suprasternal notch
          c) Radiates to neck
          d) Thrill may be felt in suprasternal notch
          e) Harsh
          f) Crescendo-decrescendo

(d) Pulmonary stenosis (PS)
    (i)   Maximal loudness at 2LSB
    (ii)   Pulmonary systolic ejection sound (click)
    (iii)   Radiates to left side of neck
    (iv)   Thrill usually felt at 2LSB
    (v)   Harsh
    (vi)   Crescendo-decrescendo
    (vii) Usually louder on inspiration
    (viii) Usually grade III–IV intensity
    (ix)   Expiratory split of S_2 – the more severe the stenosis, the more pronounced the split

(e) Interventricular septal defect
    (i)   Maximal loudness along lower sternal border
    (ii)   Radiates widely
    (iii)   Thrill usually present at lower LSB
    (iv)   Pansystolic

(f) Coarctation of aorta
    (i)   Maximal loudness over left midback between scapulae
    (ii)   Radiates to neck
    (iii)   Thrill may be felt on back
    (iv)   Systolic ejection murmur at base of heart
    (v)   Crescendo-decrescendo

(2) Diastolic
  (a) Mitral stenosis (MS)
    (i)   Mid-diastolic or presystolic
    (ii)   Often very faint in intensity
    (iii)   May be heard only when patient is lying on left side or in act of turning
    (iv)   Maximal intensity at apex
    (v)   If presystolic, usually crescendo

        (vi)   Intensity and severity have no association

        (vii)   Associated with an opening snap and accentuated S_1

        (viii) Intensity not affected by inspiration

  (b)   Tricuspid stenosis (TS)

        (i)   Maximal intensity at 4LSB

        (ii)   Radiates to apex and xiphoid area

        (iii)   May be associated with a thrill at 4LSB

        (iv)   May increase on inspiration

        (v)   Protodiastolic

        (vi)   Rumbling decrescendo

        (vii)   Intensity increased on inspiration

        (viii) May have an opening snap

  (c)   Aortic insufficiency (regurgitation) (AI)

        (i)   Maximal intensity at 3, 4 LSB and 2RSB

        (ii)   Blowing quality

        (iii)   Intensity very faint, I/VI

        (iv)   Radiates to apex

        (v)   Thrill uncommon

        (vi)   Pandiastolic

        (vii)   Decrescendo

        (viii) High-pitched

  (d)   Pulmonary insufficiency (PI)

        (i)   Maximal loudness along 2LSB

        (ii)   Radiates along LSB toward apex

        (iii)   Decrescendo

        (iv)   High-pitched

        (v)   Blowing quality

        (vi)   Sometimes increases with inspiration

  (e)   Patent ductus arteriosus (PDA)

        (i)   Maximal intensity 2LSB

        (ii)   Radiates to neck

        (iii)   Thrill at 2LSB

        (iv)   Usually continuous

        (v)   Intensity varies

        (vi)   Harsh in quality

ix. Abnormal sounds due to dysrhythmias

  (a)   RBBB

     (1)   Abnormal expiratory split of S_2

     (2)   Wider-than-normal split on inspiration

  (b)   LBBB

     (1)   Paradoxical splitting of S_2

     (2)   Split narrows on inspiration

     (3)   Heard best at 3 LSB

      (c) Complete heart block
          (1) S_1 varies in intensity
          (2) Usually associated with systolic ejection murmur
- g. Peripheral auscultation
  - i. Systemic arterial blood pressure via sphygmomanometry
  - ii. Significance of, e.g., renal artery stenosis
    - (a) Hypertension
    - (b) Hypotension, i.e., acute myocardial infarction, shock
    - (c) Pressure differences between arms (aortic aneurysm)
    - (d) Pressure differences between arms and legs (coarctation of aorta)
    - (e) Pulse pressure differences (increased in AI, decreased in AS)

DIAGNOSTIC STUDIES

1. **Laboratory**
   - a. Serum
     - i. CBC, Hb, HCT
     - ii. Clotting profile
       - (a) Prothrombin time (PT)
       - (b) Partial thromboplastin time (PTT)
       - (c) Thrombin time (TT)
     - iii. Enzymes
       - (a) Serum glutamic oxalacetic transaminase (SGOT)
       - (b) Lactic dehydrogenase (LDH)
       - (c) Creatinine phosphokinase (CPK)
       - (d) Isoenzymes (CPK-MB, LDH-1
     - iv. Serum glucose
     - v. Electrolytes
     - vi. Lipid profile
   - b. Urine
     - i. Routine urinalysis
     - ii. Electrolytes
2. **Noninvasive methods of cardiac diagnosis**
   - a. Apexcardiography records cardiac apex thrust
     - i. Used in diagnosis of aortic valve stenosis, IHSS, and mitral valve disease
     - ii. Used to determine left ventricular function
   - b. Radioisotope scanning ("Myocardial imaging") used to
     - i. Evaluate left ventricular contraction
     - ii. Evaluate ejection fraction
     - iii. Locate ventricular aneurysms
     - iv. Evaluate regional dysfunction – akinesia, dyskinesia
     - v. Evaluate pulmonary capillary perfusion

vi. Demonstrate pericardial effusion

vii. Visualize ventricular hypertrophy, aortic aneurysms. subvalvular obstructions, congenital shunting lesions

c. Echocardiography — utilizes sound waves in study of

    i. Mitral valve patterns, degree, and rate of motion permitting diagnosis of MS and its severity

    ii. Pericardial effusions

    iii. Atrial tumors

    iv. Tricuspid valve pattern, degree, and rate of motion

    v. Function of prosthetic ball valves

    vi. AS

d. Vectorcardiography

    i. Definition — a graphic representation of changing direction and magnitude of electrical forces of heart. Demonstrates more clearly phasic changes of action potentials

    ii. Purpose: to help diagnose

      (a) Ventricular hypertrophy

      (b) LBBB and RBBB

      (c) Posterior and anterior fascicular blocks

      (d) Myocardial infarction

      (e) Myocardial ischemia

      (f) Atrial enlargement

      (g) ASD

    iii. Advantages over traditional ECG

      (a) Demonstrates cardiac pathology earlier

      (b) ECGs tend to be suggestive of disease, whereas vectorcardiograms are a more definitive diagnostic tool

e. Electrocardiography

    i. General information

      (a) Measures electrical activity of heart by measuring difference in electrical potential between two points on body

      (b) Demonstrates or detects

        (1) Anatomic orientation of heart

        (2) Size of chambers and any enlargement

        (3) Disturbance of rhythm and conduction

        (4) Ischemia or infarct

        (5) Electrolyte abnormalities

        (6) Drug toxicity

      (c) ECG paper

        (1) Vertical lines measure time

          (a) Each small box = 0.04 sec

          (b) Each large box = 0.20 sec

          (c) Allows for measurement of the P, QRS, T complexes (in time), as well as P-R intervals

    (2) Horizontal lines measure voltage
        (a) Each small box = 1 mm (= 0.1 mv)
        (b) Each large box = 5 mm (= 0.5 mv)
        (c) Allows for measurement of height of P wave, QRS complex, and T wave
        (d) Useful in detection of atrial and ventricular hypertrophies

  (d) Deflections: the waves (which constitute ECG) are either above or below isoelectric line
    (1) Isoelectric line is a straight line on ECG indicating either no electrical forces or equivalent amounts of movement toward and away from positive electrode

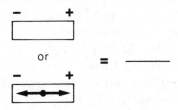

    (2) Positive deflections are produced where electrical forces are moving *toward* positive electrode

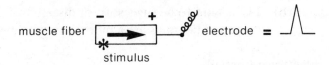

    (3) Negative deflections are produced when electrical forces are moving *away* from positive electrode (toward negative electrode)

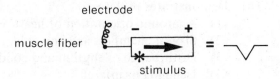

    (4) Diphasic deflections are produced when electrical forces move both *toward* and *away from* positive electrode

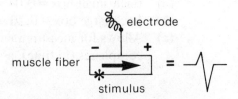

ii. Cardiac conduction cycle (Friedberg, 1969, pp. 36–37)
   (a) P wave represents atrial depolarization
      (1) First portion represents right atrial depolarization
      (2) Second portion represents left atrial depolarization
      (3) Normal height P = $<$ 3 mm
         (a) Abnormal if P wave exceeds 3 mm in height in extremity leads and exceeds 2.5 mm in precordial leads
      (4) Normal width = $<$ 0.1 seconds
      (5) Abnormalities (Goldman, 1976, p. 387)
         (a) Increased amplitude or width associated with atrial hypertrophy
         (b) Tall peaked P waves in leads II, III, aVF, and tall or diphasic P waves in V_1 are associated with right atrial enlargement
         (c) Wide, notched P waves (P-mitrale) in leads I, aVL, and V_{4-6}, and diphasic P waves with a broad negative deflection in lead V_1 are associated with left atrial hypertrophy
   (b) P-R interval (Goldman, 1976, p. 24) represents atrial depolarization and conduction through A-V node – measures atrioventricular conduction time
      (1) Measured from beginning of P wave to beginning of QRS complex
      (2) Normal – 0.12–0.20 seconds
      (3) P-R segment represents normal delay of impulse in A-V node – normally isoelectric
         (a) With abnormalities this delay prolongs P-R interval to above 0.20 seconds
            (i)   Indication of diseased A-V node or ischemia
            (ii) Called first-degree A-V block
         (b) Q wave (Goldman, 1976, p. 389) is the first negative deflection resulting from ventricular depolarization
            (i)   Abnormal if greater than 0.4 seconds wide or 25% of R wave amplitude
            (ii) Seen in myocardial infarctions, left ventricular hypertrophy (LVH), right ventricular hypertrophy (RVH), LBBB
         (c) R wave is the first positive deflection and represents atrial depolarization
            (i)   Normal – less than 13 mm amplitude
            (ii) Greater than 13 mm in aVL, greater than 27 mm in V_5 or V_6, or greater than 35 mm in V_5 plus S in V_1 indicates LVH

(d) S wave is first negative deflection of ventricular depolarization following first positive deflection (R wave)

(e) QRS complex (Goldman, p. 388)

    (i)   Measurement of total ventricular depolarization

    (ii)   Measured from onset of Q wave (or R if no Q is visible) to end of S wave

    (iii)   Normal – 0.06–0.12 seconds

    (iv)   Abnormal if greater than 0.12 sec., indicative of delayed impulse seen in bundle branch blocks and hyperkalemia

(f) T wave represents ventricular repolarization and diastole

    (i)   Negative deflection may indicate infarcts or ischemia

    (ii)   Tall, peaked T waves may indicate hyperkalemia

(g) S-T segment represents ventricular repolarization (Goldman, pp. 392–393)

    (i)   Normal – 0.32 seconds

    (ii)   Measured immediately after QRS complex to beginning of T wave

    (iii)   Prolonged S-T segment indicative of hypocalcemia

    (iv)   Elevated S-T segment (i.e., 1 mm or more above isoelectric line) may indicate pericarditis, infarcts, aneurysms (for exact leads refer to each particular entity in this chapter)

    (v)   Depressed S-T segments may indicate angina, RVH, digitalis toxicity

(h) Q-T interval – summation of depolarization and repolarization representing electrical systole; varies with heart rate

iii. ECG leads (12-lead)

(a) Bipolar leads – standard limb leads (I, II, III)

    (1)   Record electrical potential in frontal plane

    (2)   Record difference in potential between 2 limb leads

        (a)   Lead I – R arm negative, L arm positive

        (b)   Lead II – R arm negative, L leg positive

        (c)   Lead III – L arm negative, L leg positive

    (3)   Normally, all major wave forms are positive deflections in standard limb leads

(b) Unipolar leads – augmented
   (1) aVR – R arm positive electrode; normally a negative deflection
   (2) aVL – L arm positive electrode; usually a positive deflection
   (3) aVF – L leg positive electrode; usually a positive deflection
(c) Unipolar precordial leads (chest)
   (1) V_1 – 4RSB
   (2) V_2 – 4LSB
   (3) V_3 – half-way between V_2 and V_4
   (4) V_4 – 5LSB, left midclavicular line
   (5) V_5 – 5LSB, left anterior axillary line
   (6) V_6 – 5LSB, left midaxillary line
   Note: Normally, in moving from V_1 toward V_6, R waves get progressively larger and S waves get progressively smaller ("normal R wave progression")
(d) Miscellaneous leads
   (1) Lewis leads – used to amplify waves of atrial activity:
      (a) A bipolar chest lead
      (b) Amplify waves of atrial activity, i.e., P waves
      (c) R arm electrode placed in 2ICS, right of sternum. L arm electrode placed on 4ICS, right of sternum. Tracing recorded on lead I
   (2) Esophageal lead (unipolar)
      (a) Catheter lead passed via nose and connected to V_1 lead
      (b) Measured in centimeters from nares
         (i) E_{10-35} – reflects atrial area
         (ii) E_{25-35} – reflects region of atrial groove
         (iii) E_{35-50} – reflects posterior surface of left ventricle
      (c) Esophageal leads enable one to examine atrial complexes and explore posterior surface of left ventricle
iv. Electrical axis – cardiac vectors.*
v. ECG interpretation – see the bibliography for references on dysrhythmias
   (a) Analysis – each dysrhythmia should be analyzed in a systematic manner with particular attention to

---

*This aspect of electrocardiography will not be dealt with here. It is used to determine right and left axis deviations that occur in certain disease entities, such as fascicular blocks. For more information, refer to Alspach, 1979 or Goldman, 1976.

      (1)   Rate — both atrial and ventricular

      (2)   Rhythm — regular, irregular

      (3)   Identification of P waves

          (a)   Their relationship to QRS

          (b)   Consistency of configuration/morphology

          (c)   Normalcy of morphology

      (4)   Determine P-R interval

      (5)   Determine QRS interval

      (6)   Identify origin of dysrhythmia if possible

      (7)   Identify possible implications for patient

  (b) Categories of dysrhythmias

      (1)   Sinus origin

          (a)   Sinus arrhythmia

          (b)   Bradycardia

          (c)   Tachycardia

          (d)   Arrest/block

          (e)   Sick sinus syndrome

      (2)   Atrial origin

          (a)   Paroxysmal atrial tachycardia (PAT) with or without block

          (b)   Atrial tachycardia

          (c)   Premature atrial contractions (PAC)

          (d)   Wandering atrial pacemaker

          (e)   Atrial flutter

          (f)   Atrial fibrillation

      (3)   A-V junction origin

          (a)   Junctional rhythm (idiojunctional rhythm)

          (b)   Accelerated idiojunctional rhythm

          (c)   Tachycardia

          (d)   Premature junctional contractions with or without aberrancy

          (e)   Junctional escape beats

          (f)   Paroxysmal junctional tachycardia

      (4)   Ventricular origin

          (a)   Idioventricular rhythm

          (b)   Accelerated idioventricular rhythm

          (c)   Ventricular tachycardia

          (d)   Premature ventricular contractions

          (e)   Ventricular fibrillation

          (f)   Ventricular escape beats

      (5)   A-V conduction defects

          (a)   First-degree A-V block

          (b)   Second-degree — Mobitz I (Wenckebach); Mobitz II

          (c)   Third-degree — complete heart block

      (6)   Atrioventricular dissociation

          (a)   Slowing of primary pacemaker, which lets latent focus take over

(b)   Accelerated discharge of latent focus
(c)   Complete A-V block
(7)   Intraventricular conduction defects
(a)   LBBB, RBBB
(b)   Fascicular block – left anterosuperior, left posteroinferior
(c)   Bifascicular block
(d)   Trifascicular block
(8)   Ectopy versus aberrancy
(c)   ECG interpretation of ischemia, injury, infarcts – see pp. 127–129
(d)   ECG changes of pericarditis – see p. 150
(e)   ECG changes of myocardial trauma
(1)   Dysrhythmias
(2)   Pattern of pericarditis
(3)   Nonspecific S-T and T changes
(4)   Infarction pattern
(f)   ECG changes with potassium disturbances
(1)   Hypokalemia
(a)   Prominent U wave
(b)   T wave amplitude decreases
(c)   S-T segment depressed
(d)   P-R interval may be prolonged
(2)   Hyperkalemia
(a)   T wave symmetrically peaked, narrowed, elevated
(b)   P-R interval prolonged
(c)   P wave amplitude diminished
(d)   QRS widened
(g)   ECG changes with calcium disturbances
(1)   Hypocalcemia
(a)   Prolonged Q–T interval
(b)   Prolonged isoelectric S-T segment
(2)   Hypercalcemia
(a)   Shortened Q-T interval
(b)   Shortened or absent S-T segment

3. **Invasive methods of cardiac diagnosis**
a.   Purpose – general
i.   To confirm clinically suspected lesions, i.e., of arteries, valves, muscle tissue
ii.   To evaluate severity of lesions
iii. To assess pathophysiology of cardiac disorders
iv.   To provide information on left ventricular function
v.   To allow for measurement of pressures in heart
vi.   Measurement of cardiac output
vii. Measurement of blood gas content

    b. Complications of cardiac catheterization — general
       i.   Cardiac dysrhythmias
      ii.   Conduction disturbances
     iii. Arterial thrombosis
     iv. Catheter embolism
      v.   Perforation of atria, arteries, ventricle
         (a) Cardiac tamponade
         (b) Pleural effusion
         (c) Pneumothorax
     vi. Allergic reactions to contrast media

    c. Swan-Ganz catheter (Schroeder and Daily, 1976, pp. 62–79)
       i.   Allows for bedside insertion and continuous hemodynamic monitoring so that patient's vascular tone, myocardial contractility, and fluid balance can be assessed
      ii.   Measures pulmonary artery (PA) and pulmonary capillary wedge pressures (PCWP)
         (a) PA pressure reflects left heart pressures
         (b) PA systolic represents pressure produced by right ventricle (20–30 mm Hg)
         (c) PA diastolic is actually lowest pressure in PA prior to next right ventricular systole. Normal PA diastolic is less than 10 mm Hg
            (1) Reflects LVEDP (pressure in left ventricle just before systole)
               (a) Used as measure of left ventricular function and diastolic filling pressure
               (b) "The LVEDP reflects the compliance or flexibility of the ventricle, that is, the ability of the left ventricle to relax and accept blood from the atrium during diastole . . . In general, the higher the LVEDP, the more noncompliant (or resistant to filling) is the left ventricle . . ." (Schroeder and Daily, 1976, p. 63)
         (d) PA mean reflects average of PA systolic and PA diastolic pressures — normally less than 20 mm Hg
         (e) PCWP — ballon of catheter is inflated, wedging in a small branch of PA. It measures pressures distal to balloon — in lungs
            (1) Reflects left atrial pressure
            (2) Normal is 4–12 mm Hg
            (3) Mean PCWP should be roughly comparable to PA diastolic
            (4) Also reflects LVEDP
         (f) Used in differential diagnosis of cardiogenic vs hypovolemic shock (see Shock section for specific findings)

    iii. Change in pressures (indicating change in left ventricular function) are seen prior to onset of complications, and thus allow for preventive intervention

    iv. Complications associated with Swan-Ganz catheter

      (a) If balloon is left inflated after a wedge, necrosis of pulmonary tissue will ensue and cause pulmonary infarction

      (b) Balloon may rupture, causing emboli, infarcts

      (c) Sepsis

      (d) Hemorrhage

      (e) Dysrhythmias during passage of catheter

      (f) Perforation of right atrium, right ventricle, or PA

d. His bundle electrocardiography (Fowler, 1976, pp. 979–1005)

    i. Definition — electrode catheter technique that allows for recording of electrical activity of A-V junction, bundle of His, and bundle branches

    ii. Purpose — to detect precisely and locate with specificity the sites of A-V conduction delays and blocks, whether in A-V node itself, bundle of His, or bundle branch

      (a) First-degree block

      (b) Second-degree block

      (c) 2:1, 3:1 block

      (d) Complete heart block

    iii. Used clinically in studying

      (a) Atrial fibrillation

      (b) Atrial flutter

      (c) Paroxysmal tachycardia

      (d) Aberrant ventricular conductions

      (e) Ventricular tachycardias

      (f) Wolff-Parkinson-White syndrome (anomalous A-V conduction)

      (g) Drug effects

e. Intracardiac phonocardiography

    i. Relatively new technique still under investigation

    ii. Useful in defining origin of heart sounds and murmurs in patients with acquired and congenital heart disease

f. Coronary arteriography

    i. Definition — Method by which coronary arteries are made visible via injection of radiopaque contrast material

    ii. Purpose

      (a) To study extent of coronary artery disease (CAD)

      (b) To evaluate ischemic heart disease

      (c) To evaluate atypical angina

      (d) To locate areas of infarct with aid of radionuclides

      (e) To study patients with myocardial disease in order to rule out CAD

g. Ventriculography
  i. Definition — a method in which radiopaque contrast medium is injected, allowing ventricles to be visualized
  ii. Purpose
    (a) To evaluate ventricular function
    (b) To help determine prognosis in patients selected for cardiac surgery
    (c) To determine left ventricular function by measuring
      (1) End-diastolic volumes (EDV)
      (2) End-systolic volumes (ESV)
      (3) Stroke volumes; SV = EDV–ESV
      (4) Ejection fraction; EF = SV/EDV
h. Aortography
  i. Definition — opacification of lumen of aorta, valve leaflets, and all vessels arising from aorta
  ii. Purpose — to determine/diagnose
    (a) Aortic valve incompetence
    (b) Aneurysms of ascending aorta
    (c) Coarctation of aorta

_____ GENERAL PATIENT CARE MANAGEMENT _____

MAINTENANCE OF ADEQUATE CARDIAC FUNCTION AND OUTPUT

1. **Check pulse:** for rhythm, rate, volume, and jugular venous distention

2. **Compare apical and radial pulses:** note any "pulse deficit"

3. **Check for presence/absence of peripheral pulses and for bilateral equality**

4. **Monitor ECG patterns continuously:** describe dysrhythmias according to outline on pp. 113–114

5. **Evaluate circulatory pressure and volume:** by obtaining vital signs

6. **Note trends of deviation from expected normals:** document these and report to appropriate personnel

7. **Measure and record intake and output as prescribed**

8. **Assess neurologic status**

9. **Support myocardium:** through administration of pharmacologic agents and humidified oxygen as prescribed

10. **Evaluate patient's hemodynamic parameters:** by measuring intra-cardiac pressures, i.e., PAP, PCWP, CO, CVP

11. **Hemodynamic monitoring**
    a. Central venous pressure monitoring
        i.   Obtain readings according to prescribed routine, evaluating trends and reporting significant changes
        ii. Prevent complications
             (a) Thrombophlebitis caused by infection or mechanical irritation
             (b) Obstruction of fluid flow due to clot at catheter tip or kinking of catheter — maintain continuous heparinized drip; flush catheter after blood withdrawal; avoid taking BP in arm with catheter
             (c) Inaccurate readings caused by malposition of catheter, manometer, or stopcock, or lack of catheter patency — record pressures with position of patient and mano-meter the same for each reading
    b. Pulmonary artery/wedge pressure monitoring
        i.   Obtain readings according to prescribed routine, evaluating trends and reporting significant changes
        ii. Pressure readings can be obtained with patient in any position, providing that transducer is at same level of phlebostatic axis (Woods, 1976, p. 1769). Phlebostatic axis is imaginary point defined by intersection of two imaginary lines. One line is drawn from 4ICS from sternum to edge of chest, and down to side. Other line is drawn in middle of lateral chest wall from last rib to axilla. Point of intersection of these two lines is phlebostatic axis
        iii. Prevent complications
             (a) Inflamed painful area above insertion site due to thrombophlebitis — provide sterile dressing changes with appropriate skin care every 24 hours
             (b) Ventricular irritability from excess catheter in right ventricle or migration of catheter from PA to right ventricle — assess that suture attached to catheter is intact
             (c) Electrically induced ventricular fibrillation due to fluid-filled catheter serving as low resistance path of electric current to heart — avoid use of battery-operated articles; maintain grounding of electrical wiring and equipment
             (d) Pulmonary hemorrhage or infarction caused by perforation of PA, prolonged wedging, or overinflation of balloon during wedging — assure that suture attached to catheter is intact; avoid flushing in wedged position; have balloon deflated

        (e)   Thrombi formation due to stasis and clot formation cause by low cardiac output status — maintain continuous heparinized drip

  c. Intra-aortic balloon pump

      i.   Assess and document presence/absence of peripheral pulses, temperature and color of extremities

      ii.   Take precautions to prevent pressure sores

      iii.   Ensure proper functioning of all hemodynamic monitoring devices

      iv.   Monitor all hemodynamic parameters, i.e., CVP, PAP, PCWP, intake and output, lab values

      v.   Assess level of consciousness

      vi.   Elevate head of bed no greater than 30 degrees

      vii.   Patient can be turned toward side of insertion but the extremity must not be flexed

      viii.   Ensure adequate oxygenation of patient

      ix.   Change dressings over IABP insertion site daily (or according to ward procedures) and inspect the insertion site for signs of infection or hematoma

      x.   Employ measures to prevent patient disorientation

      xi.   Provide emotional support for the patient and significant others

Note: For detailed discussion of IABP refer to article in bibliography by Sue Bull.

PROMOTION OF ADEQUATE PERIPHERAL CIRCULATION

1. **Passive and active range of motion (ROM):** encourage patient to move toes, dorsiflex and hyperextend feet

2. **Encourage patient to deep-breathe**

3. **Observe lower extremities:** for color, warmth, swelling, pulses, texture, edema, ulcerations

4. **Maintain anticoagulant therapy**

REDUCTION OF WORKLOAD ON THE HEART

1. **Administer humidified oxygen**

2. **Administer tranquilizers as prescribed**

3. **Assist patient with planned, graduated levels of activity**

4. **Provide environment conducive to rest**

5. Allow patient to rest between nursing activities

6. Provide for rest period after meals

7. Make provisions for adequate bowel elimination

8. Anticipate and meet patient needs promptly

MAINTENANCE OF FLUID AND ELECTROLYTE BALANCE

1. Administer IV therapy as prescribed

2. Maintain and record accurate intake and output

3. Weigh patient daily and record

4. Monitor fluid and sodium restrictions (if appropriate)

5. Observe for presence or absence of edema

6. Assess hydration status

7. Monitor serum and urine electrolytes, BUN and creatinine laboratory results: report significant deviations

8. Monitor ECG pattern for signs of electrolyte imbalance: report significant deviations

PROMOTION OF PHYSICAL AND MENTAL REST TO INCLUDE RELIEF OF PAIN

1. Observe patient for verbal and nonverbal expression of pain or discomfort

2. Provide environment conducive to rest, whenever possible

3. Plan nursing activities around patient's rest periods

4. Maintain calm, confident attitude

5. Administer narcotics and analgesics per order: record observed results

6. Provide adequate oral hygiene

7. Postion patient to provide comfort and support

8. Answer patient's questions in detail appropriate to individual situation

9. Provide emotional support to family members

PREVENTION AND DETECTION OF INFECTION

1. Inspect skin for redness, extreme warmth, or drainage from incision or IV site(s)
    a. Culture drainage
    b. Culture catheter tip if catheter discontinued

2. Administer antibiotics as prescribed

3. Report elevation in temperature and changes in laboratory data indicative of infectious process: i.e., increased WBC with increased neutrophils

4. Use aseptic technique when handling IV lines

5. Change IV and IV tubing every 24 hours: or as hospital policy indicates

6. Change dressings every 24 hours and PRN

7. Remove mucus and secretions from respiratory tract

8. Encourage deep breathing and coughing

9. Assist patient to change position on a regular basis
    a. Provide water or air mattress, especially if patient is elderly
    b. Give gentle massages to bony prominences

10. Perform aseptic urinary catheter care every shift

11. Monitor urine for color, consistency, odor

12. Discontinue all catheters, IV lines, drains as soon as possible

MAINTENANCE OF ADEQUATE NUTRITION

1. Insure availability of progressive therapeutic diet: e.g., liquid, soft, low calorie, sodium-restricted, cholesterol-restricted

2. Ascertain patient's food preferences: attempt to comply with requests

3. Monitor intake of fluids and foods

4. Provide effective oral hygiene

PROMOTION OF REHABILITATION

1. Encourage patient decision-making during routine care activities

2. Plan day's activities with patient

3. Prepare patient for discharge from critical care setting

4. Plan for coordination and follow-up of patient care after discharge

EDUCATION OF PATIENT AND FAMILY

1. **Teaching**: provide information to meet individual patient and family needs: details will vary

2. Explain treatments, unit protocols, machinery, etc., used in patient's care

3. Use principles of adult teaching/learning, stress theory, and crisis intervention

4. Ascertain patient/family's expectations for hospitalization

——— PATHOLOGIC CONDITIONS AND MANAGEMENT ———

ARTERIOSCLEROSIS

1. **Definition**: "a chronic disease of the arteries characterized by abnormal thickening and hardening of the vessel walls resulting in loss of elasticity." (Andreoli, 1975, p. 8)

2. **Types**
   a. Intimal atherosclerosis — tunica intima (inner muscle layer of artery) thickens; plaques of fatty acids and cholesterol form, and can either partially or totally occlude lumen of artery; affects mostly large vessels
   b. Medial sclerosis — tunica media (middle layer of artery) of middle-sized arteries calcifies and hypertrophies; again, diameter of lumen is decreased
   c. Arteriolar sclerosis — affects small arteries; there is hypertrophy of tunica media and thickening of intima

3. **Conditions that show high correlations to development of arteriosclerosis:** possible etiologic factors, risk factors
    a. Heredity
    b. Arterial hypertension (positive correlations exist that show increased incidence of coronary artery disease in patients with hypertension.
    c. Diabetes mellitus — patients with DM are five times more likely to develop coronary artery disease (CAD) than those without DM
    d. Age — most prevalent in older age-groups, 55 and over
    e. Sex — more prevalent in men than in women (prior to menopause years)
    f. Race — most often seen in Caucasians
    g. Cigarette smoking — increased incidence associated with smoking
    h. Hyperlipidemia — controversial, but high levels of cholesterol, in particular, have been associated with arteriosclerosis
    i. Obesity
    j. Emotional tension — increased stress, type A personality
    k. Sedentary life style
    l. Gout
    m. Soft water (Ariela, 1975, p. 91) — those who drink soft water rather than hard are more likely to develop arteriosclerosis

4. **Pathologic results of arteriosclerosis**
    a. Angina
    b. Ischemia
    c. Myocardial infarction
    d. CHF
    e. Sudden death

ANGINA PECTORIS

1. **Definition:** the chest pain associated with myocardial ischemia (Berne, 1977, p. 230)

2. **Pathophysiology**
    a. Etiologic factors lead to decreased blood flow and oxygen supply to cardiac muscle
    b. Imbalance between oxygen supply and myocardial oxygen demand
    c. Ischemia leading to angina pectoris

3. **Etiologic factors** (Fowler, 1976, p. 635)
    a. Atherosclerotic heart disease
    b. Hypertension
    c. Aortic valvular disease

    d. Anemia

    e. Dysrhythmias (especially tachydysrhythmias)

    f. Thyrotoxicosis

    g. Shock

    h. CHF

    i. Aortitis

4. **Precipitating factors**

    a. Physical activity — not necessarily strenuous; brushing teeth may induce angina

    b. Emotional excitement

    c. Nocturnal angina, when patient is in recumbent position. This position decreases cardiac output and coronary perfusion, subsequently causing decreased myocardial oxygen supply and resulting angina

    d. Smoking — increases myocardial oxygen demands and interferes with oxyhemoglobin relationship, lowering oxygen transport

    e. Heavy meals

5. **Clinical presentation**

    a. Pain — location usually

        i. Precordial

        ii. Middle or lower sternum or retrosternal

        iii. May radiate to shoulders, arms, jaw, neck, epigastrum

    b. Quality of pain (as described by patients)

        i. Burning

        ii. Squeezing/aching

        iii. Heaviness

        iv. Smothering

        v. Heavy weight

    c. Other characteristics of pain

        i. Usually begins on exertion and subsides with rest

        ii. *Gradually* subsides

        iii. Usually lasts for 1–4 minutes and subsides when precipitating factor is removed

        iv. Relieved with nitroglycerin, usually within 45–90 seconds; if not, is less likely to be angina

    d. Medical management

        i. Patient must adjust life style so that physical activity does not exceed pain threshold, but graded exercise is recommended

        ii. Administer nitroglycerin PRN and prophylactically

        iii. Surgical intervention necessary for severe CAD

        iv. Preventive measures to decrease risk factors must be instituted

        v. Provide adequate rest — 8–10 hours per day

6. **Varieties of angina**
    a. Nocturnal
    b. Prinzmetal's – patient has chest discomfort, usually at rest, less likely with activity, and often at night

7. **Diagnostic aids**
    a. History – presence of risk factors
    b. ECG changes – S-T segment depression seen during attack
    c. Positive stress test
    d. Coronary arteriography

ACUTE CORONARY INSUFFICIENCY: Synonyms: pre-infarction angina, unstable angina, impending infarction.

1. **Pathologic, etiologic, and precipitating factors:** same as angina pectoris

2. **Major difference:** symptoms may be more prolonged and attacks more frequent than with angina pectoris; however, there is no evidence of an infarct

MYOCARDIAL INFARCTION: Death of myocardial tissues due to deprivation of blood supply. (In this section MI will be used to mean myocardial infarction.)

1. **Etiologic and precipitating factors:** same as for arteriosclerosis
    a. Arteriosclerosis present in 90% of cases
    b. Coronary artery embolism
    c. Coronary artery spasms – usually cause of MI in patients without CAD

2. **Clinical presentation**
    a. Signs and symptoms
        i. Chest pain
            (a) Differs from angina
                (1) Constant
                (2) Not relieved with rest or nitrates
                (3) Duration 30 minutes and more
                (4) Similar to angina in location, but more severe
                (5) Pain not affected by lying down or deep breathing
        ii. Nausea and vomiting
        iii. Dyspnea, orthopnea
        iv. Anxiety, severe apprehension
        v. Diaphoresis
        vi. Cyanosis
        vii. Dysrhythmias
        viii. Weakness

b. Diagnostic findings
   i. History indicative of MI
   ii. Physical examination — any of the following may be found, alone or in combination
      (a) Inspection
         (1) Shortness of breath
         (2) Cyanosis
         (3) Anxiousness
      (b) Palpation — thrills, heaves, abnormal PMI
      (c) Auscultation
         (1) Presystolic gallop (S_4)
         (2) Precordial friction rubs
         (3) Murmurs
         (4) Rales
         (5) Split S_1, S_2
         (6) Extracardiac sounds

3. **Laboratory findings**
   a. Increased leukocyte count
   b. Increased sedimentation rate
   c. Increased serum enzymes*

ENZYME	ONSET	PEAK	RETURN TO NORMAL
1. CPK	2–5 hours	24 hours	2–3 days
2. SGOT	6–8 hours	24–48 hours	4–8 days
3. LDH	6–12 hours	48–72 hours	7–10 days
4. HBD	12 hours	48–72 hours	1–3 weeks

   d. Isoenzymes are more specific for cardiac muscle damage
      i. CPK-MB
      ii. LDH-1

4. **Pathologic changes found on ECG** (Goldman, 1976, p. 142)
   a. Ischemia
      i. S-T segment depression
      ii. T wave inversion
      iii. Both changes above may be found in leads 1, aVL or aVF, and in leads V_{4-6}
   b. Injury (Marriot, 1977, p. 232) — a stage beyond ischemia, but still reversible.
      i. S-T elevation — epicardial injury and ischemia
      ii. T elevation — epicardial injury and ischemia

---

*An increase in the enzymes is not diagnostic of MI, but may be caused by other conditions.

    iii. S-T segment returns to isoelectric position within a few days

c. Infarction (Goldman, 1976, pp. 152–153)

    i. Q waves — pathologic, must be 0.04 mm wide or 25% of the R wave in depth in certain leads

    ii. S-T segment changes

      (a) Elevated in lead over or facing infarcted area

      (b) Reciprocal changes (S-T depression) will be found in leads 180° from area of infarction

    iii. T wave changes

      (a) May occur hours to weeks after infarct

      (b) In leads with S-T depression, T waves are tall and very symmetrical

      (c) In leads with S-T elevation, T wave is inverted

      (d) In some leads with an isoelectric S-T segment, T wave may be inverted

      (e) May last for weeks and return to normal, or remain inverted for rest of patient's life

    iv. ECG changes associated with various sites of infarct — indicative changes: Q, S-T elevation, T wave inversion

      (a) Acute anterior infarction (Marriott, 1977, p. 238)

        (1) Indicative changes in leads I, aVL, and pre-cordial leads of anterior chest

        (2) Reciprocal changes in leads II, III, aVF and pre-cordial leads of posterior chest

      (b) Anterolateral MI (Fowler, 1976, p. 676)

        (1) Q waves in leads I, II, V_{4-6}

        (2) Negative T waves in same leads

        (3) Changes in leads V_{1-6} will be found with extensive anterolateral MI

      (c) Anteroseptal MI (Marriott, 1977, p. 251)

        (1) Indicative changes found in one or more of leads V_{1-4}

      (d) Inferior wall MI (diaphragmatic) (Marriott, 1977, p. 238)

        (1) Indicative changes in leads II, III, aVF, and precordial leads of posterior chest

        (2) Reciprocal changes seen in leads I, aVL, and precordial leads of anterior chest

      (e) Posterior wall MI (Marriott, 1977, p. 235)

        (1) No leads truly reflect posterior surface of the heart

        (2) Diagnosis of infarct is inferred from reciprocal changes seen in anterior chest leads V_{1-3}

        (3) Abnormally tall R waves seen in V_1 and V_2 (Goldman, 1976, p. 174)

      (f) Lateral wall MI (Marriott, 1977, p. 251)

        (1) Indicative changes seen in leads I and aVL

    (g) Inferolateral MI
        (1) Indicative changes seen in leads II, III, aVF, and leads V_{5-6}
        (2) Reciprocal changes in leads I, aVL
    (h) Subendocardial MI (Goldman, 1973, p. 178) — infarcts of endocardial surface do not produce abnormal Q waves in facing leads since part of myocardium is still electroactive
        (1) No abnormal Q waves seen
        (2) S-T depression and T wave inversion in leads facing epicardial surface overlying infarct
        (3) Reciprocal changes — S-T elevation and upright T waves in opposite leads

5. **Complications**
   a. Dysrhythmias of all types
   b. CHF, pulmonary edema
   c. Cardiogenic shock
   d. Conduction system defects
   e. Thromboembolism
   f. Papillary muscle rupture, mitral insufficiency
   g. Pericarditis
   h. Ventricular aneurysm
   i. Ventricular rupture
   j. Dressler's syndrome
   k. Emotional responses
   l. Sudden death

6. **Specific patient care**
   a. Prevention and early detection of complications
      i. Monitor ECG in CCU
      ii. Hemodynamic monitoring as indicated
   b. Bed rest 24–48 hours (depending on individual case)
   c. Emotional rest — adequate sleep
      i. Tranquilizers
      ii. Sedatives
   d. Relief from pain
      i. Morphine
      ii. Dilaudid
      iii. Demerol
   e. Diet
      i. Low sodium — progressing from liquids to regular diet
      ii. Decaffeinated drinks
   f. Oxygen therapy
   g. Elimination
      i. Straining must be avoided
      ii. Stool softeners

    h. Prevention of venous stasis
        i.   Passive/active range of motion
        ii. Elastic bandages, support hose, etc.*

Note: The following section on Pacemaker Therapy is in sequence with the above information on myocardial infarction, but is set up in this way to facilitate inclusion of all the material.

MANAGEMENT OF SYSTEM CONDUCTION DEFECTS WITH ARTIFICIAL PACING

1. **Temporary pacing**
   a. Therapeutic indications
       i.   A-V block following acute inferior MI, if
            (a) Adequate ventricular rate cannot be maintained with drug therapy
            (b) Mobitz II block is present (very rare in inferior wall MI)
            (c) Symptomatic third-degree A-V block is present with wide QRS complexes unresponsive to drug therapy
            (d) Symptomatic bradydysrhythmias
       ii. Anterior wall MI under following circumstances
            (a) complete RBBB with left anterior hemiblock
            (b) complete RBBB with left posterior hemiblock
            (c) complete RBBB with first-degree A-V block
            (d) complete LBBB and first-degree A-V block with P-R interval greater than 0.22 sec
            (e) complete LBBB alternating with complete RBBB
            (f) Mobitz II A-V block
            (g) Complete heart block
       iii. Emergency treatment for Adams-Stokes syndrome
       iv. Before and during insertion or implantation of permanent pacemaker
       v.   Before or during change of pulse generator that has failed
       vi. CHF with medically unresponsive, slow ventricular rates
       vii. Symptomatic bradyarrhythmias
       viii. Drug-refractory tachyarrhythmias
       ix. High degree or complete A-V block during cardiac surgery
       x.   Symptomatic, digitalis-induced, high degree, or complete A-V or S-A block
   b, Diagnostic indications
       i.   Atrial pacing in patients with CAD as a form of stress test
       ii. Atrial pacing with His bundle recordings to assess effect of changes in heart rate on A-V conduction

---

*Do not encourage patient to use foot board for exercises. Current research indicates that this form of isometric exercise increases secretion of catecholamines in blood. These catecholamines injure lining of arterial blood vessels, inducing platelet aggregations and thus thrombus formation (Haft, 1976, p. 257; Constantinides, 1976, p. 422).

    iii. Sudden cessation of rapid atrial pacing to assess intrinsic S-A node pacemaking function

    iv. Delivering premature stimuli during tachyarrhythmias to support re-entry versus automaticity as cause of arrhythmia

2. **Permanent pacing**
   a. Symptomatic, acquired, chronic heart block
      i. Etiology
         (a) Nonspecific, degenerative, fibrotic, and sclerotic changes account for half the instances of heart block
         (b) Acute myocardial infarction accounts for one fourth of cases of permanent block requiring a pacemaker
         (c) Remaining one-fourth of cases with heart block due to
            (1) Rheumatic heart disease
            (2) Cardiomyopathies
            (3) Surgical and other trauma
            (4) Sarcoidosis
            (5) Parasitic infection
            (6) Other unusual lesions
      ii. Clinical features
         (a) Syncopal attacks with or without convulsions
         (b) Dizziness or weakness
         (c) Caused by
            (1) Bradycardia and resultant decrease in cardiac output
            (2) Intermittent failure of idioventricular pacemaker
      iii. Prognosis
         (a) Course of heart block unpredictable and highly lethal
         (b) Drug therapy not satisfactory for long-term treatment
         (c) Without pacemaking, mortality rate at end of first year is 50–60%
      iv. Variants of heart block requiring permanent pacing
         (a) Complete heart block
         (b) A-V block – symptomatic Mobitz II block
         (c) A-V block, atrial fibrillation, and slow ventricular response
         (d) Bifascicular intraventricular block
            (1) RBBB with left anterior hemiblock
               (a) With syncope
               (b) Onset during acute myocardial infarction
               (c) Associated with additional conduction system disease
               (d) Changing pattern of block; or dysrhythmia
            (2) RBBB with left posterior hemiblock
         (e) Bilateral BBB and transient complete heart block during hospitalization for acute myocardial infarction
   b. Intractable CHF associated with bradycardia and refractory to medical management
   c. Cerebral or renal insufficiency improved by temporary pacing

    d. Sick sinus syndrome
       i. Sinus bradycardia unresponsive to atropine therapy or exercise
      ii. S-A block or arrest with long pauses in ventricular response
     iii. Alternating bradycardia and tachycardia
    e. Hypersensitive carotid sinus syndrome
    f. Recurrent refractory tachyarrhythmias in which temporary pacing has been effective

PACEMAKER INSERTION

1. **Equipment**
    a. Pulse generator
       i. External
      ii. Implantable
    b. Leads (catheters)
       i. Types
         (a) Myocardial (epicardial)
         (b) Endocardial
    c. Electrodes
       i. Unipolar (one electrode)
         (a) Catheter must be connected to indifferent electrode elsewhere
           (1) Small metal needle in skin connected to positive terminal of pulse generator
           (2) Negative terminal of pulse generator connected to catheter electrode; or
           (3) Electric circuit completed through body tissues to metal plate on pulse generator, or by metallic housing of pulse generator itself
         (b) Generates larger pacemaker artifact (spike) on ECG than do bipolar electrodes
           (1) Pacing artifact immediately precedes P wave when atrium is paced, or QRS complex when ventricle is paced
           (2) Larger artifact signal improves sensing by pacemaker
      ii. Bipolar (two electrodes)
         (a) More commonly used
         (b) Positive and negative terminals on, or in, heart
         (c) If one electrode fails, can be converted to unipolar system by adding skin electrode
         (d) Generate smaller pacemaker artifact on ECG than does unipolar electrode

2. **Temporary pacemaker insertion**
   a. Epicardial pacing routine after cardiac surgery
      i. Atrial and ventricular wires placed during surgery come out through chest wall ready to attach to pulse generator
      ii. Wires easily pulled out when no longer needed
   b. Transvenous endocardial pacing most common method
      i. Catheter inserted percutaneously or by venous cutdown
         (a) Routes — antecubital, femoral, jugular, subclavian veins
         (b) Monitoring
             (1) Antecubital insertion with electrocardiographic or fluoroscopic control
             (2) Femoral insertion with fluoroscopic guidance
         (c) Placement of catheter tip
             (1) Ventricular pacing — tip wedged between trabeculae of right ventricular apex
             (2) Atrial pacing — tip lodged in atrial appendage or coronary sinus
         (d) Electrodes attach to external pulse generator
             (1) Part of monitoring unit
             (2) Self-contained battery unit
         (e) Pacing threshold measurement
             (1) Minimal intensity of pacing stimulus that maintains continuous capture of heart
             (2) Used to verify adequate electrode placement
             (3) Gradually decreased until capture is lost; increased until QRS complex follows each pacing impulse
             (4) Amount of current when 1:1 capture first occurs is stimulation threshold
             (5) If exceeds 1.5 milliamps (ma), lead is in unsatisfactory position
             (6) Setting for stimulus current should be at least twice pacing threshold
             (7) Stable pacing position confirmed after having patient deep breathe, cough, and shift slightly
         (f) Sensitivity threshold
             (1) Measure to confirm adequate sensing of intrinsic cardiac activity if demand pacing is used
             (2) Rate dial turned below patient's heart rate
             (3) Sensitivity dial turned to most sensitive demand position
             (4) Sense/Pace indicator should deflect toward "Sense"

(5) Turn dial to middle of sensitivity range
(6) If pacemaker does not sense R wave, lead should be repositioned
   c. Emergency pacing
      i. Large needle used to insert electrodes directly into ventricle via chest wall
         (a) Risks include coronary artery trauma, pericardial tamponade, or dysrhythmias
         (b) Preferred to external pacemaker
      ii. External pacemaker
         (a) Delivers regular shock of 50–150 volts directly to chest wall via electrodes over precordium
         (b) Painful and, if prolonged, may burn skin
         (c) Least effective approach

3. **Permanent pacemaker insertion**
   a. Transvenous endocardial pacing
      i. Advantages
         (a) Can be applied in any hospital where facilities for minor surgery are available
         (b) Does not require a thoracotomy
         (c) Can be performed in individuals who would be poor risks for general anesthesia
      ii. Disadvantages (complications)
         (a) Catheter dislodgement
         (b) Right ventricular perforation
         (c) Diaphragmatic stimulation
         (d) Pulmonary embolism (rare)
         (e) Air embolism
         (f) Infection
   b. Thoracotomy epicardial pacing
      i. Advantages
         (a) Reliability of pacing
         (b) Necessary approach with synchronous atrial pacing
         (c) Indicated for young people who have not attained full growth
         (d) Eliminates dangers of bacterial endocarditis and peripheral embolization
      ii. Disadvantages (complications)
         (a) Risks of major surgery in elderly population
         (b) Carries significant morbidity and mortality
         (c) Infection
   c. Subxiphoid, transxiphoid, transmediastinal epicardial pacing
      i. Advantages
         (a) No chest tubes or long postoperative recovery
         (b) Facilitates use of screw electrodes
         (c) Reliability of pacing

(d) Eliminates dangers of bacterial endocarditis and peripheral embolization

TYPES OF PACEMAKERS

1. **Basic features**
   a. Asynchronous (fixed rate) pacing
      i.   Operate at a set rate; unable to respond to physiologic demands
      ii. Stimulus can be directed to atrium, ventricle, or both
      iii. Independent of intrinsic cardiac activity
      iv. Can be competitive with spontaneous ventricular activity
   b. Demand (programmed) pacing
      i.   Senses spontaneous cardiac activity
      ii. Can be used in atrial and ventricular pacing, or both
      iii. Avoids generating competitive rhythms
   c. Effects on ECG
      i.   Ventricular pacemaker
         (a) Pacing stimulus artifact accompanied by prolonged QRS
         (b) Transvenous endocardial pacing of right ventricle results in LBBB pattern (development of RBBB pattern suggests either perforation of IVS or migration of pacemaker electrode tip to coronary sinus)
         (c) Epicardial transthoracic pacing of left ventricle results in RBBB pattern
      ii. Atrial pacemaker
         (a) Pacing stimulus artifact accompanied by P wave
         (b) Contour of pacemaker-induced P wave differs from spontaneously generated P waves
   d. Automatic interval
      i.   Interval between two consecutive pacing stimuli
      ii. Automatic interval (pacing rate) selected by physician
   e. Capture
      i.   When depolarization takes place due to pacemaker stimulus
      ii. When pacemaker stimulates every beat, called "complete capture"
   f. Escape interval
   g. Hysteresis

2. **Ventricular pacemakers**: stimulation of ventricles
   a. Continuous asynchronous ventricular pacemaker (fixed rate) (rarely used)
      i.   Features
         (a) Only has a stimulating mechanism
         (b) Delivers stimuli continuously to ventricles
         (c) Discharge rate adjusted to clinical situation
         (d) Discharge rate unaffected by spontaneous beats

    ii. Disadvantages

        (a) When natural beats appear, summated heart rates result from sum of natural beats and artificial beats

        (b) When stimuli fall during vulnerable period, repetitive ventricular beats may occur

        (c) Pacemaker rate cannot respond to physiologic demands such as fever or increased activity

        (d) Lack of sequential A-V contraction eliminates effectiveness of atrium as booster pump

b. QRS-inhibited ventricular pacemaker (demand)

    i. Features

        (a) Stimulation and sensing accomplished via ventricular electrode

        (b) If natural beat is sensed, pacemaker output is suppressed or inhibited

        (c) Pacing stimulus emitted only after preselected escape interval

        (d) When natural rate falls below escape rate of pacemaker, pacemaker depolarizes ventricle at fixed continuous rate

    ii. Advantage: eliminates competition

    iii. Disadvantage: during periods of inhibition, difficult to evaluate stimulating property of unit

c. QRS-triggered ventricular pacemaker (standby)

    i. Features

        (a) Stimulation and sensing accomplished via ventricular electrode

        (b) Programmed to deliver electrical stimulus during formation of natural QRS complexes when natural rate exceeds pacemaker rate

        (c) Natural QRS triggers pacemaker to fire in synchrony with inherent rhythm

        (d) Pacemaker fires after preset escape interval that corresponds to rate of pacemaker

        (e) When natural rate falls below escape rate of pacemaker, pacemaker depolarizes ventricle at fixed continuous rate

    ii. Disadvantages

        (a) Stimulus artifact distorts natural QRS morphology

        (b) Difficulty in interpreting ECG in certain acute dysrhythmias

d. P-wave-triggered ventricular pacemaker (P-wave synchronous)

    i. Features

        (a) Atrial sensing circuit and ventricular stimulating circuit provided by separate atrial and ventricular electrodes

        (b) Sensing electrode detects P wave; after a delay corresponding to normal P-R interval, ventricle is stimulated

        (c)   P wave triggers release of ventricular stimulus

        (d)   If a P wave fails to appear after a preset escape interval, ventricular pacemaker will escape and fire at fixed rate

        (e)   If atrial rate becomes excessively rapid, ventricular pacemaker will induce 2:1 or greater block between sensed P waves and ventricular stimulation

    ii.   Advantages

        (a)   Enables atria to vary ventricular rate according to physiologic demands

        (b)   Reduces competition

        (c)   Preserves sequential A-V contraction ("atrial kick")

    iii.   Disadvantages

        (a)   Complex circuitry

        (b)   Frequent need for thoracotomy to achieve stable sensing and pacing

        (c)   Short battery life

        (d)   Precipitation of other dysrhythmias

3. **Atrial pacemakers**: stimulation of atria
   a. Basic requirements
      i.   A-V conduction must be intact
      ii.   No persistent atrial flutter or fibrillation present
   b. Advantages
      i.   Provides electrical and hemodynamic benefits of normal atrioventricular contraction
      ii.   Reduces dangers of ventricular competition
   c. Continuous asynchronous atrial pacemaker (fixed rate)
      i.   Atrial electrode delivers stimuli continuously to atria
      ii.   Discharge rate adjusted to clinical situation
      iii.   Discharge rate unaffected by spontaneous atrial beats
   d. P-wave-inhibited atrial pacemaker (demand)
      i.   Stimulation and sensing accomplished via atrial electrode
      ii.   If atrial depolarization is sensed, pacemaker output is suppressed or inhibited
      iii.   Pacing stimulus emitted only after preselected escape interval
      iv.   When natural rate falls below escape rate of pacemaker, pacemaker depolarizes atria at fixed continuous rate
   e. P-wave-triggered atrial pacemaker
      i.   Stimulation and sensing accomplished via atrial electrode
      ii.   Programmed to deliver electrical stimulus during formation of natural P wave when natural rate exceeds pacemaker rate
      iii.   Natural P wave triggers pacemaker to fire in synchrony with inherent atrial rhythm
      iv.   Pacemaker fires after preset escape interval that corresponds to rate of pacemaker

      v. When natural rate falls below escape rate of pacemaker, pacemaker depolarizes atria at fixed continuous rate
- f. QRS-inhibited atrial pacemaker
  - i. Faster ventricular rates suppress output of pacemaker
  - ii. Pacemaker atrial escapes occur when a QRS complex fails to appear before a preset interval

4. **Atrial and ventricular pacemakers**
   - a. Continuous sequential atrial and ventricular pacemaker
     - i. Stimulation accomplished via atrial and ventricular electrodes
     - ii. Continuous stimuli delivered to atria and ventricles in sequence
     - iii. Sequential delay between two stimuli equal to normal P-R interval
     - iv. Potential problem: competitive rhythms
   - b. QRS-inhibited sequential atrial and ventricular pacemaker (bifocal demand)
     - i. Stimulation accomplished via atrial and ventricular electrodes
     - ii. Sensing accomplished via ventricular electrode
     - iii. When natural QRS is sensed, both atrial and ventricular pacemaker stimuli are suppressed or inhibited
     - iv. Escape interval
       - (a) Shorter for atrial pacemaker than for ventricular pacemaker
       - (b) Time difference between two escape intervals defines A-V sequential interval, i.e., P-R interval
     - v. Pacemaker may stimulate atria and ventricles in sequence, or only atria, or may remain dormant when regular sinus rhythm returns

COMPLICATIONS

1. **Pacemaker malfunction**
   - a. Inadequate stimulus release
     - i. Causes
       - (a) Battery failure
       - (b) Component failure (lead, electrode)
       - (c) Disconnections within or between catheter and pulse generator
       - (d) Sensing malfunction
       - (e) Electromagnetic interference
     - ii. Clinical manifestations
       - (a) Slowing of pacing rate or variations in rate of stimulus discharge
       - (b) Intermittent, or complete absence of, stimulus artifact on ECG

(c) Runaway pacemaker — acute emergency requiring immediate disconnection of pacing unit and provision of pacing by another means

b. Failure to capture (stimulate)

   i. Causes

     (a) Low voltage

     (b) Faulty connection between pulse generator and catheter

     (c) Faulty connection between catheter and bridging cable

     (d) Improper position of catheter

     (e) Catheter wire fracture

     (f) Fibrosis at catheter tip

   ii. Clinical manifestations

     (a) Slowing of atrial or ventricular rate

     (b) Pacing artifact does not produce a P wave or QRS on ECG (artifact must fall outside absolute refractory period of atria or ventricle for capture to occur)

     (c) Chest x-ray confirms displacement of catheter

   iii. Intervention

     (a) Check connections between catheter and battery pack

     (b) Reposition patient or patient's arm

     (c) Increase milliamps or voltage and check response

     (d) Record ECG and obtain chest x-rays to check catheter position

c. Failure to sense (relates to QRS-inhibited ventricular pacemaker)

   i. Causes

     (a) Faulty sensing mechanism

     (b) Improper position of catheter

     (c) Poor intracavitary signals in area of electrode placement

     (d) Battery failure

   ii. Clinical manifestations

     (a) Competition

       (1) Stimulus artifact may fall during vulnerable period of T wave and induce repetitive ventricular beats

         (a) Occurs when there is a reduction in threshold for ventricular tachycardia or ventricular fibrillation, as seen with

           (i) Acute myocardial ischemia or infarction

           (ii) Cardioactive drug overdose or sensitivity

           (iii) Electrolyte imbalance, especially hypokalemia

           (iv) Increased catecholamine excretion

           (v) Hypoxic states

           (vi) Chronic severe heart disease

              (b) Hazard is remote in stable patients in whom electrode has matured and stimulation threshold has increased by appearance of fibrotic tissue at site of insertion

        (b) Summated heart rates

            (1) Palpitations

            (2) Lightheadedness, angina (depending on underlying clinical state)

  iii. Intervention (depends on underlying rhythm)

        (a) If patient's natural rhythm is adequate, pacemaker may be turned off

        (b) If patient's rhythm is inadequate

            (1) Increase pacer rate to overdrive

            (2) Administer lidocaine if unsensed natural beat is ventricular in origin

            (3) Increase sensitivity

            (4) Reposition patient

            (5) Unipolarize a bipolar system

        (c) If pacemaker is set on asynchronous or continuous pacing, turn to demand mode

        (d) Replace battery pack

2. Electrical complications of pacemaking

  a. Leakage of 60-cycle current from line-powered equipment

    i. In contact with myocardial pacing lead, can cause ventricular fibrillation

    ii. Always a threat with temporary electrodes that traverse the skin

    iii. Cautionary measures

        (a) Only battery-powered pacemakers should be used on myocardial electrodes

        (b) Terminals and connections on unit must be shielded against accidental contact with sources of 60-cycle currents

        (c) If monitoring device is used on myocardial electrode, instrument should be the only one in contact with patient, or instruments should be connected to one power receptacle

        (d) With completely implanted devices, safe to use line-powered electrocardiographs and monitoring instruments

        (e) All room equipment should be grounded

        (f) "Tingling" sensations emitted from electrical equipment in patient's room should be reported

        (g) Rubber gloves should be worn when adjusting electrodes of battery temporary pacemaker

        (h) Intracavitary lead should be connected to V lead of ECG machine, since this circuit has high electrical resistance in relation to ground

b. Hazards arising from external electrical fields
    i.   Asynchronous pacemakers insensitive to most environ-
mental electrical fields
   ii.   Ventricular programmed pacemakers more sensitive to
electrical fields
    (a)   In presence of strong alternating conduction currents
or magnetic fields, demand pacemaker will revert to
fixed operation
    (b)   Extremely low conducted currents and magnetic
fields can cause either reversion to lower-than-normal
stimulation rate or complete inhibition
        (1)   Interferences affect pacemaker temporarily, while
wearer is in direct contact with source
        (2)   Normal operation of pacemaker will resume as
soon as contact is broken or wearer withdraws
from close proximity
    (c)   Cautionary measures
        (1)   Pacemaker wearers should be discouraged from
operating appliances such as
            (a)   Magnetic tape erasers
            (b)   Tool demagnetizers
            (c)   Large transformer-driven devices
            (d)   Arc welding machines
        (2)   Diathermy should never be used on body areas
overlying implanted pacemaker
        (3)   Electroconvulsive therapy interferes with pace-
maker
        (4)   Electrosurgical apparatus should be used in
bursts separated by several seconds; pulse should
be monitored manually
        (5)   Cautery and cutting instruments should not be
used within 2 inches of implanted pacemakers
        (6)   Wearers should inform physicians, dentists, and
physical therapists that they have a pacemaker
        (7)   Wearers should use electrical devices that are
properly grounded and in good repair
        (8)   Wearers should never use an electrical device in
damp or wet areas
        (9)   Electric hair clippers and shavers should not be
repeatedly turned on and off or operated directly
over implanted area
      (10)   Wearers should avoid working directly over
ignition systems in operation (cars, lawnmowers,
boat motors, etc.)
      (11)   Wearers should avoid direct close contact with store
theft prevention devices and microwave ovens

NURSING CARE OF PATIENT WITH TEMPORARY PACEMAKER

1. **Preoperative care**
   a. Explain procedure to patient and family in view of emergency time frame
   b. Obtain signature on operative permit
   c. Administer sedation if necessary
   d. Prepare for potential emergency
      i. Establish IV line
      ii. Make defibrillator available
      iii. Make drugs available — lidocaine, atropine, isoproterenol

2. **Postoperative care**
   a. Record date, site of pacemaker insertion, and following pacemaker settings: rate, milliamps, fixed rate or demand
   b. Shield or protect pacemaker dials, and instruct patient not to touch unit
   c. Stabilize arm, catheter, and pacemaker to arm, or place pacemaker at bedside
   d. Avoid electrical hazards
      i. Cover exposed pacemaker terminals with rubber gloves
      ii. Wear rubber gloves when connecting or disconnecting pacemaker or adjusting terminals
      iii. Ensure that there is no radio broadcasting equipment, electric shavers, or other superfluous electric items in vicinity
   e. Periodically check ECG and compare it to tracing taken at time of pacemaker insertion
   f. Using sterile technique, cleanse area of catheter insertion daily, and observe for infection and inflammation
   g. Monitor pacemaker function and report significant variations
      i. Observe monitored cardiac rhythm
      ii. Check pacing current and sense/pace indicator regularly
      iii. Observe for pacemaker malfunction
         (a) Improper stimulus release
         (b) Failure to capture
         (c) Failure to sense (QRS-inhibited ventricular pacemaker)
   h. Monitor vital signs and evaluate patient complaints
   i. Continue to reassure and counsel patient and family
   j. In the event of cardiac arrest
      i. If pacemaker is off
         (a) Turn it on
         (b) Increase milliamps, e.g., from 3 to 5, since patient's threshold may have increased
         (c) Increase rate to 60 if below 60
         (d) Observe pacemaker function: sense/pace indicator, ECG, patient's pulse

       ii.   If pacemaker is on and patient requires defibrillation
          (a) Turn pacemaker off
          (b) If time allows, disconnect both wires from pacemaker
               terminals
               (1) Prevents diversion of current from its cardiac
                    pathway
               (2) Prevents possible pacemaker damage, even though
                    most pacemakers are made to withstand shocks of
                    up to 400 watt seconds
   k. To discontinue pacemaker, turn it off and leave catheter in place
      for prescribed period
       i.   Monitor natural cardiac activity
       ii.   Reassure patient and family

NURSING CARE OF PATIENT WITH PERMANENT PACEMAKER

1. **Preoperative care**
   a. Monitor temporary pacemaker routinely used preoperatively and
      during surgery
   b. Reassure and explain procedure to patient and family, depending
      on site of surgery, including
       i.   Benefits of pacemaker
       ii.   Skin discoloration
       iii. Skin pouch
       iv. Discomforts
       v.   Nursing care
   c. Describe postoperative period and what patient should expect

2. **Postoperative care**
   a. Surgical approach (transvenous, thoracotomy, subxiphoid)
      determines emphasis of patient care
       i.   Post-thoracotomy patients require more physical care, and
          risk more physical complications
       ii.   Routine postoperative care specific to surgical approach
   b. Care specific to pacemaker
       i.   Record date, site of insertion, type of pacemaker
       ii.   Obtain and record baseline values of pacemaker function
          including:
          (a) Escape interval
          (b) Continuously discharging interval (both spontaneous
              and magnet-induced)
          (c) Refractory period
          (d) Sensed P to QRS stimulus interval (synchronous atrial
              pacing)
          (e) Sensed QRS (demand ventricular pacemaker)
          (f) Current or voltage delivered
          (g) Artifact size
          (h) Stimulation threshold

     iii. Obtain baseline ECG, and posteroanterior and lateral chest x-ray films

     iv. Evaluate stimulation function in demand or synchronous ventricular pacemakers

       (a) Vagal stimulation to slow sinus rate or induce A-V block

       (b) Magnet on skin overlying pacemaker actuates a switch that causes it to revert to continuously discharging mode

     v. Restrict activity of patients with transvenous pacemaker for a few days to reduce risk of catheter dislodgement

     vi. Care for surgical site

       (a) Check site for bleeding, swelling, pain, infection

       (b) Apply sterile dressings over site

       (c) Administer prescribed antibiotics for initial 5 to 7 days

       (d) Prepare for removal of sutures 7 to 10 days after surgery

     vii. Implement passive ROM exercises to arm on side of operation

     viii. Monitor cardiac rhythm

       (a) Observe for competition with fixed rate pacemakers

         (1) Pacemaker is initially set to deliver a large amount of energy to myocardium, since fibrosis around electrodes will eventually occur and dissipate this energy to a degree. A week or more is required for adequate fibrosis to occur

         (2) A new, stiff catheter may produce a certain amount of injury to myocardium that may result in PVCs

3. Rehabilitation planning

   a. Psychologic factors

     i. Assess patient's attitudes toward pacemaker, including

       (a) Dependency on it for life

       (b) Fear of sudden death from pacemaker failure

       (c) Fear of a "fragile" heart

       (d) Concerns about physical exertion or exercise

       (e) Preoccupation with pacemaker's function

     ii. Intervention

       (a) Encourage patient to ventilate; reassure and counsel accordingly

       (b) Encourage patient and family to talk with pacemaker wearers who are adjusted

   b. Patient teaching program

     i. Review how heart works; how patient's own heart was failing to work; how pacemaker can help

ii. Involve family in teaching program
iii. Stress importance of patient carrying an identification card at all times, showing his name; his physician's name, address, phone number; type of pacemaker
iv. Teach patient to check pacemaker function
    (a) Count pulse daily for a full minute at same time every day; if rate slows 5 or more beats, check again and if still slow, call physician
    (b) Immediately report dizziness, fainting spells, prolonged weakness or fatigue, palpitations, prolonged hiccoughing
v.   Teach patient to report other symptoms, including
    (a) Swelling of legs, ankles, arms, or wrists
    (b) Chest pain, difficulty in breathing
    (c) Fever with redness, swelling or drainage at surgical scar
vi. Review therapeutic program
    (a) Emphasize any changes in diet, and assist in menu planning
    (b) Discuss prescribed medications – purpose, dosages, times to be taken, side effects that should be reported
vii. Ensure that following points are included in program
    (a) Travel or relocating
        (1) Inform physician before traveling and carry list of physicians or hospitals in localities, with a medical summary to give them
        (2) In event of a move, ask physician to recommend a new physician to whom records can be sent
    (b) Return to work
        (1) Physician will recommend appropriate time to return
        (2) If job must be less strenuous, plan modifications or alternatives
    (c) Driving a car usually resumed after a month
    (d) Exercise
        (1) Physician should advise time to begin exercise
        (2) Regular, moderate exercise is recommended
        (3) Body contact sports should be avoided
    (e) Sexual relations
        (1) Patient can return to degree of activity desired and that he is able to tolerate
        (2) A young woman with pacemaker can tolerate pregnancy
    (f) Clothing – some guidance should be offered in selection of comfortable clothing and underwear
    (g) Electrical precautions (see p. 141)

   c. Followup care
- i. Patient at home
  - (a) Should have daily pulse counts
  - (b) Should report unusual symptoms
  - (c) May have instrument to measure pulse width or rate
- ii. Pacemaker clinic
  - (a) Provides continuing contact with physician and nurse at monthly or annual intervals
  - (b) Pacemaker can be checked by:
    - (1) ECG
    - (2) Pulse width measuring device
    - (3) Pacer analyzer
    - (4) X-rays
    - (5) Spike analysis on an oscilloscope
  - (c) Other cardiac problems (e.g., hypertension, CHF, coronary artery or valvular disease) can be evaluated and treated
  - (d) Patient should be encouraged to call when problems arise
- iii. Telephone monitoring
  - (a) Between clinic visits, telephone checkups can monitor pacemaker function
  - (b) Patient must have own transmitter to engage in telephone checking service
  - (c) Telephone transmission of ECGs has reliably predicted impending battery failure

   d. Pulse generator replacement
- i. Indications
  - (a) Battery failure (most common indication)
  - (b) Component failure
  - (c) Wire fracture
  - (d) High threshold
  - (e) Infection/extrusion
- ii. Battery failure
  - (a) Knowledge of mode of battery exhaustion of every pacemaker model in followup is needed to form broad judgment on replacement timing
  - (b) Time of failure is spread over large portion of total longevity of any pulse generator model; hence, importance of followup
  - (c) Elective replacement of pulse generator has been abandoned
  - (d) Indications of end of battery life include
    - (1) Drop of rate
    - (2) Compensatory increase of pulse width
- iii. Replacement procedure
  - (a) Under local anesthesia, pulse generator is replaced with a new one

(b) Patient's cardiac rhythm is observed for a few days to ensure proper pacemaker function

CONGESTIVE HEART FAILURE/PULMONARY EDEMA: "A state in which the cardiac output is insufficient to meet the metabolic needs of the body." (Andreoli, 1975, p. 58)

1. **Pathophysiology:** left heart failure to right heart failure
   a. Diseased left ventricular myocardium cannot pump blood returning from lungs into systemic circulation — this decreases cardiac output
   b. Pressure increases in lungs owing to accumulation of blood in lungs
       i.   If pressure exceeds pulmonary capillary oncotic pressure (30 mm Hg), fluid will leak into pulmonary interstitial space, resulting in pulmonary edema
       ii. Oxygen/carbon dioxide exchange is impeded
   c. As pressure continues to increase in lungs, pressure in right heart increases (due to backflow of pressure in pulmonary vasculature)
   d. Right heart cannot pump its blood into pulmonary system owing to this backflow of pressure
   e. Venous return is impeded
   f. Pressure continues to back up, and eventually organs become congested with venous blood

2. **Etiology or precipitating factors**

Left heart failure	Right heart failure
i. Atherosclerotic heart disease	i. Left heart failure
ii. Acute myocardial infarction	ii. Atherosclerotic heart disease
iii. Tachycardia/ bradycardia	iii. Acute myocardial infarction
iv. Myocarditis	iv. Tachycardia/ bradycardia
v. Increased circulating volume	v. Pulmonary embolism
vi. Valvular disease	vi. Fluid overload/excess sodium intake
	vii. COPD — pulmonary hypertension (cor pulmonale)
	viii. Valvular disease

3. **Clinical presentation**

Left heart failure	Right heart failure
i. Anxiety	i. Hepatosplenomegaly with or without pain
ii. Air hunger	ii. Dependent pitting edema
iii. Nocturnal dyspnea, dyspnea on exertion, orthopnea	iii. Venous distention, jugular venous distention, HJR

3. **Clinical presentation** *(Continued)*

Left heart failure	Right heart failure
iv. Cough with frothy sputum	iv. Bounding pulses
v. Tachycardia	v. Oliguria
vi. Diaphoresis	vi. Dysrhythmias
vii. Basilar rales	vii. Elevated CVP – right atrial pressures
viii. Bronchial wheezing	
ix. Cyanosis or pallor	
x. Hypoxia, respiratory acidosis	
xi. Gallop rhythm	
xii. Insomnia	
xiii. Elevated PA diastolic and PCWP	
xiv. Palpitations	
xv. Hyperventilation	
xvi. Pulmonary hypertension	
xvii. Pulsus alternans	

4. **Diagnostic findings**
   a. History and physical examination (see Clinical presentation)
      i. Weight gain
      ii. Upper abdominal pain (hepatosplenomegaly)
      iii. Nocturia (increased cardiac output due to rest causes diuresis)
      iv. Anorexia and nausea (edema of bowel)
   b. Radiologic examination – chest x-ray
      i. Pulmonary clouding – interstitial density
      ii. Cardiac hypertrophy
   c. Liver function tests may be abnormal owing to hepatic venous congestion.
   d. Swan-Ganz findings will be dependent on location and degree of failure

5. **Complications**
   a. Progressive deterioration of cardiac and pulmonary function
   b. Serious cardiac dysrhythmias
   c. Potential complications of therapy
      i. Fluid and electrolyte imbalance
      ii. Opiate overdosage
      iii. Digitalis toxicity
      iv. Oxygen toxicity

6. **Specific patient care**
   a. Maintenance of adequate ventilation and respiration to improve gas exchange
      i. Administer humidified oxygen

       ii.   Administer IPPB treatments with bronchodilator therapy as indicated
      iii.   Position patient to encourage maximal inflation of lungs
      iv.   Check arterial blood gases to monitor ventilatory status
       v.   Encourage coughing and deep breathing

b. Reduction of pulmonary venous congestion and blood volume
       i.   Administer diuretics as prescribed and record observed effects
      ii.   Maintain fluid and sodium restrictions
      iii.   Manage rotating tourniquets
      iv.   Assist with phlebotomy
       v.   Assist patient to maintain position that enables him to breathe more easily

c. Improvement of myocardial contractility with the use of inotropic agents

d. Monitor hemodynamics in order to assess fluid balance and cardiac function

PERICARDITIS

1. **Pathophysiology**
   a. Inflammation of pericardium
   b. Fibrinous deposits on serous pericardium
   c. Effusion into pericardium and cardiac tamponade

2. **Etiology or precipitating factors**
   a. Idopathic – nonspecific
   b. Acute myocardial infarction
   c. Trauma (penetrating or nonpenetrating)
   d. Postcardiotomy or post-thoracotomy
   e. Collagen diseases
   f. Infection
          i.   Bacterial
         ii.   Viral
         iii.   Fungal
         iv.   Protozoal
   g. Neoplasms
   h. Dissecting aortic aneurysms
   i. Radiation therapy
   j. Uremia
   k. Drugs
          i.   Procainamide
         ii.   Hydralazine
         iii.   Diphenylhydantoin
         iv.   Adriamycin
   l. Tuberculous

3. **Clinical presentation**
   a. Cough
   b. Precordial or pleuritic chest pain
   c. Hemoptysis
   d. Dyspnea
   e. Mental confusion
   f. Tachycardia
   g. Fever
   h. Pericardial friction rub
   i. Accentuated pulmonary S_2
   j. Cyanosis
   k. Pallor
   l. Pulsus paradoxus
   m. Dysrhythmias
   n. Jugular venous congestion

4. **Diagnostic findings**
   a. History
      i. Specific complaint of chest pain
         (a) Increased pericardial pain (i.e., "pleuritic") with deep inspiration or turning of thorax
         (b) Increased pain with lying down
         (c) Relieved by sitting up or leaning forward
         (d) Pain very similar to that in myocardial infarction, but in myocardial infarction the pain generally is not positional
      ii. Nonspecific complaints — upper respiratory infection, fever, joint discomfort, fatigue — suggest a systemic disease causing pericarditis
   b. Physical examination
      i. Palpation — tachycardia, HJR
      ii. Auscultation — heart sounds normal except muffled/ distant with effusion; pericardial friction rub, pulsus paradoxus
      iii. Inspection — cyanosis, pallor, distended neck veins, dyspnea
   c. Diagnostic studies
      i. ECG changes
         (a) S-T elevation in two or three limb leads
         (b) S-T elevation in precordial leads
         (c) S-T depression in V_1 and aVR
         (d) T inverted after S-T is isoelectric again
      ii. Laboratory findings
         (a) Leukocytosis
         (b) SGOT may be elevated but is usually normal
      iii. Radiologic examination — chest x-ray may be normal or may show cardiac dilatation, pericardial effusion
      iv. Echocardiography — may show pericardial effusion

    v. Cardiac catheterization used to
- (a) Evaluate severity of constriction
- (b) Check need for pericardiotomy
- (c) Differentially diagnose pericarditis from restrictive cardiomyopathy

5. Complications
a. Cardiac tamponade
b. Dysrhythmias

6. Specific patient care
a. Relief of cardiac tamponade — assist with pericardiocentesis
b. Reduction of inflammation in heart — administer steroids or salicylates as prescribed
c. Monitor hemodynamics via Swan-Ganz and ECG
d. Control bleeding tendencies — administer anticoagulants as ordered
e. Relief of fever — administer antipyretics as prescribed, and record effects

HYPERTENSIVE CRISIS (Moser, 1975; Onesti, 1973)

1. Pathophysiology
a. Accelerated/malignant hypertension (a severe acceleration of hypertension in association with other primary diseases)
    i. Diastolic BP reaches "critical" level (individualized reaction)
    ii. Necrotizing arteriolitis appears in arterial wall
    iii. Renal-pressor system theory — arterial wall changes → renin release → production and release of angiotensin → excessive secretion of aldosterone (see Renal section for details of these mechanisms)
b. Hypertensive encephalopathy — excessive elevation of blood pressure → dysfunction of cerebral autoregulation → increased cerebral blood flow → increased capillary pressure → cerebral edema and hemorrhage

2. Etiology or precipitating factors
a. Untreated or inadequately treated essential hypertension
b. Poor compliance with antihypertensive medication treatment plan
c. Essential hypertension — highest incidence in black females
d. Renal diseases such as acute/chronic glomerulonephritis, chronic pyelonephritis, collagen vascular disease, renal vascular disease
e. Toxemia of pregnancy
f. Concurrent intake of catecholamine precursors and monoamine oxidase (MAO) inhibitor drugs

      g. Pheochromocytoma
      h. Polycythemia
      i. Pituitary tumors
      j. Coarctation of aorta
      k. Adrenocortical hyperfunction
      l. Acromegaly
      m. Cushing's syndrome

3. **Clinical presentation** (Onesti, 1973, pp. 207–210)
    a. Accelerated malignant hypertension
      i. Severe fixed hypertension – diastolic blood pressure greater than 120 mm Hg
      ii. Severe retinopathy with exudates, hemorrhage, and papilledema
      iii. Severe impairment of renal function
      iv. Headache
      v. Restlessness
      vi. Epistaxis
    b. Hypertensive encephalopathy
      i. Complication of accelerated/malignant hypertension, usually associated with renal disease
      ii. Sudden excessive rise in BP above previous level in accelerated/malignant hypertension
      iii. Severe headache
      iv. Nausea, vomiting
      v. Mental confusion increasing to stupor, coma
      vi. Convulsions
      vii. Transitory focal neurologic signs, e.g., nystagmus
      viii. Visual disturbances
      ix. Localized weakness

4. **Diagnostic findings**
    a. History
      i. Acute rise in BP
      ii. Complaints of severe suboccipital or occipital headaches in morning upon arising, nausea and vomiting, dizziness, shortness of breath on exertion, "anginal" pain, visual changes
    b. Physical examination – findings consistent with target organ affected
      i. Palpation –delayed or absent femoral pulses, prominent left ventricular impulse, tachycardia, dependent edema
      ii. Auscultation – diastolic BP 120–140 mm Hg or above, rales, S_3 and S_4, faint murmur of aortic insufficiency, bruit over flanks or anteriorly over renal vasculature, postural hypotension, BP in legs may be lower than in arms
      iii. Inspection – retinopathy with hemorrhage, exudate, papilledema

c. Diagnostic studies
   i. Laboratory (Laragh, 1974, pp. 692–696) – purpose is to find cause of hypertension if possible and its effects on end organs
      (a) CBC – HCT is decreased in renal failure and polycythemia in association with hypertension
      (b) Serum potassium – used to rule out primary aldosteronism, which causes hypokalemia and hypertension
      (c) Serum BUN or creatinine clearance used to assess kidney function (elevated in renal disease – a possible cause of hypertension)
      (d) Serum glucose elevated in Cushing's syndrome, pheochromocytoma, and diabetes – all possible causes of hypertension
      (e) Urinalysis – routine; especially important is presence of proteinuria and red blood cells
         (1) Proteinuria indicates renal disease, which may be causing the hypertension
         (2) Hematuria also indicates renal disease, i.e., malignant nephrosclerosis
      (f) Urinary vanillylmandelic acid (VMA) – catecholamines – are elevated in pheochromocytoma (an etiologic factor in hypertension)
      (g) Serum uric acid – hyperuricemia is associated with hypertension
   ii. Radiologic
      (a) Renal arteriography – used to show renal artery stenosis as a cause of hypertension
      (b) Timed sequence intravenous pyelogram – only indicates presence of kidney disease; cannot differentiate types of kidney disease, i.e., renal artery stenosis, chronic pyelonephritis, nephrosclerosis.
      (c) Chest x-ray – may indicate cardiomegaly
   iii. Miscellaneous
      (a) ECG – may reveal signs of left ventricular hypertrophy, ischemia, effects of hypertension on myocardium

5. **Complications**: complications in this section are different from other core sections. For this disease entity, they constitute the course of the disease (Moser, 1975, pp. 151–153)
   a. Accelerated/malignant
      i. Untreated – death within months due to cerebral infarcts, myocardial infarcts, renal disease, dissection of aorta
      ii. Treated – without coexisting severe renal damage, may have alleviation of crisis and long-term survival
   b. Hypertensive encephalopathy
      i. Untreated – can lead to death

  ii. Treated promptly – progression of symptoms can be reversed

 6. **Specific patient care**: prompt reduction of BP
  a. Administer parenteral antihypertensive medications as ordered
  b. Ascertain BP on specialized schedule on initiation of antihypertensive therapy – e.g., every 5 minutes for 15 minutes, every 15 minutes for 1 hour, and every hour until stable
  c. Understand actions and side effects of antihypertensive medications used in hypertensive crisis
   i. Diazoxide (Hyperstat)
   ii. Sodium nitroprusside (Nipride)
   iii. Hydralazine (Apresoline)
   iv. Pentolinium tartrate
   v. Trimethaphan camsylate (Arfonad)
   vi. Reserpine
   vii. Methyldopa
   viii. Phentolamine (Regitine)
   ix. Guanethidine

SHOCK: A circulatory disturbance characterized by an acute reduction of blood flow and inadequate perfusion of the tissues (Anderson and Kissane, 1977, p. 157).

 1. **Pathophysiology**
  a. Physiologic initiators of shock
   i. Decrease in venous return to heart because of decrease in effective circulating blood volume
    (a) Diminished blood or plasma volume (e.g., hemorrhage, dehydration)
    (b) Vasodilatation in peripheral vascular bed resulting in reduction of effective circulating volume without actual blood loss (e.g., anaphylaxis, anesthesia)
    (c) Postcapillary vasoconstriction in peripheral vascular bed resulting in pooling and stasis of blood in capillary bed (e.g., septic shock)
   ii. Decrease in ability of heart to pump blood
    (a) Deficient filling (e.g., cardiac tamponade)
    (b) Deficient emptying (e.g., myocardial infarction)
  b. Hemodynamic mechanism of shock (Anderson and Kissane, 1977, p. 158)
   i. Reduction of effective circulating volume
   ii. Decreased venous return to heart
   iii. Decreased cardiac output
   iv. Reduced blood flow
   v. Reduced delivery of oxygen to tissues

Note: The hemodynamic mechanism is the same for all types of shock, regardless of etiology.

    c.   Compensatory mechanisms of shock. These attempt to prevent deterioration of circulation during shock. Recovery from moderate degrees of shock is influenced by negative feedback control mechanisms that attempt to return cardiac output and arterial pressure to normal limits

        i.   Baroreceptor reflex (see also p. 90 in section on Cardio-vascular Physiology). A drop in mean arterial pressure or pulse pressure results in decreased stretching of arterial baroreceptors and loss of their inhibitory effect on vaso-motor center. This sympathetic vasomotor stimulation causes secretion of norepinephine at endings of vasocon-strictor nerves, and stimulation of vasoconstrictors through-out body and heart, resulting in

           (a)   Arteriolar constriction

           (b)   Venous constriction

           (c)   Increased force and rate of cardiac contraction

Note: Sympathetic stimulation does not cause significant constriction of cerebral arterioles. The coronary vessels dilate because of increased myocardial metabolism secondary to tachycardia.

       ii.   Norepinephrine-epinephrine vasoconstrictor mechanism – stimulation of vasomotor center also stimulates adrenal medulla to secrete norepinephrine and epinephrine, further assisting vasoconstriction throughout body

      iii.   CNS ischemic response – when mean arterial pressure drops below 50 mm Hg, ischemia and resultant elevated CO_2 levels in vasomotor center cause extremely powerful sympathetic stimulation. Degree of vasoconstriction caused by this response is so severe that peripheral vessels may become totally occluded

      iv.   Widespread reflex venoconstriction – intense vasoconstric-tion in splanchnic area, subcutaneous and pulmonary veins help maintain filling pressure of heart (not clear which receptors are responsible for this)

       v.   Constriction of afferent and efferent arterioles of kidneys – reduced renal arterial pressure results in renal arteriolar constriction, causing decreased glomerular filtration and renal plasma flow, and resulting in decrease in urine output and increase in sodium retention

      vi.   Activation of renin-angiotensin system – reduced renal afferent arteriolar pressure stimulates baroreceptors in juxtaglomerular cells and activates the renin-angiotensin system, assisting in elevation of arterial pressure, and causing

           (a)   Vasoconstriction of arterioles, and to a lesser extent veins

           (b)   Increased tubular reabsorption of sodium and water

        (c)   Stimulation of adrenal cortex to increase production of aldosterone, which causes retention of renal sodium, thereby expanding extracellular fluid volume

   vii. Shifting of tissue fluid into capillaries — because of decrease in capillary hydrostatic pressure from arteriolar constriction and decreased venous pressure, fluid moves into capillaries from interstitial and intracellular spaces

d. Failure of compensatory mechanisms of shock — if underlying cause of shock is not corrected or self-limiting, circulatory system compensatory mechanisms begin to deteriorate. Poor tissue perfusion and progressively diminishing cardiac output results

    i. Myocardial depression — when arterial pressure falls below level required to maintain coronary blood flow, myocardial ischemia and depression occur, further dereasing cardiac output and blood flow

   ii. Vasomotor center depression — severe cerebral ischemia leads to depression of vasomotor center and elimination of sympathetic stimulation, resulting in pooling of blood in periphery, further reducing venous return and cardiac output

  iii. Vascular failure — arterial and venous dilatation can occur from decrease in nutrients to vessels during shock, causing decrease in blood flow to vital organs and pooling of blood in venous bed

   iv. Thrombosis of minute vessels — minute plugs in small vessels may form because of continued tissue metabolism in presence of sluggish blood flow. Agglutination of erythrocytes, leukocytes, and platelets may be precipitated by

        (a)   Platelet aggregation by catecholamines

        (b)   Damage to endothelial lining of small vessels, with subsequent deposition of fibrin and accumulation of microthrombi

        (c)   Hypoxia increasing the rigidity of red cells

        (d)   Release of vasoactive peptides and anaphylatoxins as a result of complement activation

    v. Release of toxins by ischemic tissues

        (a)   Myocardial toxic factor (MTF) depresses myocardial contractility by interfering with function of calcium ions in excitation-contraction coupling process. It is thought that pancreatic ischemia causes release of proteolytic enzymes, which either stimulate release of MTF or alter plasma proteins to form new toxic substance

        (b)   Endotoxin is relased from bodies of dead gram-negative bacteria in intestines. Diminished blood flow and depression of normal antibacterial defense mechanism of reticuloendothelial system enhance its absorption. Endotoxin causes vascular dilatation and cardiac depression. The importance of this factor in all types of shock is not clear

   vi. Cellular deterioration
     (a) Active transport of sodium and potassium through cell membrane is reduced
     (b) Mitochondrial activity is depressed
     (c) Loss of integrity of lysosome membranes causes release of acid hydrolases that degrade protein, carbohydrates, and fats
     (d) Cellular metabolism of nutrients is depressed

  vii. Acidosis — inadequate tissue perfusion leads to increased anerobic glycolysis and production of lactic acid. Resulting lactic acidosis depresses myocardium and decreases peripheral vascular responsiveness to catecholamines

 viii. Tissue necrosis — prolonged diversion of blood from kidneys, liver, GI tract, etc., contribute to increasing anaerobic metabolism in these areas, resulting in cell death and tissue necrosis

   ix. Deterioration of microcirculation — spasm of precapillary sphincters and venules is compensatory mechanism of shock, but when vasoconstriction is prolonged, continued ischemia and local acidosis cause dilatation of precapillary sphincters, while more resistant venules remain constricted. Blood enters capillaries, but pools and stagnates. This continual increase in capillary hydrostatic pressure causes fluid to leave vascular system in increasing amounts. Capillary walls eventually lose their integrity, and slough

   x. Depletion of cellular high energy phosphate reserves — anaerobic metabolism of shock results in decreased production of ATP and rapid degrading of creatinine phosphate and sarcoplasmic ATP. Depression of protein synthesis and derangement of active transport mechanism and cell membrane permeability result.

2. **Etiology or precipitating factors**
  a. Hypovolemic shock — loss of blood plasma to exterior or into tissues, leading to decreased circulating blood volume and venous return, reduced cardiac output, and inadequate tissue perfusion
    i. Causes
     (a) Hemorrhage
     (b) Burns
     (c) Trauma
     (d) Surgery
     (e) Dehydration
     (f) Intestinal obstruction
     (g) Diabetes mellitus

      (h)   Diabetes insipidus

      (i)   Diuretic therapy

      (j)   Peritonitis

      (k)   Pancreatitis

      (l)   Cirrhosis

      (m) Hemothorax

      (n)   Hemoperitoneum

b. Neurogenic shock — generalized vasodilation because of decreased vasomotor tone. Blood volume is within normal limits, but capacity of blood vessel is increased; consequently, peripheral pooling occurs, resulting in diminished venous return and reduced cardiac output

    i.   Causes

      (a)   General anesthesia

      (b)   Spinal anesthesia

      (c)   Epidural block

      (d)   Spinal cord injury

      (e)   Ganglion-blocking or other antihypertensive drugs

      (f)   Ingestion of barbiturates or phenothiazines

      (g)   Orthostatic hypotension

      (h)   Vasovagal syncope

      (i)   Direct damage to vasomotor center of medulla

      (j)   Altered function of vasomotor center in response to low blood glucose (insulin shock)

      (k)   Anaphylaxis (etiologic classification of anaphylaxis varies considerably from author to author)

c. Septic shock — inadequate tissue perfusion, usually following bacteremia with gram-negative enteric bacilli

    i.   Causes

      (a)   Overt infection

      (b)   Localized infection gaining entry into systemic circulation

      (c)   Urinary tract infection

      (d)   Postabortion and postpartum infection

      (e)   Immunosuppressant therapy

      (f)   Severe underlying disease

    ii. Mechanism

      (a)   Release of endotoxin from organism's cell wall into circulation

      (b)   Endotoxin, directly or indirectly causes vasoconstriction of pre- and postcapillary sphincters

      (c)   Local acidosis develops and promotes relaxation of precapillary sphincters while postcapillary sphincters remain constricted

      (d)   Blood pools in capillary bed, hydrostatic pressure increases, and intravascular fluid leaks into interstitial spaces

    (e)   There is a resultant decrease in effective circulating volume and a decrease in cardiac output

d. Cardiogenic shock — inadequate cardiac pumping resulting in decreased stroke volume and cardiac output, and inadequate tissue perfusion

    i.   Causes

       (a)   Myocardial infarction

       (b)   Dysrhythmias

       (c)   CHF with decreased cardiac output

       (d)   Pulmonary embolism

       (e)   Tension pneumothorax

       (f)   Cardiac tamponade

       (g)   Dissecting aortic aneurysm

       (h)   Atrial myxoma

       (i)   Surgical or spontaneous damage to valves

       (j)   Myocarditis

       (k)   Any form of severe myocardial injury

3. Clinical presentation

a. Common clinical presentation

    i.   Hypotension usually results owing to decrease in stroke volume and cardiac output (BP initially may be normal or high because of sympathetic stimulation)

    ii.   Tachycardia with weak thready pulse is result of sympathetic vasoconstriction

    iii.   Decreased pulse pressure results from decrease in stroke volume

    iv.   Tachypnea initially is the result of chemoreceptor stimulation from reduced arterial pressure, but as shock progresses it is result of medullary respiratory stimulation from metabolic acidosis

    v.   Cool, pale, clammy skin is result of peripheral vasoconstriction from sympathetic stimulation

    vi.   Cyanosis occurs owing to excessive concentration of reduced hemoglobin in blood

    vii.   Oliguria and anuria result from decreased renal perfusion

    viii.   Extreme thirst occurs because of decrease in extracellular fluid volume

    ix.   Hypothermia (except in septic shock) is result of decreased metabolism

    x.   Irritability and anxiety may occur in early shock because of increased secretion of epinephrine from sympathetic stimulation or from hypoxia

    xi.   Apathy, lethargy, confusion, and coma occur as shock progresses, because of acidosis and decreased cerebral blood flow

          xii. Angina may occur in patient with intrinsic coronary artery disease

    b. Clinical presentation specific to hypovolemic shock

        i. Decreased CVP

        ii. Decreased cardiac output

        iii. Decreased PAP

        iv. Decreased PCWP

    c. Clinical presentation for neurogenic shock — similar to that for hypovolemic shock

    d. Clinical presentation specific to septic shock

        i. Early signs are those of bacteremia: hyperthermia, chills, nausea, vomiting, and diarrhea. Cardiac output tends to be greater than normal because of increased metabolic and febrile state

        ii. Subtle warning signs include hyperventilation and diminished sensorium, ranging from restlessness and confusion to obtundation

        iii. As septic shock develops from bacteremia, presentation becomes similar to that in all types of shock

    e. Clinical presentation specific to cardiogenic shock

        i. Elevated CVP, decreased cardiac output (these values may be normal depending on duration of shock and durability of reflex compensatory mechanisms)

        ii. Elevated PAP

        iii. Elevated PCWP

        iv. Pulmonary congestion

        v. Peripheral edema

        vi. Distended neck veins when CVP is elevated

4. **Diagnostic findings**

    a. Common diagnostic findings

        i. Respiratory alkalosis progressing to metabolic acidosis. This occurs initially as compensatory mechanism to blow off CO_2 because of increasing lactic acidosis. As shock progresses, metabolic acidosis develops

        ii. In presence of volume depletion, HCT is elevated (hemoconcentration) but drops (hemodilution) as volume deficit is replaced

        iii. Decreased serum bicarbonate

        iv. Elevated serum lactate

        v. Elevated BUN

        vi. Elevated creatinine

        vii. Hyperkalemia due to oliguria and inadequate tissue perfusion

        viii. Elevated urine specific gravity

        ix. Elevated urine osmolality

        x. Decreased urine creatinine clearance

b. Diagnostic findings specific to septic shock
   i. Leukocytosis usually occurs with a shift to left (refers to increased production of neutrophils, an indicator of acute infection)
   ii. Thrombocytopenia usually seen
   iii. Abnormal PT, PTT, reflecting deficiency in clotting factors
   iv. Blood cultures identifying causative pathogen (cultures may be negative because bacteremia can be intermittent or patient may already have received antibiotic therapy, thereby masking diagnosis)

5. **Complications**
   a. Adult respiratory stress syndrome (shock lung) (see ARDS in Pulmonary section — shock affects lung by producing endothelial damage in capillary bed or precapillary arterioles, and results in increased resistance to blood flow, systemic hypoxia, and interstitial pulmonary edema
   b. Renal failure may occur because of inadequate renal perfusion. Prolonged hypoperfusion can result in acute tubular necrosis or renal cortical necrosis
   c. Cardiac failure may occur because of myocardial damage from decrease in coronary artery blood flow, or from decreased myocardial contraction due to acidosis and release of MTF. Functionally, this is indicated by increase in LVEDP
   d. Liver dysfunction — decreased perfusion to liver during shock results in damage to its reticuloendothelial cells. As a result, patients sustaining shock are more susceptible to overwhelming infections
   e. Disseminated intravascular coagulation — excessive consumption of clotting factors that can occur following shock state, multiple injuries, massive bleeding, and septic shock may result in deficiency of several clotting factors and activation of clotting system by factor XII (Hageman factor)
   f. Gastrointestinal ulcerations — most likely with septic shock. Etiology not clearly defined, but may be related to reduction in blood flow to splanchnic area and gastric mucosa, increased production of acid, and stimulation of sympathetic nervous system
   g. Cerebral infarction
   h. Myocardial infarction
   i. Dysrhythmias

6. **Specific patient care**
   a. General management
      i. Expand blood volume by administration of blood, plasma expanders, albumin, and electrolyte solutions
      ii. Provide adequate ventilation and prevent pulmonary complications

      (a) O_2 therapy essential
      (b) Auscultation for evaluation of breath sounds
      (c) Frequent stimulation to cough
      (d) Suction
      (e) Turn patient
      (f) Postural drainage
      (g) Humidification of inspired air
      (h) Chest physiotherapy
      (i) Avoid excessive administration of parenteral fluids

iii. Maintain adequate circulation
      (a) ECG monitoring for evaluation of rate and rhythm
      (b) Mean arterial pressure monitoring provides indication of tissue blood flow
      (c) CVP provides index of absolute and relative blood volume
      (d) PAP
      (e) PCWP reflects LVEDP
      (f) Check cardiac output
      (g) Evaluate cutaneous vasoconstriction as clue to peripheral resistance
      (h) Change in mental status may indicate decline in cerebral blood flow
      (i) Avoid overheating and resultant vasodilatation
      (j) Do not further compromise circulation by allowing patient to sit or stand
      (k) Sedatives and other CNS depressants should be used sparingly because they depress discharge of vasomotor center
      (l) Patient should be placed in horizontal position with legs slightly elevated. Extreme forms of this position cause abdominal viscera to press on diaphragm, making adequate ventilation difficult to maintain

iv. Monitor urinary output
      (a) Indwelling catheter indicated for accurate monitoring
      (b) Measure output q. 1 h. — output of less than 30 ml/hr is indicator of inadequate arterial pressure and renal perfusion

v. Correct acid-base disturbances (shock produces complex abnormalities due to hypoxia, tachypnea, hypocapnia, lactic acidosis)
      (a) Metabolic acidosis treated with sodium bicarbonate, fluids, and improvement of perfusion
      (b) Respiratory acidosis treated with endotracheal suctioning and mechanical ventilation
      (c) Respiratory alkalosis treated with sedation and adjustment of ventilator volume, and increase in dead space

      (d) Metabolic alkalosis treated with ammonium chloride (Berk et al., 1976, p. 232)

  b. Management specific to hypovolemic shock — vasopressors generally are contraindicated because normal sympathetic response is capable of producing maximal tolerable vasoconstriction. Used, however, when volume replacement and sympathetic response are inadequate

  c. Management specific to septic shock

     i. Administer prescribed antibiotics — the longer they are used, the greater the chance of overgrowth of resistant organisms and drug toxicity

    ii. Administer beta-receptor stimulants, which have positive inotropic effect on heart and vasodilate microcirculation

      (a) Dopamine

      (b) Isoproterenol

   iii. Vasopressors that stimulate alpha-adrenergic receptors are contraindicated

   iv. Administer digoxin and diuretics in presence of elevated CVP and oliguria

    v. Administer steroids during early phase of shock — major beneficial effect is stabilization of lysosomal membrane

  e. Management specific to cardiogenic shock

     i. Administer vasopressors

      (a) Beta-adrenergic stimulators

        (1) Dopamine — has positive inotropic and chronotropic effect at low doses

        (2) Isoproterenol — has positive inotropic effect that increases myocardial oxygen requirement. Also causes coronary artery dilatation, which improves coronary perfusion but also increases myocardial oxygen requirement

      (b) Alpha-adrenergic stimulator

        (1) Norepinephrine (Levophed) — has positive inotropic effect and is peripheral vasoconstrictor (increases afterload)

    ii. Administer vasodilators

      (a) Sodium nitroprusside — reduces arterial pressure (afterload reducer)

      (b) Nitroglycerin IV (afterload reducer)

   iii. Monitor BP continuously via an arterial line, with appropriate drug titration — mandatory during administration of vasoactive drugs

Note: Cardiac and Vascular Surgery (not pathologic conditions) are included at this point to amplify surgical therapy for the pathologic conditions just discussed.

CARDIAC SURGERY (ADULTS)

1. **Pathophysiology**
   a. Indications for surgery
      i. Coronary artery disease resulting in partial or total occlusion of coronary vessels
      ii. Valvular disease resulting in calcification, partial fusion of commissures, or dilatation of valve rings
      iii. Congenital abnormalities
      iv. Septal defects from cardiac disease and congenital defects
      v. Ventricular aneurysm, infarction
   b. Classification of surgical procedures
      i. Myocardial revascularization
      ii. Septal closure
      iii. Valvular repair/replacement
      iv. Correction of congenital malformations
      v. Aneurysmal excision
      vi. Any combination of above

2. **Etiology or precipitating factors**
   a. Acute myocardial infarction
   b. CHF
   c. Rheumatic fever
   d. Syphilis
   e. Congenital abnormalities

3. **Clinical presentation and diagnostic findings:** these differ for each pathologic condition requiring cardiac surgery. See bibliography for specific information

4. **Complications:** resulting from defect or surgical procedure and after pump procedure
   a. Cardiac
      i. Dysrhythmias
      ii. Conduction defects
      iii. Shock
      iv. Tamponade
   b. Respiratory
      i. Atelectasis
      ii. Pneumonitis
      iii. Pneumonia
      iv. Embolism
      v. Acidosis/alkalosis
      vi. Pulmonary edema
      vii. Pneumothorax
   c. Metabolic
      i. Acidosis
      ii. Hypokalemia – after pump procedure
      iii. Hyponatremia/hypernatremia

    d. Vascular
       i. Thrombus formation
      ii. Hemorrhage
     iii. Embolism
     iv. Clotting defects
    e. Cerebral
       i. Psychic disturbances
      ii. Cerebral vascular accident
     iii. Cerebral edema
    f. Renal
       i. Oliguria
      ii. Acute tubular necrosis
    g. Infections
    h. Psychologic

5. **Specific patient care**
    a. Maintenance of patent airway and adequate ventilation (see section on Pulmonary System) — maintain patency of mediastinal chest tubes
    b. Monitoring of physiologic parameters (usually via transducers) — record and report measurements being monitored
       i. Arterial pressure
      ii. PAP
     iii. PCWP
     iv. Left atrial pressure
      v. CVP
    c. Prevention and detection of clotting problems
       i. Monitor laboratory results and report significant changes immediately
      ii. Check dressings and mediastinal chest tube drainage for excessive bleeding
     iii. Administer blood or components as prescribed
     iv. Observe for blood in urine or feces

VASCULAR SURGERY

1. **Pathophysiology**
    a. Sequence
       i. Atheromatous plaques build up in arteries at levels of branching and division — most commonly in carotid, renal, popliteal, aortoiliac, and femoral arteries
      ii. Plaques alter composition of vessel wall
     iii. Bleeding occurs into vessel
     iv. Thrombus forms and either partially or totally occludes vessel
      v. Aneurysms may form along vessel wall owing to weakness of wall pressure on it

    b. Classification of surgical procedures
       i. Endarterectomy or resection and graft replacement (e.g., carotid, aortoiliac)
      ii. Aneurysmal resection with graft replacement of patch graft (e.g., thoracic)

2. **Etiology or precipitating factors:** same as those for arteriosclerosis

3. **Clinical presentation and diagnostic findings:** these differ for each pathologic condition requiring vascular surgery. See bibliography for specific information

4. **Complications**
    a. Clotting of graft with cyanosis and possible loss of extremity
    b. Bleeding from graft site
    c. Acute renal failure
    d. Hypertension
    e. Infection
    f. Cerebral vascular accident

5. **Specific patient care**
    a. Maintenance of patent vessels or grafts
       i. Administer antihypertensive medications as ordered, and record effects
      ii. Check pulses distally to incision site on a scheduled basis, comparing equality of pulses bilaterally
     iii. Observe color and check temperature of extremities, comparing equality bilaterally
     iv. Position patient so that graft and knees are not bent.
      v. Avoid IPPB for patients with carotid endarterectomy for first 48 hours postoperatively
     vi. Wrap extremities with ace bandages or elastic stockings, rewrapping on a regular schedule (at least every 8 hours) and PRN

THE CARDIOVASCULAR SYSTEM

General References

Alspach, J.: Electrical axis: how to recognize deviations on the EKG and interpret them. Am. J. Nurs. *79:* 1976–1983, 1979.

Andreoli, K. G., Fokes, V. H., Zipes, D. P., and Wallace, A. G.: Comprehensive Cardiac Care, 3rd ed. C. V. Mosby Co., St. Louis, 1975.

Baigrie, R.S., and Morgan, C.D.: Hemodynamic monitoring: catheter insertion techniques, complications and troubleshooting. Can. Med. Assoc. J. *121 (7):* 885–892, 1979.

Bain, B.: Pacemakers and the people who need them. Am. J. Nurs. *71:*1582–1585, 1971.

Barstow, R. E.: Nursing care of patients with pacemakers, Cardiovasc. Nurs. *8:* 7–10, 1972.

Behrendt, D. M., and Austin, W. G.: Patient Care in Cardiac Surgery. Little, Brown & Co., Boston, 1972.

Berne, R. M., and Levy, M. N.: Cardiovascular Physiology, 3rd ed. C. V. Mosby Co., St. Louis, 1977.

Brener, E. R.: Surgery for coronary artery disease. Am. J. Nurs. 72:469–473, 1972.

Brenner, A. S., et al.: Transvenous, transmediastinal, and transthoracic ventricular pacing. Circulation 49:407–414, 1974.

Brunner, L. S., and Suddarth, D. S.: The Lippincott Manual of Nursing Practice. J. B. Lippincott Co., Philadelphia, 1980.

Bull, S.: Intra-aortic balloon pump. Crit. Care Update 3:5–21, 1976.

Cameron, A., et al.: Aortocoronary bypass surgery: a seven year follow up. Cardiovasc. Surg. 60:9–13, 1979.

Clark, N. F.: Pump Failure. Nurs. Clin. North Am. 7:529–539, 1972.

Conn, H. L., et al.: Cardiac and Vascular Diseases. Vol. 1: pp. 123–138, 182–287. 301–424, 425–481, 577–589, 686–746. Vol. II: pp. 1463–1472. Lea & Febiger, Philadelphia, 1971.

Constantinides, P.: Cellular pathophysiology of coronary atherosclerosis. In Russek, H. I. (ed.): Cardiovascular Problems. University Park Press, Baltimore, 1976.

Door, K. S.: The intra-aortic balloon pump. Am. J. Nurs. 75:52–55, 1975.

Dorland's Illustrated Medical Dictionary, 25th ed. W. B. Saunders Co., Philadelphia, 1974.

Dubin, D.: Rapid Interpretation of EKG's, 3rd ed. Cover Publishing Co., Tampa, 1976.

Escher, D. J.: Medical aspects of artificial pacing of the heart. Cardiovasc. 8:1–5, 1972.

Foster, S. B.: Pump Failure. Am. J. Nurs. 74:1830–1834, 1974.

Fowler, N. O.: Cardiac Diagnosis and Treatment, 2nd ed. Harper & Row, New York, 1976.

Friedberg, C.: Diseases of the Heart, 3rd ed. W. B. Saunders Co., Philadelphia, 1966.

Ganong, W. F.: Review of Medical Physiology. Lange Medical Publications, Los Altos, CA, 1977.

Germain, C. P.: Helping your patient with an implanted pacemaker. RN 37: 30–35, 1974.

Goldberger, E.: Treatment of Cardiac Emergencies, C. V. Mosby Co., St. Louis, 1974.

Goldman, M. J.: Principles of Clinical Electrocardiology, 9th ed. Lange Medical Publications, Los Altos, CA, 1976.

Green, H. L.: Hazards of electronic equipment in critical care areas: a research approach. Cardiovasc. Nurs. 9:7–12, 1973.

Grossman, W.: Cardiac Catheterization and Angiography. Lea & Febiger, Philadelphia, 1976.

Guyton, A. C.: Textbook of Medical Physiology, 5th ed. W. B. Saunders Co., Philadelphia, 1976, pp. 160–383.

Haapaniemi, J., et al.: Massive hemoptysis secondary to flow-directed thermodilution catheters. Cathet. Cardiovasc. Diagn. 5:151–157, 1979.

Haft, J.: Relationship of stress and microvascular platelet aggregation in the heart. In Russek, H. I. (ed.): Cardiovascular Problems. University Park Press, Baltimore, 1976.

Hathaway, R.: The Swan-Ganz catheter: a review. Nurs. Clin. North Am. 13: 389–407, 1978.

Heart and Lung: All issues have current and pertinent articles on the cardiovascular system.

Hoffman, I.: XYZ is the ABC of EKG. Year Book Medical Publishers, Inc., Chicago, 1972.

Hollander, W.: Antihypertensive drugs in the prevention and treatment of complications of essential hypertension. Cardiovasc. Med. 2:83–96, 1977.

Humphries, J. O'N.: Selection of therapy for angina pectoris: medical versus surgical. Cardiovasc. Med. 2:1097–1105, 1977.

Hurst, J. W., et al.: The Heart, 3rd ed. McGraw-Hill Book Co., New York, 1974.

Kane, P. B., et al.: Artifacts in the measurement of pulmonary wedge pressure. Crit. Care Med. 6:36–38, 1978.

King, E. G.: Influence of mechanical ventilation and pulmonary disease on pulmonary artery pressure monitoring. Can. Med. Assoc. J. 6:121(7):901–904, 1979.

Kintzel, K. C., et al.: Advanced Concepts in Clinical Nursing. J. B. Lippincott Co., Philadelphia, 1972, pp. 68–81, 144–206.

Kory, R. C.: Cardiac catheterization and related procedures. Cardiovasc. Nurs. 4:17–22, 1969.

Krasnow, N., and Stein, R. A.: Evaluating cardiac murmurs and valvular heart disease: use and abuse of echocardiogram. Cardiovasc. Med. 3:797–816, 1978.

Kubler, A.: Monitoring pulmonary artery pressure in critically ill patients. Resuscitation 6:43–46, 1978.

Laragh, J. H.: Hypertension Manual. Yorke Medical Books, New York, 1974.

Lefkowitz, R. J.: Biochemical properties of alpha and beta adrenergic receptors and their relevance to the clinician. Cardiovasc. Med. 2:573–588, 1977.

Lehmann, J., Sr.: Auscultation of heart sounds. Am. J. Nurs. 72:1242–1246, 1972.

Long, M. L., Scheuling, M. A., and Christian, J. L.: Cardiopulmonary bypass. Am. J. Nurs. 74:860–862, 1974.

Marriott, H. L.: Practical Electrocardiography, 6th ed. Williams & Wilkins Co., Baltimore, 1977.

Meltzer, L. E., et al.: Textbook of Coronary Care. Charles Press Publishers, Inc. Philadelphia, 1973.

Merck, Sharp, & Dohme, West Point, PA: The Electrocardio Guide.

Michaelson, S. P., and Wolfson, S.: Role of propranolol in the treatment of angina pectoris. Cardiovasc. Med. 3:331–342, 1978.

Morse, D., et al.: The modern choice and followup of cardiac pacemakers. Cardiol. Dig. 10:19–27, 1975.

Moser, M.: Hypertension: A Practical Approach. Little, Brown & Co., Boston, 1975.

Nichols, W. W., et al.: Complications associated with ballon-tipped, flow directed catheters. Heart Lung 8:503–506, 1979.

Noble, B.: Cardiopulmonary bypass: the pump and oxygenator. Am. J. Nurs. 74:862–868, 1974.

Onesti, G., et al. (eds.): Hypertension: Mechanisms and Management. Grune & Stratton, New York, 1973.

Parsonnet, V.: Followup of implanted pacemakers: an evaluation of methods. Cardiol. Dig. 11:18–19, 23, 26, 1976.

Phillips, R. E., and Feeney, M. K.: The Cardiac Rhythms. W. B. Saunders Co., Philadelphia, 1973, pp. 277–315.

Pinneo, R., et al.: Cardiac monitoring. Nurs. Clin. North Am. 7:457, 1972.

Prior, J. A., and Silberstein, J.S.: Physical Diagnosis, 5th ed. C. V. Mosby Co., St. Louis, 1977.

Roche Laboratories: Cardiac Auscultation Series. New Jersey, 1968.

Rodman, T., Myerson, R. M., Lawrence, T., Gallagher, A. P., and Kaspat, A. J.: The Physiologic and Pharmacologic Basis of Coronary Care Nursing. C. V. Mosby Co., St. Louis, 1971.

Ross, J., Jr.: Effects of afterload of impedance on the heart: afterload reduction in the treatment of cardiac failure. Cardiovasc. Med. 2:1115–1132, 1977.

Rubler, S.: Cardiac manifestations of diabetes mellitus. Cardiovac. Med. 2:823–835, 1977.

Samet, P.: Cardiac Pacing. Grune & Stratton, Inc., New York, 1972.

Schroeder, J. S., and Daily, E. K.: Techniques in Bedside Hemodynamic Monitoring. C. V. Mosby Co., St. Louis, 1976.

Seymour, F., and Escher, D. J. W.: Transtelephone pacemaker monitoring. Ann. Thorac. Surg. 20:326–336, 1975.

Shearer, J. K., and Caldwell, M.: Use of sodium nitroprusside and dopamine hydrochloride in the post operative cardiac patient. Heart Lung 8:302–307, 1979.

Shinn, A. F., Collins, D. N., and Hoopes, E. J.: Drug interactions of common coronary care unit medications. Am. J. Nurs. 74:1442–1446, 1974.

Smith, A. M., Thierer, J. A., and Huang, S. A.: Serum enzymes in myocardial infarction. Am. J. Nurs. *73*:277–279, 1973.

Stemerman, M. B.: Atherosclerosis: the etiologic role of blood elements and cellular changes. Cardiovasc. Med. *3*: 17–36, 1978.

Stephenson, H. E., Jr.: Immediate Care of the Acutely Ill and Injured. C. V. Mosby Co., St. Louis, 1974, pp. 43–60.

Stude, C.: Cardiogenic Shock. Am. J. Nurs. *74*:1636–1640, 1974.

Thorpe, C. J.: A nursing care plan — the adult cardiac surgery patient. Heart Lung *8*:690–698, 1979.

Tilkian, M. S., et al.: Clinical Implications of Laboratory Tests. C. V. Mosby Co., St. Louis, 1979.

Twerski, A. J.: Psychological considerations on the coronary care unit. Cardiovasc. Nurs. *7*:65–68, 1971.

Ungvarski, P. J., Argondizzo, N. T., and Boos, P. K.: CPR: current practice revised. Am. J. Nurs. *75*:236-247, 1975.

Verderber, A.: Cardiopulmonary bypass: postoperative complications. Am. J. Nurs. *74*:868–869, 1974.

Vinsant, M. O., Spence, M. I., and Chappell, D. E.: A Common Sense Approach to Coronary Care: A Program. C. V. Mosby Co., St. Louis, 1972.

Weinstein, J., et al.: Temporary transvenous pacing via the percutaneous femoral vein approach. Am. Heart J. *85*:695–705, 1973.

Wilson, R. F.: Principles and Techniques of Critical Care. Upjohn Co. Kalamazoo, 1977.

Winslow, E. H.: Digitalis. Am. J. Nurs. *74*:1062–1065, 1974.

Winslow, E. H., and Marino, L. B.: Temporary cardiac pacemakers. Am. J. Nurs. *75*:586–591, 1975.

Wintrobe, M., et al.: Harrison's Principles of Internal Medicine, 6th ed. McGraw Hill Book Co., New York, 1970.

Woodburne, R. T.: Essentials of Human Anatomy, 4th ed. Oxford University Press, New York, 1969.

Woods, S. L.: Monitoring pulmonary artery pressures. Am. J. Nurs. *76*:1765, 1976.

Wright, K. E., and McIntosh, H. D.: Artificial pacemakers, indications and management. Circulation *67*:1108-1118, 1973.

Zalis, E. G., and Conover, M. H.: Understanding Electrocardiography: Physiological and Interpretive Concepts. C. V. Mosby Co., St. Louis, 1972.

Pacemaker Therapy

Abernathy, W. S., and Crevey, B. J.: Right bundle branch block during transvenous ventricular pacing. Am. Heart J. *90*:774–776, 1975.

Andreoli, K. G., et al.: Comprehensive Cardiac Care, 4th ed. C. V. Mosby Co., St. Louis, 1979.

Barold, S. S.: Modern concepts of cardiac pacing. Heart Lung *2*:238–252, 1973.

Beller, B. M., et al.: The use of ventricular pacing for suppression of ectopic ventricular activity. Am. J. Cardiol. *25*: 467–473, 1970.

Brenner, A. S., et al.: Transvenous, transmediastinal, and transthoracic ventricle pacing. Circulation *49*:407–414, 1974.

Chardack, W. M.: Cardiac pacemakers and heart block. *In* Sabiston, D. C., and Spencer, F. C. (eds.): Gibbon's Surgery of the Chest, 3rd ed. W. B. Saunders Co., Philadelphia, 1976, pp. 1252–1300.

Dorney, E. R.: The use of cardioversion and pacemakers in the management of arrhythmias. *In* Hurst, J. W., et al. (eds.): The Heart. McGraw-Hill Book Co., New York, 1974, pp. 558–569.

Escher, D. J. W.: Medical aspects of artificial pacing of the heart. Cardiovasc. Nurs. *8*:1–5, 1972.

Escher, D. J. W., and Furman, S.: Emergency treatment of cardiac arrhythmias: emphasis on use of electrical pacing. J.A.M.A. *214*:2028-2034, 1970.

Fruehan, C. T., et al.: Refractory paroxysmal supraventricular tachycardia. Am. Heart J. *87*:229–237, 1974.

Mansour, K. A., et al.: Screw-in electrode eases pacemaker implantation. J.A.M.A. *223*:963, 1973.

Morse, D., et al.: The modern choice and followup of cardiac pacemakers. Cardiol. Dig. *10*:19–27, 1975.

Parsonnet, V.: Followup of implanted pacemakers: an evaluation of methods. Cardiol. Dig. *11*: 18–19, 23, 26, 1976.

Parsonnet, V., et al.: The natural history of pacemaker wires. J. Thorac. Cardiovasc. Surg. *65*:315–322, 1973.

Pennock, R. S., et al.: Long-term monitoring of patients with implanted cardiac pacemakers. Heart Lung *1*:227–232, 1972.

Phillips, R. E., and Feeney, M. K.: The Cardiac Rhythms. W. B. Saunders Co., Philadelphia, 1973, pp. 277–315.

Preston, T. A., and Yates, J. D.: Management of stimulation and sensing problems in temporary cardiac pacing. Heart Lung *2*:533–538, 1973.

Rossel, C. L., and Alyn, I. B.: Living with a permanent cardiac pacemaker. Heart Lung *6*:273–279, 1977.

Samet, P.: Cardiac Pacing. Grune & Stratton, New York, 1972.

Schnitzler, R. N., et al.: Floating catheter for temporary transvenous ventricular pacing. Am. J. Cardiol. *31*:351–354, 1973.

Seymour, F., and Escher, D. J. W.: Transtelephone pacemaker monitoring. Ann. Thorac. Surg. *20*:326–336, 1975.

Spence, M. I., and Lemberg, L.: Cardiac pacemakers. I. Modalities of pacing. Heart Lung *3*:820–827, 1974.

Spence, M. I., and Lemberg, L.: Cardiac pacemakers. II. Indications for pacing. Heart Lung *3*:989–995, 1974.

Spence, M. I., and Lemberg, L.: Cardiac pacemakers. III. Pacemakers in the management of reciprocating tachycardias. Heart Lung *4*:128–133, 1975.

Spence, M. I., and Lemberg, L.: Cardiac pacemakers. IV. Complications of pacing. Heart Lung *4*:286–295, 1975.

Tyers, G. F. O., et al.: The advantages of transthoracic placement of permanent cardiac pacemaker electrodes. J. Thorac. Cardiovasc. Surg. *69*:8–16, 1975.

Tzivoni, D., and Shlomo, S.: Pacemaker implantation based on ambulatory ECG monitoring in patients with cerebral symptoms. Chest *67*:274–278, 1975.

Waugh, R. A., et al.: Immediate and remote prognostic significance of fascicular block during acute myocardial infarction. Circulation *67*:765–775, 1973.

Weinstein, J., et al.: Temporary transvenous pacing via the percutaneous femoral vein approach. Am. Heart J. *85*:695–705, 1973.

Winslow, E. H., and Marino, L. B.: Temporary cardiac pacemakers. Am. J. Nurs. *75*:586–591, 1975.

Wright, K. E., and McIntosh, H. D.: Artificial pacemakers. Indications and management. Circulation *67*:1108–1118, 1973.

Shock

Alpert, J., and Francis, G.: Manual of Coronary Care. Little, Brown, and Co., Boston, 1977.

Anderson, W., and Kissane, J.: Pathology. C. V. Mosby Co., St. Louis, 1977.

Barker, A.: Clinical implications of laboratory test. Crit. Care Q. *II*:1–16, 1979.

Berk, J. L., et al.: Handbook of Critical Care. Little, Brown, and Co., Boston, 1976.

Burrell, Z. L., and Burrell, L. O.: Critical Care. C. V. Mosby Co., St. Louis, 1977.

Ganong, W. F.: Review of Medical Physiology. Lange Medical Publications, Los Altos, 1977.

Groer, M., and Shekleton, M. E.: Basic Pathophysiology: A Conceptual Approach. C. V. Mosby Co., St. Louis, 1979.

Guyton, A. C.: Textbook of Medical Physiology. W. B. Saunders Co., Philadelphia, 1976.

Guyton, A. C.: Basic Human Physiology: Normal Function and Mechanisms of Disease. W. B. Saunders Co., Philadelphia, 1977.

Jennings, B.: Improving your management of DIC. Nursing 79 *IX*:60–67, 1979.

Kapoor, A., and Dang, N.: Reliance on physical signs in acute myocardial infarction and its complications. Heart Lung 7:1020–1024, 1978.

Kelman, G. R.: Physiology: A Clinical Approach. Churchill-Livingstone, New York, 1975.

Luckmann, J., and Sorenson, K.: Medical-Surgical Nursing: A Psychophysiologic Approach. W. B. Saunders Co., Philadelphia, 1980.

Meltzer, L., et al.: Concepts and Practices of Intensive Care for Nurse Specialists. Charles Press Pub., Bowie, 1976.

Nunn, J. F.: Applied Respiratory Physiology. Butterworths, Inc., Boston, 1977.

Palmer, R. F., et al.: Drug therapy: sodium nitro-prusside. N. Engl. J. Med. *292*: 294–297, 1975.

Robbins, S., and Angell, M.: Basic Pathophysiology. W. B. Saunders Co., Philadelphia, 1976.

Shumer, W., and Nyhus, L.: Treatment of Shock: Principles and Practice. Lea and Febiger, Philadelphia, 1974.

Thorn, G. W., et al.: Harrison's Principles of Internal Medicine. McGraw Hill Book Co., New York, 1977.

Tramont, E. C.: Current concepts, the diagnosis and treatment of septic shock. Milit. Med. *144*:153–157, 1979.

THE
NERVOUS
SYSTEM

prepared by
DIANA L. NIKAS, R.N., M.N., CCRN, CNRN

BEHAVIORAL OBJECTIVES

Functional Anatomy

1. Describe the function(s) of the cells that comprise the nervous system.
2. Identify the anatomic divisions of the central nervous system (CNS) and the structures included in each.
3. Describe the functions of each CNS structure.
4. Describe the cerebral circulation, describing the areas of the brain that each major vessel supplies.
5. Diagram the circulation of cerebrospinal fluid (CSF).
6. Describe the function, normal values, and properties of CSF.
7. Describe the function of the major ascending and descending spinal cord tracts.
8. Describe the specific functions of the components of each division of the peripheral nervous system.

Physiology

1. Describe the salient features of cerebral metabolism.
2. Identify the effects of disrupted metabolism on cerebral functioning.
3. Compare and contrast the transmission of impulses between neurons with that at the neuromuscular junction.
4. Identify the major differences between monosynaptic and polysynaptic reflex arcs.

Assessment

1. Describe the assessment of each of the following: general cerebral functions, speech, head and face, cranial nerves, motor and sensory systems.
2. Describe the neurologic examination of a patient with an altered state of consciousness.
3. Describe the rationale for the use of selected neurologic diagnostic studies.

General Patient Care Management

1. Analyze the physiologic basis of the symptoms of increased intracranial pressure.
2. Identify the nursing responsibilities involved in caring for patients who require intracranial pressure monitoring.
3. Describe the methods used to control increased intracranial pressure (ICP).
4. Identify the patient care appropriate to the diagnostic procedure.
5. Identify the pertinent aspects of care for a postoperative craniotomy patient.
6. Describe the fluid and electrolyte problems frequently encountered in the neurologically ill patient.
7. Incorporate the care of other body systems into the management of the neurologically ill patient.

Pathologic Conditions and Management

For each of the following: cerebrovascular accident, intracranial hematomas, closed head injuries, skull fractures, acute spinal cord injury, meningitis, Guillain-Barré syndrome, myasthenia gravis, seizures, status epilepticus, and intracranial aneurysms:

1. Describe the pathogenesis and specific physiologic derangement of each disorder.

2. Describe a systematic approach to the diagnosis of each disorder based on its clinical presentation, the presence of etiologic or precipitating factors, and the diagnostic findings.

3. Describe the treatment modalities used in the management of each disorder.

4. Outline the specific patient care designed to meet the needs of patients with the above disorders.

(THE NERVOUS SYSTEM)

FUNCTIONAL ANATOMY

SCALP

1. **Galea aponeurotica:** freely movable, dense, fibrous tissue that covers skull and absorbs force of external trauma

2. **Fatty and vascular layer:** subcutaneous layer between skin and galea containing blood vessels that contract poorly when injured

3. **Subaponeurotic space:** space beneath galea that contains diploic and emissary veins

SKULL

1. **Bones:** frontal, parietal, temporal, and occipital.

2. **Rigid cavity:** houses and protects brain and has volume of 1400–1500 ml

3. **Composition:** an inner table and an outer table, separated by diploic space (cancellous bone) — this arrangement provides maximal strength with an economy of weight

4. **Fossae:** three depressions in base of skull — anterior, middle, and posterior

MENINGES

1. **Dura mater**
   a. Outermost covering of brain consisting of two layers of tough fibrous tissue
      i. Outer layer is periosteum of bone
      ii. Inner layer forms falx cerebri and tentorium cerebelli
   b. Meningeal arteries and venous sinuses lie within clefts formed by separation of inner and outer layers of dura

2. **Arachnoid mater**
   a. Fine, fibrous, elastic layer that lies between dura mater and pia mater
   b. Subarachnoid space
      i. Lies between arachnoid mater and pia mater
      ii. Separates widely at base of brain to form subarachnoid cisterns

      iii. Contains larger blood vessels of brain

      iv. Contains CSF, which completely surrounds brain and spinal cord and acts as shock absorber

  c. Arachnoid villi — processes of arachnoid mater that serve as channels for absorption of CSF into venous system (pacchionian bodies are large arachnoid villi distributed along superior sagittal sinus)

3. Pia mater
  a. Delicate layer that adheres to surface of brain and spinal cord

  b. Follows sulci and gyri of brain, and carries branches of cerebral arteries with it

  c. Blood vessels of pia form choroid plexus

VERTEBRAL COLUMN

1. Composed of 33 vertebrae
  a. Cervical

      i. 7 vertebrae that support muscles of head and neck

      ii. Smallest of all vertebrae

      iii. Atlas — first cervical vertebra — articulates with occipital bone superiorly and with axis inferiorly

      iv. Axis — second cervical vertebra

        (a) Articulates with atlas and allows for rotation of head

        (b) Odontoid process (dens) — a projection of axis that articulates with atlas

  b. Thoracic

      i. 12 vertebrae

      ii. Articulate with ribs and support muscles of chest

  c. Lumbar

      i. 5 vertebrae that support back muscles

      ii. Largest and strongest of vertebrae

      iii. Site of most herniated intervertebral discs

  d. Sacral — 5 vertebrae fused to form a large triangular bone called the sacrum

  e. Coccygeal — 4 rudimentary vertebrae with rudimentary bodies, articulating facets, and transverse processes

2. Typical vertebra
  a. Body — solid portion of vertebra, lying anteriorly

  b. Arch — made up of

      i. Spinous process

      ii. Transverse processes, one on either side of spinous process

      iii. Lamina that connects spinous process to transverse processes

  c. Articular processes — portions of vertebra that come into contact with vertebrae above and below

    d. Intervertebral foramina — openings through which spinal nerves pass
    e. Spinal foramina — openings through which spinal cord passes
    f. Intervertebral disc
       i. Layer of fibrocartilage found between bodies of adjoining vertebrae
      ii. Acts as shock absorber
     iii. Composed of anulus fibrosus (tough outer layer) and nucleus pulposus (gelatinous inner layer)

CELLS OF NERVOUS SYSTEM

1. **Neurons:** transmitters of nerve impulses (information)
    a. 10 billion in CNS
    b. Functions include
       i. Receiving input from other neurons, primarily via dendrites and cell body
      ii. Summation of inhibitory or excitatory postsynaptic potentials, eventually leading to an action potential (AP)
     iii. Conducting action potentials along axon to axon terminal
     iv. Transferring information by synaptic transmission to other neurons, muscle cells, or gland cells
    c. Components of each are
       i. Cell body (soma or perikaryon) — carries out metabolic functions of cell; contains nucleus and cytoplasmic organelles (i.e., neurofibrils, neurofilaments, microtubules, Nissl material, mitochondria, Golgi apparatus)
      ii. Dendrites — extensions of cell body that conduct impulses toward cell body; dendritic zone — receptive area of neuron. Each neuron may have numerous dendrites
     iii. Axon hillock — thickened area of cell body from which axon originates
     iv. Axon — conducts impulses away from cell body. Usually myelinated. Outside of brain, axons are also covered with neurilemma. Each neuron possesses one axon
      v. Myelin sheath — a white protein-lipid complex that surrounds some axons; laid down by Schwann cells in peripheral nervous system and by oligodendrocytes in CNS
     vi. Nodes of Ranvier — periodic constrictions along axon where it is not covered by myelin. Impulse is conducted from node to node (saltatory conduction) and thus is speeded up
    vii. Synaptic knobs (terminal buttons or axon telodendria) — contain vesicles in which neurotransmitter substances are stored

2. **Neuroglial cells:** these form supporting structure for nervous system
    a. About ten times as numerous as neurons

    b. Four types
        i.   Microglia — no special function known under normal conditions, but they phagocytize tissue debris when nervous tissue is damaged
       ii.   Oligodendroglia — responsible for myelin formation. Seem to have a symbiotic relationship with nerve cells within CNS
     iii.   Astrocytes — function uncertain. Send many end feet to blood vessels, may provide nutrients for neurons, or may be basic structure of blood-brain barrier. Constitute structural and supporting framework for nerve cells and capillaries
     iv.   Ependyma — specialized glial tissue lining ventricles of brain and central canal of spinal cord

DIVISIONS OF THE BRAIN

1. **Cerebrum:** consists of
    a. Telencephalon — two cerebral hemispheres separated by longitudinal fissure; joined by corpus callosum
        i.   Functional localization in cortex
           (a) Frontal lobe — responsible for voluntary motor function (origin of pyramidal motor system) and higher mental functions such as judgment and foresight, affect, and personality
           (b) Temporal lobes — responsible for hearing, speech in dominant hemisphere, vestibular sense, behavior, emotion
           (c) Parietal lobe — responsible for sensory function, sensory association areas, higher level processing of general sensory modalities, e.g., stereognosis
           (d) Occipital lobe — responsible for vision
           (e) Corpus callosum — commissural fibers that transfer learned discriminations, sensory experience, and memory from one cerebral hemisphere to the other
           (f) Cerebral dominance. In right-handed and some left-handed people, left cerebral hemisphere is dominant for verbal, linguistic, arithmetical, calculating, and analytic functions. Nondominant hemisphere is generally thought to be concerned with geometric, spatial, visual, pattern, and musical functions
       ii.   Basal ganglia (also called basal nuclei)
           (a) Includes caudate nucleus, putamen, globus pallidus, claustrum, subthalamic nucleus, and substantia nigra
           (b) Exerts regulating and controlling influences on motor integration; suppresses muscle tone; influences postural reflexes. A major center of the extrapyramidal motor system

b. Diencephalon – consists of
  i.   Thalamus – anatomically forms lateral walls of third
       ventricle. Subdivided into several nuclei on basis of fiber
       connections and phylogenetic connections
       (a) Certain nuclei receive specific sensory input for general
            senses, taste, vision, and hearing, and relay it to cerebral
            cortex
       (b) Other nuclei participate in affective aspects of brain
            function; are functionally related to association areas of
            cortex; or have a role in motor function and ascending
            reticular activating system
  ii. Hypothalamus – forms ventral part of diencephalon, facing
       third ventricle medially. Hypothalamic nuclei interconnect
       with each other and with limbic system, midbrain, thalamus,
       and pituitary gland. Functions include
       (a) Temperature regulation (anterior and posterior
            hypothalamus)
       (b) Regulation of food and water intake (ventromedial and
            lateral regions)
       (c) Behavior – as part of limbic system, it is concerned
            with aggressive and sexual behavior. May be involved
            with sleep along with other CNS structures
       (d) Autonomic responses – parasympathetic responses are
            elicited by stimulation of anterior hypothalamus;
            sympathetic responses may be elicited by stimulation
            of posterior and lateral hypothalamic nuclei
       (e) Control hormonal secretion of pituitary gland (see
            Endocrine section)
            (1) Posterior pituitary (neurohypophysis) – stores
                 and releases antidiuretic hormone (ADH) and
                 oxytocin, which are produced by the supraoptic
                 and paraventricular nuclei, respectively, of
                 hypothalamus
                 (a) Increased serum osmolarity or decreased
                      extracellular fluid volume stimulates ADH
                      synthesis and release. ADH causes increased
                      reabsorption of water from distal tubule and
                      collecting duct of nephron
                 (b) Oxytocin stimulates contraction of uterus
                      under appropriate circumstances, and
                      ejection of milk from lactating breast
            (2) Anterior pituitary (adenohypophysis) – hormonal
                 secretion from anterior pituitary is under control
                 of pituitary releasing/inhibiting factors produced
                 in hypothalamus and transported to anterior
                 pituitary via a pituitary portal system. Hormones
                 thus influenced are
                 (a) Follicle-stimulating hormone (FSH)

      (b)   Luteinizing hormone (LH)
      (c)   Prolactin
      (d)   Thyroid-stimulating hormone (TSH)
      (e)   Adrenocorticotropic hormone (ACTH)
      (f)   Somatotropic hormone (STH) or growth hormone (GH)

  c. Limbic system

     i.   Composed of the cingulate and parahippocampal gyri, hippocampal formation, part of amygdaloid nucleus, hypothalamus, and anterior nucleus of thalamus

     ii. Responsible for affective aspect of emotional behavior as well as visceral responses accompanying them. Also involved in some aspects of memory

2. Brain stem

  a. Midbrain (mesencephalon) – located between pons and diencephalon

     i.   Contains nuclei of third (oculomotor) and fourth (trochlear) cranial nerves

     ii. Contains motor and sensory pathways

     iii. Tectal region (inferior and superior colliculi) is concerned with visual and auditory systems

     iv. Connected to cerebellum via superior cerebellar peduncle

  b. Pons – located between midbrain and medulla; on ventral surface appears to form a bridge connecting right and left cerebellar hemispheres

     i.   Contains nuclei of fifth (trigeminal), sixth (abducens), and seventh (facial) cranial nerves. Some nuclei of eighth cranial nerve (acoustic) are found in pons

     ii. On basal portion of pons, middle cerebellar peduncle provides extensive connections between cerebral cortex and cerebellum, thus ensuring maximal motor efficiency

     iii. Contains motor and sensory pathways

  c. Medulla – located between pons and spinal cord

     i.   Contains nuclei of the eighth (acoustic), ninth (glossopharyngeal), tenth (vagus), eleventh (spinal accessory), and twelfth (hypoglossal) cranial nerves

     ii. Motor and sensory tracts of spinal cord continue into medulla

     iii. Attached to cerebellum via inferior cerebellar peduncle

  d. Reticular formation – diffuse cellular network of brain stem with axons projecting to thalamus, cortex, spinal cord, and cerebellum

     i.   Ascending reticular activating system is essential for arousal from sleep, alert wakefulness, focusing of attention, perceptual association. Destructive lesions of upper pons and midbrain produce coma

     ii. Descending reticular system may inhibit or facilitate activity of motor neurons controlling skeletal musculature

e. Respiratory and cardiovascular centers have been identified within brain stem in experimental animals

3. **Cerebellum:** lies in posterior fossa posterior to brain stem. Separated from cerebrum by tentorium cerebelli
    a. Influences muscle tone in relation to equilibrium, locomotion, and posture, and nonstereotyped movements
    b. Especially important in synchronization of muscle action
    c. Input is from spinal, brain stem, and cerebral centers; output is via descending pathways, e.g., corticospinal, vestibulospinal, and reticulospinal tracts

CEREBRAL BLOOD SUPPLY

1. **Arterial:** supplied by two paired systems of vessels, the internal carotid and vertebral artery systems
    a. Internal carotid system — internal carotid arteries arise from common carotid arteries. Branches of this system include
        i.   Anterior cerebral arteries — supply medial aspect of frontal and parietal lobes and corpus callosum
        ii. Anterior communicating artery — connects right and left anterior cerebral arteries
        iii. Middle cerebral arteries — supply most of lateral surfaces of frontal, temporal, and parietal lobe; largest, most important branch of internal carotid
        iv. Posterior communicating arteries — connect posterior cerebral arteries with internal carotid arteries
    b. Vertebral system — vertebral arteries arise from subclavian arteries and join at lower border of pons to form basilar artery. Branches of this system include
        i.   Posterior inferior cerebellar arteries — branches of vertebral arteries that supply posterior and inferior portion of cerebellum
        ii. Anterior spinal artery — supplies anterior half of spinal cord and medial aspect of brain stem
        iii. Posterior cerebral arteries — branches of basilar artery that supply posterior parietal lobe and inferior portion of temporal and occipital lobes
        iv. Superior cerebellar and anterior inferior cerebellar arteries are branches of basilar artery that supply cerebellum. Branches of these two arteries in turn supply brain stem
    c. Circle of Willis — anastomosis of arteries at base of brain formed by short segment of internal carotid and anterior and posterior cerebral arteries, which are connected by an anterior communicating artery and two posterior communicating arteries
    d. Meningeal arteries — branches of external carotid arteries that supply dura mater
        i.   Anterior meningeal artery — supplies anterior portion of dura, over frontal tips

ii. Middle meningeal artery — supplies most of dura, i.e., posterior portion of frontal area, all of temporal and parietal, and part of occipital

iii. Posterior meningeal artery — supplies occipital area of dura

iv. Pia and arachnoid derive their blood supply from internal carotid and vertebral arteries

2. **Venous:** cerebrum has external veins that lie in subarachnoid space on surfaces of hemispheres, and internal veins that drain the central core of cerebrum and lie beneath corpus callosum

a. Both external and internal venous systems empty into venous sinuses that lie between dural layers

i. Superior sagittal sinus — lies in attached border of falx cerebri. Superior cerebral veins empty into it

ii. Inferior sagittal sinus — lies along free border of falx cerebri. Receives blood from medial aspects of hemispheres

iii. Straight sinus — lies in attachment of falx cerebri to tentorium. Drains system of internal cerebral veins

iv. Transverse sinus — lies in bony groove along fixed edge of tentorium cerebelli. Usually continuous with straight sinus

v. Other sinuses include cavernous, circular, superior petrosal, inferior petrosal, basilar, sphenoparietal and occipital

vi. Emissary veins — connect dural sinuses with veins outside cranial cavity

b. Internal jugular veins — collect blood from dural venous sinuses

VENTRICULAR SYSTEM AND CEREBROSPINAL FLUID (CSF)

1. **Communicating system within brain:** composed of four cavities containing CSF

a. Lateral ventricles — the largest of the ventricles; one lies in each cerebral hemisphere. Anterior horn of lateral ventricles lies in frontal lobe; body extends back through parietal lobe to posterior horn, which extends into occipital lobe. Inferior horn transverses temporal lobe

b. Third ventricle — lies in midline between two lateral ventricles. Lateral walls are formed by the two thalami, which are connected by band of gray matter called massa intermedia

c. Fourth ventricle — lies in posterior fossa, and is continuous with aqueduct of Sylvius superiorly and central canal inferiorly

2. **Function**

a. CSF cushions brain and spinal cord, and decreases their effective weight

b. Displacement of CSF out of cranial cavity (and, to an extent, increased reabsorption of CSF) compensates for changes in intracranial volume/pressure

c. Role in metabolism is uncertain

3. **Properties**
    a. Clear, colorless, odorless
    b. Specific gravity – 1.007
    c. pH – 7.35
    d. Chloride – 120–130 mEq/liter
    e. Sodium – 142–150 mEq/liter
    f. Glucose – 60% of serum glucose level
    g. Protein
        i.   Lumbar – 15–45 mg/dl
        ii. Cisternal – 10–25 mg/dl
        iii. Ventricular – 5–15 mg/dl
    h. Ventricular system and subarachnoid space contain approximately 125–150 ml of CSF; rate of synthesis is estimated to be 500 ml per day. CSF is distributed
        i.   90 ml in lumbar subarachnoid space
        ii. 25 ml in ventricles
        iii. 35 ml in rest of subarachnoid space
    i. Pressure – 80–180 mm water with patient in side-lying position

4. **Formation**
    a. Choroid plexus – tuft of capillaries covered by epithelial cells. Principal source of CSF; found within all ventricles
    b. Majority (95%) of CSF produced in lateral ventricles. Remainder formed in third and fourth ventricles
    c. Small amounts may be produced by blood vessels of brain and meningeal linings
    d. Process of osmosis across walls of choroid plexus believed to be responsible for most CSF produced, although the composition differs from a simple ultrafiltrate of plasma

5. **Circulation**
    a. CSF circulates from lateral ventricles through interventricular foramen (foramina of Monro) to third ventricle, and via aqueduct of Sylvius to fourth ventricle
    b. From fourth ventricle, CSF circulates to cisterns and subarachnoid space via foramina of Luschka and Magendie

6. **Absorption**
    a. Most CSF is absorbed via arachnoid villi which project from subarachnoid space into dural sinuses
    b. Pacchionian bodies are relatively large arachnoid villi located along superior sagittal sinus. They are also responsible for absorption of CSF
    c. Hydrostatic pressure gradient between CSF and venous sinus is one factor that determines CSF absorption

SPINAL CORD

1. **Location:** extends from superior border of atlas (first cervical vertebra) to upper border of second lumbar vertebra
   a. Continuous with medulla oblongata
   b. Conus medullaris — caudal end of spinal cord
   c. Central canal — opening in center of spinal cord which contains CSF and is continuous with fourth ventricle
   d. Filum terminale — non-neural filament that extends from conus medullaris to its attachment to first coccygeal segment; has no known functional significance

2. **Meninges:** continuous with those covering brain
   a. Pia mater — vascular, attached to spinal cord, spinal roots, and filum terminale
   b. Arachnoid mater — extends to second sacral level where it merges with filum terminale
      i. Subarachnoid space — filled with CSF, surrounds spinal cord
      ii. Lumbar cistern — subarachnoid space between conus medullaris and second sacral level
   c. Dura mater — surrounds arachnoid and merges with filum terminale. Ends as blind sac at second sacral vertebra

3. **Gray matter**
   a. H-shaped internal mass of gray substance surrounded by white matter
   b. Anterior gray column (anterior horn) — contains cell bodies of efferent or motor fibers
   c. Lateral column — contains preganglionic fibers of autonomic nervous system. Prominent in upper cervical, thoracic, and midsacral regions
   d. Posterior gray column (posterior horn) — contains cell bodies of afferent or sensory fibers

4. **White matter**
   a. Composed of three longitudinal columns (funiculi) — anterior, lateral, posterior columns
   b. Contains mostly myelinated axons
   c. Funiculi contain tracts (fasciculi) that are functionally distinct (i.e., have same or similar origin, course, and termination), and are classified as
      i. Ascending or sensory tracts — pathways to brain for impulses entering cord via dorsal root of spinal nerves
      ii. Descending or motor tracts — transmit impulses from brain to motor neurons of spinal cord and exit via ventral root of spinal nerves

   iii. Short ascending and descending fibers that begin in one area of spinal cord and terminate in another

 d. Each tract is named to indicate

   i. Column in which it travels

   ii. Location of its cells of origin

   iii. Location of axon termination

 e. Ascending tracts of clinical significance

   i. Fasciculus gracilis and fasciculus cuneatus

    (a) Fibers enter the dorsal root of the spinal nerve and ascend in posterior funiculus

    (b) Convey position and vibratory sense, joint and two-point discrimination

   ii. Lateral spinothalamic tract

    (a) Originates in posterior horn; crosses over via anterior white commissure to contralateral anterolateral funiculus before ascending to thalamus

    (b) Conveys pain and temperature sensation

   iii. Anterior spinothalamic tract

    (a) Originates in posterior horn; crosses over to opposite side of cord via anterior white commissure, and ascends to thalamus in anterolateral funiculus

    (b) Conveys light touch, pressure and sensation

   iv. Dorsal and ventral spinocerebellar tracts

    (a) Originate in posterior horn; ascend to cerebellum via lateral funiculus. Dorsal is uncrossed tract; ventral is crossed tract

    (b) Convey proprioceptive data influencing muscle tone and synergy

   v. Spinotectal tract

    (a) Originates in cells of posterior horn

    (b) Transmits general sensory information to tectum (roof) of midbrain

 f. Descending tracts of clinical significance

   i. Rubrospinal tract

    (a) Originates in red nucleus of midbrain; receives fibers from cerebellum, and descends in lateral funiculus

    (b) Conveys impulses to control muscle tone and synergy

   ii. Ventral and lateral corticospinal tracts

    (a) Originate in cerebral cortical motor areas, and descend in lateral and anterior funiculi

    (b) Carry impulses for voluntary movement

   iii. Tectospinal tract

    (a) Originates in superior colliculus; descends in anterior funiculus

    (b) Mediates optic and auditory reflexes, e.g., reflex head turning in response to visual or auditory stimuli

PERIPHERAL NERVOUS SYSTEM

1. **Spinal nerves**
    a. 31 symmetrically arranged pairs — a sensory (dorsal) root and a motor (ventral) root: 8 cervical pairs, 12 thoracic pairs, 5 lumbar pairs, 5 sacral pairs, 1 coccygeal
    b. Fibers of spinal nerve
        i.   Meningeal branches: carry sensory and vasomotor innervation to spinal meninges
        ii. Motor fibers: originate in anterior gray column of spinal cord, form ventral root of spinal nerve, and pass to skeletal muscles
        iii. Sensory fibers: orginate in spinal ganglia of dorsal roots; peripheral branches distribute to visceral and somatic structures as mediators of sensory impulses to CNS
        iv. Autonomic fibers
             (a) Sympathetic
                  (1) Originate from cells that lie between posterior and anterior gray columns from first thoracic to second lumbar cord segment
                  (2) Innervate viscera, blood vessels, glands, and smooth muscle
             (b) Parasympathetic
                  (1) Arise from neurons of the third, seventh, ninth, and tenth cranial nerves, and sacral cord segments 2 to 4
                  (2) Pass to pelvic and lower abdominal viscera, and smooth muscles and glands of head
    c. Cauda equina — spinal nerves arising from lumbosacral portion of spinal cord contained within lumbar cistern
    d. Dermatomes — area of skin supplied by dorsal roots (sensory innervation) of a single spinal nerve
    e. Plexuses — network of spinal nerve roots
        i.   Cervical
             (a) Composed of anterior rami of C_{1-4}
             (b) Has cutaneous, motor, and phrenic branches
        ii. Brachial
             (a) Composed of anterior rami of C_{5-8} and T_1
             (b) Nerves arising from here include circumflex, musculocutaneous, ulnar, median, and radial
        iii. Lumbar
             (a) Composed of anterior rami of L_{1-4}
             (b) Branches are lateral femoral cutaneous, femoral, and genitofemoral

iv. Sacral
   (a) Composed of anterior rami of $L_{4,5}$ and S_{1-4}
   (b) Branches include sciatic and pudendal

2. **Cranial nerves**
   a. Olfactory (I)
      i. Receptors are located in nasal mucosa. Fibers pass through cribriform plate to olfactory bulb, which, in turn, forms olfactory tract. Peripheral and central connections of this nerve are numerous and complex
      ii. A sensory nerve responsible for smell
   b. Optic (II)
      i. Fibers originate from ganglion cells of retina. At optic chiasm, fibers from nasal half of retina cross; those from temporal half do not. Fibers continue as optic tracts to lateral geniculate bodies, and then to occipital cortex
      ii. A sensory nerve concerned with vision
   c. Oculomotor (III)
      i. Nuclei are located in midbrain. Preganglionic parasympathetic fibers originate in Edinger-Westphal nucleus and accompany other oculomotor fibers into orbit, where they terminate in ciliary ganglion. Postganglionic fibers pass to constrictor pupillae and ciliary muscles of eye to cause pupillary constriction in response to light
      ii. Motor fibers supply extraocular muscles — inferior rectus (depresses and adducts eye), medial rectus (adducts eye), superior rectus (elevates and adducts eye), inferior oblique (elevates and abducts eye), levator palpebrae (raises upper eyelid)
   d. Trochlear (IV)
      i. Originates caudal to oculomotor nucleus in midbrain. Only cranial nerve to originate from dorsal aspect of brain stem
      ii. Supplies superior oblique muscle, which abducts and depresses eye
   e. Trigeminal (V)
      i. Sensory fibers arise from cells in semilunar or gasserian ganglion. Nerve is attached to lateral aspect of pons. Motor fibers leave pons ventromedial to sensory roots
      ii. Three sensory divisions
         (a) Ophthalmic branch provides sensation to forehand, eyes, nose, temples, paranasal sinuses, and part of nasal mucosa
         (b) Maxillary branch provides sensation to upper jaw, teeth, lip, cheeks, hard palate, maxillary sinuses, and nasal mucosa

        (c)   Mandibular branch provides sensation to lower jaw, teeth, lip, buccal mucosa, tongue, and part of external ear, auditory meatus, and meninges

    iii. Motor fibers innervate muscles of mastication

f.   Abducens (VI)

    i.   Emerges at caudal border of pons near midline. Enters orbit with cranial nerves III and IV

    ii. Supplies lateral rectus muscle, which abducts eye

g. Facial (VII)

    i.   Fibers originate in caudal portion of pons at junction of pons and medulla, lateral to cranial nerve VI

    ii. Motor portions of nerve innervate all muscles of facial expression, plus salivary and lacrimal glands. Sensory portion of nerve conveys taste from anterior two-thirds of tongue

h. Acoustic (VIII) (vestibulocochlear nerve)

    i.   Emerges from brain stem at pontomedullary junction; has two divisions

        (a)   Cochlear nerve — fibers from cells in spiral ganglion end either in organ of Corti (peripheral fibers) or ventral and dorsal cochlear nuclei in medulla (central fibers). Fibers from these nuclei proceed to inferior colliculi and then to medial geniculate nuclei of thalamus, before ending on auditory cortex of temporal lobe

        (b)   Vestibular nerve — fibers from cells in vestibular ganglion pass to semicircular canals and maculas and vestibular nuclei in brain stem

    ii. Cochlear nerve is responsible for hearing; vestibular nerve aids in maintaining equilibrium, and coordinating head and eye movements

i.   Glossopharyngeal (IX)

    i.   Sensory fibers arise from cells at back of tongue, pharynx, and palate, and enter medulla behind facial nerve. Motor fibers originate from nucleus in medulla to innervate stylopharyngeus muscle

    ii. Sensory fibers provide sensation to pharynx, soft palate, and posterior third of tongue. They also supply special receptors in carotid body and carotid sinus concerned with reflex control of respiration, blood pressure, and heart rate

    iii. Motor fibers participate with those of vagus nerve in swallowing mechanism

j.   Vagus (X)

    i.   Sensory fibers orginate in cells in ganglia just below jugular foramen, and enter medulla just behind glossopharyngeal nerve. Motor fibers leave medulla and join sensory part of nerve. Parasympathetic fibers are distributed to abdominal and thoracic viscera

    ii. Sensory fibers provide sensation to palate and pharynx (along with IX) and to larynx (X alone)

    iii. Motor fibers innervate palatal muscles, pharyngeal muscles (along with IX), and laryngeal muscles

    iv. Postganglionic parasympathetic fibers inhibit heart rate and adrenal secretion; they stimulate gastrointestinal peristalsis and gastric, hepatic, and pancreatic glandular secretion

k. Spinal accessory (XI)

    i. Motor fibers arise from lateral surface of medulla and upper cervical spinal cord

    ii. Supplies trapezius (elevates shoulders) and sternocleidomastoid muscles (tilts, turns, and thrusts head forward)

l. Hypoglossal (XII)

    i. Motor fibers originate in ventromedial sulcus of medulla

    ii. Innervates muscles of tongue

3. **Autonomic nervous system (ANS)**

  a. Structure

    i. Composed of two neuron chains

    ii. Preganglionic cell bodies are located within lateral gray column of spinal cord or homologous motor nuclei of cranial nerves

    iii. Most preganglionic axons are myelinated, and synapse on cell bodies of postganglionic neurons located outside CNS

    iv. Axons of postganglionic neurons terminate on visceral effectors

  b. Divisions

    i. Sympathetic (thoracolumbar)

      (a) Preganglionic axons leave spinal cord in ventral roots of T_1 to L_2 and pass to

        (1) Paravertebral sympathetic ganglion chain via white rami communicantes, ending on cell bodies of postganglionic neurons

        (2) Collateral ganglia, ending on postganglionic neurons close to viscera

      (b) Postganglionic axons pass to

        (1) Viscera via sympathetic nerves

        (2) Gray rami communicantes, and are distributed to autonomic effectors in areas supplied by these spinal nerves

      (c) Segmental distribution of sympathetic fibers

        (1) T_1 – up sympathetic chain to head

        (2) T_2 – into neck

        (3) T_{3-6} – thorax

        (4) T_{7-11} – abdomen

        (5) $T_{12}, L_{1,2}$ – legs

      (d) Functions
          (1) Generally antagonistic to parasympathetic activity
          (2) Can synapse with many postganglionic fibers
          (3) Sympathetic stimulation dilates pupils and bronchioles, relaxes smooth muscles of GI tract, increases blood pressure by constricting blood vessels, increases heart rate, increases secretion of adrenal medulla
          (4) Brought into widespread activity under emergency conditions, and gives rise to mass responses of body systems

ii.   Parasympathetic (craniosacral)
      (a) Preganglionic cell bodies are in gray matter of brain stem and middle three segments of sacral cord
      (b) Preganglionic fibers end on short postganglionic neurons located on or near visceral structures
      (c) Supplies visceral structures in head via oculomotor, facial, and glossopharyngeal nerves, and those in thorax and upper abdomen via vagus nerves
      (d) Sacral outflow supplies pelvic viscera via pelvic branches of S_{2-4}
      (e) Gives rise to localized reactions, rather than mass action of sympathetic stimulation
      (f) Parasympathetic stimulation constricts pupils; contracts smooth muscle of stomach, intestine, and bladder; slows heart rate; stimulates secretion of most glands

c. Chemical mediation — ANS is divided into cholinergic and adrenergic divisions based on chemical mediator, i.e., neurotransmitter substance liberated
    i.   Cholinergic neurons release acetylcholine, and include
       (a) All preganglionic neurons except sympathetic preganglionic neurons to adrenal medulla
       (b) Parasympathetic postganglionic neurons
       (c) Sympathetic postganglionic neurons to sweat glands and skeletal muscle blood vessels (vasodilator)
    ii. Adrenergic neurons release norepinephrine, and include
       (a) Sympathetic postganglionic endings, except as noted above
       (b) Sympathetic preganglionic neurons to adrenal medulla
       (c) Constrictor fibers of skeletal muscle blood vessels

_____ PHYSIOLOGY _____

BRAIN METABOLISM

1. **Carbohydrate**
    a. Brain has high metabolic energy requirements and utilizes glucose as its principal source of energy in production of ATP necessary in cellular processes
    b. Although glycogen is present in small amounts, glycolysis is not sufficient to maintain adequate production of ATP
    c. Glucose serves as major contributor in building amino acids and fatty acids, and is source of CO_2, which helps regulate pH
    d. Hypoglycemia depresses cerebral metabolism and may lead to convulsions, coma, and death
    e. Hyperglycemia has no known direct effect on nervous system function

2. **Oxygen**
    a. O_2 consumption averages about 49 ml per minute, or about 20% of total body resting O_2 consumption
    b. Constant supply of oxygen is essential to normal brain function; cytotoxic cerebral edema results within seconds of anoxia
    c. Energy for metabolic activities of brain is normally produced by oxidative metabolism of glucose, but rate of glycolysis increases markedly during hypoxia

3. **Cerebral blood flow (CBF)**
    a. CBF varies with changes in cerebral perfusion pressure (difference between mean arterial pressure and intracranial pressure) and diameter of cerebrovascular bed
    b. CBF remains constant owing to autoregulation, an alteration in diameter of resistance vessels (arterioles) that maintains constant blood flow over a range of perfusion pressures
    c. Hypercapnia (Pa_{CO_2} greater than 45 mm Hg), and to a lesser extent hypoxia (Pa_{O_2} must fall below 50 mm Hg), lead to arteriolar dilatation and increased CBF

4. **Blood-brain barrier:** special permeability characteristics of brain capillaries and choroid plexus that act to limit transfer of certain substances into extracellular fluid (ECF) or CSF of brain. Thought to be due to unique membranous ultrastructure with "tight" junctions of endothelial cells of brain
    a. Water, CO_2, O_2, and glucose cross cerebral capillaries with ease. Uptake of other substances, such as ions, is much slower in comparison to uptake by other organs. These substances may be transported by stereospecific transport systems

    b. Functions to maintain homeostatic environment of neurons in CNS by determining level of metabolism and ionic composition of tissue fluids

    c. Of clinical significance in treating and diagnosing disease of CNS — blood-brain barrier is often disrupted in injured tissue leading to increased permeability

    d. Blood-CSF barrier permits selective transport from blood to ventricular system. Substances placed into CSF diffuse readily into interstitial fluid of brain

5. **Vitamins:** several vitamins are essential for normal CNS functioning. Because these vitamins function as co-enzymes for enzyme systems, deficiencies cause neurologic symptoms, probably by reducing activity of one or more enzyme systems

    a. Thiamine (vitamin B_1) — important in formation of compounds of Krebs cycle. Deficiencies cause necrosis of cell bodies of cranial nerve nuclei in brain stem. May also affect areas of diencephalon

    b. Vitamin B_{12} — deficiencies lead to combined subacute degeneration of spinal cord and peripheral nerves, although exact mechanism not clearly established

    c. Pyridoxine — a coenzyme for a variety of enzymatic reactions. Seizures appear to be principal reaction to deficiencies

    d. Nicotinic acid — required for enzymatic synthesis of coenzymes. Deficiencies cause pellagra, characterized by dermatitis and disturbances in mentation

6. **Cerebral neurotransmitters:** chemical mediators of nerve impulse transmission

    a. Acetylocholine (ACh) —found in cholinergic fibers of ANS and nerves to skeletal muscles. May also be involved in drinking behavior

    b. Norepinephrine (NE) — found in adrenergic fibers of ANS. Produced in locus coeruleus nucleus of brain stem. Also implicated in feeding behavior, temperature control, and sleep, particularly paradoxical (REM) sleep

    c. Dopamine (DA) — found in substantia nigra and corpus striatum. Acts as an inhibitory transmitter: e.g., inhibits release of prolactin. Found in decreased amounts in Parkinson's disease. Also associated with eating and drinking behavior, and possibly with sexual behavior

    d. Gamma-aminobutyric acid (GABA) — found at some synaptic junctions and in substantia nigra. Acts as an inhibitory transmitter. Found in decreased amounts in Huntington's chorea

    e. Serotonin (5-HT) — produced in raphe nuclei of brain stem. Also found in high concentrations in hypothalamus, midbrain, and caudate nucleus. Implicated in sleep behavior, particularly slow wave, and possibly in REM sleep

SYNAPTIC TRANSMISSION OF IMPULSES

1. **Nerve impulse:** transient change in physiochemical state of cell membrane

2. **Synapse:** a junction between one neuron and the next that permits unidirectional conduction of an impulse from presynaptic to postsynaptic neurons

3. **Excitatory neurotransmitter:** a substance secreted by presynaptic knobs or vesicles (usually located at axon terminal) that excite a postsynaptic neuron. Released when cell membrane is depolarized by nerve impulse

4. **Depolarization:** causes increase in permeability of cell membrane, resulting in intracellular flow of sodium ions
   a. Increased levels of intracellular Na^+ cause decrease in resting membrane potential (RMP)
   b. RMP is voltage difference across a cell membrane with inside negative to outside
   c. Change in RMP is called the excitatory postsynaptic potential (EPSP)

5. **Action potential:** if transient voltage change that occurs with depolarization is of sufficient magnitude, i.e., threshold level, an action potential occurs. Once initiated, it is self-propagated and spreads like a wave over membrane

6. **Summation:** simultaneous excitation of successively greater numbers of excitatory presynaptic terminals (or rapidly successive discharges from same presynaptic terminal) which cause progressive increase in postsynaptic potential
   a. Facilitation — if summated postsynaptic potential is less than its threshold for excitation, neuron is said to be facilitated but not excited. No action potential occurs
   b. Rate of discharge of neuron is dependent on summated postsynaptic potential in relation to threshold for excitation
      i. Complete refraction (neuron is incapable of producing an action potential) limits the frequency of impulses a cell can generate
      ii. Relative refraction means that neuron can be excited again, but only with summation above threshold

7. **Repolarization**
   a. At peak of action potential, cell membrane again becomes impermeable to Na^+, and RMP returns toward normal
   b. Cell also becomes more permeable to K^+, and RMP returns to normal with aid of $Na^+ - K^+$ pump, which pumps Na^+ out of cell and K^+ into cell

8. Inhibition
    a. Inhibitory postsynaptic potential (IPSP)
        i. Hyperpolarization of cell membrane is caused by secretion of an inhibitory transmitter (perhaps GABA) by presynaptic terminals of inhibitory neurons
        ii. Results in increase in negativity of RMP caused by increased permeability of cells to K^+ and Cl^-
        iii. This causes decreased excitability and inhibition of impulse transmission
    b. Presynaptic inhibition – causes inhibition by reducing amount of neurotransmitter substance released from excitatory presynaptic endings, and thus reducing to subthreshold levels the magnitude of EPSP they produce

NEUROMUSCULAR TRANSMISSION

1. **Physiologic anatomy**
    a. Motor end plate (neuromuscular junction) – a specialized region where motor axon loses its myelin sheath and splays out in a flattened plate close to muscle fiber membrane
    b. Synaptic cleft – space between nerve terminal and muscle fiber membrane
    c. Synaptic gutter – area of muscle fiber membrane characterized by numerous folds, which increase surface area available for neurotransmitter substance to act
    d. Vesicles – structures of nerve terminal that store and release neurotransmitter substance, ACh

2. **Release of ACh:** when action potential reaches neuromuscular junction, vesicles release ACh into synaptic cleft. Amount released depends on magnitude of action potential and presence of calcium. ACh attaches to receptor sites on postjunctional muscle-membrane and increases its permeability to Na^+ and K^+

3. **End-plate potential:** motor-nerve action potential caused by depolarization owing to Na^+ influx and K^+ efflux. Differs from action potential in that it is local, i.e., non-propagated and is graded rather than all-or-nothing

4. **Muscle contraction:** action potentials subsequently are formed on either side of end plate and conducted in both directions along muscle fiber, initiating a series of events that result in muscle contraction

5. **Acetylcholinesterase:** catalyzes hydrolysis of ACh to choline and acetic acid, and thus limits duration of ACh action on end plate and ensures production of only one action potential. ACh is then resynthesized in presence of choline acetylase and coenzyme A acetate

REFLEXES

1. **Monosynaptic reflex arc**
   a. Stimulation of large Group I afferent nerve fibers sends impulses to spinal cord through dorsal roots of spinal nerve
   b. Impulse synapses with anterior motoneurons, sending out an efferent discharge that is confined to axons supplying muscle from which afferent impulse originated

2. **Polysynaptic reflex arc**
   a. Stimulation of smaller afferent axons of muscle nerves causes synapses with interneurons, leading to asynchronous discharge of motoneurons
   b. Polysynaptic discharge is distributed in motor axons supplying ipsilateral flexor muscles and contralateral extensor muscles

3. **Law of reciprocal innervation:**   impulses that excite motoneurons supplying a particular muscle also inhibit motoneurons of antagonistic muscles

_____ ASSESSMENT _____

HISTORY

1. **Medical:** current and significant past medical history of all major systems, including traumatic injury
   a. Childhood diseases
   b. Pertinent family history — diabetes mellitus, hypertension, cardiac or vascular disease

2. **Signs and symptoms:** altered functioning of
   a. Cerebrum — e.g., personality changes, altered states of consciousness, speech disturbances
   b. Cranial nerves — e.g., pupillary changes, loss of gag/swallow reflex, facial asymmetry
   c. Cerebellum — e.g., uncoordinated movements
   d. Motor system — e.g., decreased muscle size, tone, or strength, abnormal movements
   e. Sensory system — e.g., decreased appreciation of light touch, pinprick, positional or vibratory sense
   f. Reflexes — e.g., abnormal increase or decrease of muscle stretch reflexes, presence of abnormal reflexes, e.g., Babinski's sign

3. **Medication history:** current
   a. Tranquilizers, sedatives
   b. Anticoagulants
   c. Aspirin

    d. Anticonvulsants
    e. Alcohol
    f. Drug abuse
    g. Other

PHYSICAL EXAMINATION

1. **General cerebral functions:** mental status examination
   a. General behavior and appearance – dress, grooming, demeanor
   b. Sensorium – level of consciousness or awareness, attention span, memory, insight, orientation, calculation
   c. Intellectural capacity – bright, average, dull, demented, retarded
   d. Emotional state – mood and affective responses
   e. Thought content, judgment – illusions, hallucinations, delusions
   f. Stream of talk – conversation

2. **Speech:** evaluate patient for
   a. Dysphonia – difficulty producing sound
   b. Dysarthria – difficulty with articulation
   c. Dysprosody – difficulty with stress of syllables, inflections, pitch of voice, rhythm
   d. Dysphasia – difficulty in expression or understanding of words

3. **Head and face**
   a. Inspection – check
      i. Facial gestalt, motility, emotional expression
      ii. Eyes for ptosis, width of palpebral fissures
      iii. Contour of nose, mouth, chin, ears
      iv. Hair of scalp, eyebrows, beard
      v. Head for abnormalities in shape and symmetry
   b. Palpate skull for lumps, depression, tenderness if patient palpate carotid and temporal arteries
   c. Percuss sinuses and mastoid processes for tenderness if patient complains of headaches
   d. Auscultate great vessels, eyes, temples, and mastoid processes for bruits

4. **Cranial nerves**
   a. Olfactory (I) – testing each nostril separately, ask patient to identify familiar nonirritating odors such as cloves, coffee, perfume. Loss of sense of small is called anosmia
   b. Optic (II)
      i. Visual acuity may be tested with a Snellen chart, or more grossly with newsprint
      ii. Inspect optic fundi ophthalmoscopically
      iii. Determine visual fields by confrontation. Ask patient to fixate, and bring finger from periphery into patient's field of

vision. By positioning yourself directly in front of patient, you can compare his visual fields with yours. Test each eye individually

c. Oculomotor (III), trochlear (IV), and abducens (VI)
    i. Examine size and shape of pupils, pupillary light reflexes — direct, consensual, and accommodation
        (a) Direct light reflex — constriction of pupil when stimulated by light
        (b) Consensual light reflex — constriction of opposite pupil when light stimulates only one eye
        (c) Accommodation reflex — adaptation of eyes for near vision. Involves pupillary constriction, convergence, and lens thickening
    ii. Check range of ocular movements by having patient's eyes follow your finger through all fields of gaze. Observe for nystagmus at rest and during ocular movements

d. Trigeminal (V)
    i. Sensory
        (a) Test forehead, cheeks, and jaw on each side of face. Use wisp of cotton for light touch, pin for pinprick, test tubes of hot and cold water for temperature
        (b) Corneal reflex — touch cornea with wisp of cotton. Observe for reflex blinking. This tests the afferent arc of V and efferent arc of VII
    ii. Motor — ask patient to clench his teeth and palpate masseter and temporal muscles. Assess ability to chew

e. Facial (VII)
    i. Ask patient to raise his eyebrows, frown, smile, open eyes against resistance. Note strength and symmetry of facial muscles
    ii. Test taste on anterior two-thirds of tongue by applying salt and sugar to both sides of tongue

f. Acoustic (VIII)
    i. Cochlear (hearing)
        (a) Hearing acuity — cover one ear and test the other with watch or whisper. If deficit is suggested, proceed to (b) and (c) below
        (b) Weber's test — place stem of tuning fork on midline vertex of skull. Normally, there is no lateralization of sound. When sound is referred to better hearing ear, decreased hearing is due to impaired function of cochlear nerve
        (c) Rinne's test — place tuning fork on mastoid bone and, when sound is no longer heard, place in front of ear. Since air conduction is normally greater than bone conduction, middle ear disease is suspected in patients in whom this is not true

      ii. Vestibular

        (a) Patient complaints of vertigo, nausea, anxiety; signs of nystagmus, postural deviation, pallor, sweating, hypotension, vomiting all may indicate vestibular nerve dysfunction

        (b) Caloric test – position patient in 30° sitting position to bring semicircular canals to a vertical plane. After checking to ensure an unoccluded ear canal and an intact tympanic membrane, irrigate canal with cold water. Normal response produces nausea, horizontal nystagmus (fast component) and vertigo toward unirrigated side, postural deviation and past-pointing to irrigated side (DeMyer, 1980)

g. Glossopharyngeal (IX) and vagus (X)

    i. Ask patient to open his mouth and say "Ah"; observe for symmetric elevation of palatal arch

    ii. Gag reflex – stroke palatal arch with a tongue blade. Palate should elevate. This tests afferent arc of IX and efferent arc of X

    iii. Speech – appraise articulation. If defect is suspected, having patient say "Kuh, Kuh, Kuh," "La, La, La," and "Mi, Mi, Mi" tests competency of soft palate, tongue, and lips respectively

    iv. Swallowing – if patient is dysarthric or dysphagic, ask him to swallow water. If unable to follow commands, observe how he handles secretions

    v. Carotid sinus reflex – pressure over carotid sinus normally produces slowing of heart rate and fall in BP

    vi. Hoarseness – may indicate damage to vagal nerve. Laryngoscopic examination may be indicated

h. Spinal accessory (XI)

    i. Inspect sternocleidomastoid (SCM) and trapezius muscles for size and symmetry

    ii. Ask patient to turn head and not allow you to force it back toward midline. Palpate opposite SCM muscle

    iii. Ask patient to shrug shoulders upward against resistance of your downward pressure on his shoulders. Note strength and contraction of trapezius muscles

    iv. Ask patient to push head forward against your hand. Assess strength of both SCM muscles

i. Hypoglossal (XII)

    i. Inspect tongue for atrophy while at rest

    ii. Have patient protrude tongue and push it to right and left. Have patient press tongue against inside of cheek while you assess its strength

    iii. Check alignment of tongue when protruded by comparing median raphe with notch between medial incisors

5. **Motor system**
    a. Inspection — check
        i. Size and contour of muscles — note atrophy, hypertrophy, asymmetry, joint malalignments
        ii. Involuntary movements — fasciculations, tics, tremors, or abnormal positions
    b. Palpate muscles if tenderness or spasm is suspected, or if they seem atrophic or hypertrophic
    c. Strength testing
        i. Shoulder girdle — press down on patient's arms after he abducts them to shoulder height. Check for scapular winging
        ii. Upper extremities — test biceps, triceps, wrist dorsiflexion, hand grasps, strength of finger abduction and extension
        iii. Lower extremities — test hip flexors, abductors and adductors, knee flexors and extensors (deep knee bend), foot dorsiflexors, invertors, evertors
        iv. Abdominal muscles — observe for umbilical migration as patient does a sit-up
        v. Note whether weakness follows a distributional pattern such as proximal-distal, right-left, or upper-lower extremity. Grade strength as normal, minimal, moderate, severe weakness, or paralysis
    d. Muscle tone — note whether rigidity, spasticity, or clonus is elicited by passive motion
    e. Muscle stretch reflexes (deep tendon reflexes) — elicited by percussing a tendon with a reflex hammer, which causes stretch of muscle spindles and subsequent contraction of muscle fibers. Compare response on one side with the other.
        i. Jaw reflex (cranial nerve V)
        ii. Biceps reflex (C_{5-6})
        iii. Brachioradialis (C_{5-6})
        iv. Triceps (C_{7-8})
        v. Finger flexion (C_7-T_1)
        vi. Quadriceps (patellar) (L_{2-4})
        vii. Achilles (ankle jerk) (L_5-S_{1-3})
    f. Superficial reflexes — tested by stroking skin with moderately sharp object
        i. Upper abdominal (T_{7-9}) and lower abdominal (T_{11-12}) — umbilicus normally deviates toward quadrant tested; this response is absent with upper motoneuron lesions
        ii. Cremasteric (L_{1-2}) — stroking thigh causes elevation of ipsilateral testicle; this response is absent with upper motoneuron lesions
        iii. Plantar (S_{1-2})
            (a) Stroking lateral aspect of sole of foot causes flexion of great toe

        (b)   An abnormal response, seen with upper motoneuron lesions, is extension of great toe — Babinski sign

        (c)   There are other methods to elicit extensor plantar response, but all indicate same pathology

    iv.   Other abnormal reflexes that indicate diffuse cerebral dysfunction

        (a)   Grasp reflex — patient grasps when something is placed in his hand, and does not release on command

        (b)   Snout reflex — pursing of lips when side of mouth is touched

        (c)   Glabellar reflex — repeated blinking in response to tapping on forehead

6. **Cerebellar function**

    a. Testing adequacy depends on ability of patient to perform volitional movements, i.e., motor system related to area being tested must be intact — e.g., hemiplegic or comatose patient cannot perform cerebellar function tests because of inability to perform voluntary movements, not because of cerebellar dysfunction

    b. Four major clinical signs of dysfunction and tests used to detect them, are

      i.   Dystaxia (intention tremor or incoordination of volitional movements)

        (a)   Inspect patient for swaying when standing with his feet together, first with his eyes open, then closed (Romberg's test)

        (b)   Gait dystaxia — detected by observing patient for a wide-based gait while walking, and assessing ability to perform tandem (heel-to-toe) walking.

        (c)   Arm dystaxia — detected by finger-to-nose test (asking patient to touch his nose, then the examiner's finger), and rapid-alternating movement test (asking patient to slap his thigh first with palm and then with back of his hand in quick alternating movements)

        (d)   Leg dystaxia — detected by heel-to-shin test (patient is asked to run his heel from opposite knee down his shin)

      ii.   Hypotonia (lack of muscle tone)

        (a)   Inspect patient for rag doll postures and gait

        (b)   Feel for muscular resistance when passively moving patient's extremity

        (c)   In patients with cerebellar dysfunction, leg continues to swing like a pendulum after tendon reflex is elicited

        (d)   Postural dysequilibrium may be elicited by rebound tests—wrist-slapping and arm-pulling

    iii. Nystagmus (jerky, oscillatory eye movements)
      (a) Inspect and have patient follow your finger through fields of gaze
      (b) Nystagmus results from lesions of eye, cerebellum, vestibular system, or their brain stem pathways, and have different clinical characteristics. Interpretation of findings thus may require consultation
    iv. Dysarthria (inability to articulate speech sounds) — see test for cranial nerves IX and X

7. **Sensory system**
   a. Tested with patient's eyes closed — one side of body is compared to the other
   b. Determine if the distribution of sensory loss is dermatomal, related to peripheral nerve(s) or central pathway, or nonorganic
   c. Broad dermatomal areas are
       i. C_{3-4} — "cape" area of shoulders
       ii. C_5-T_1 — surface of arms
       iii. T_2 abuts on C_4 over "cape" area of shoulders
       iv. T_4 — nipple line
       v. T_{10} — umbilicus
       vi. L_5 — great toe
       vii. S_1 — small toe
       viii. S_{4-5} — perianal area
   d. Superficial sensory modalities
       i. Light touch — touch hands, trunk, and feet with wisp of cotton
       ii. Pain — using a pin, gently touch hands, trunk, and feet. Ask patient to identify when being touched by sharp and dull ends of pin.
       iii. Temperature — ask patient to discriminate between hot and cold test tubes of water touched to hands, trunk, and feet
   e. Deep sensory modalities
       i. Vibration — apply vibrating tuning fork to bony prominences and soft tissue and ask patient to report when he feels vibration. Apply fork to a toe or finger and place your finger under the digit. Patient should report feeling vibration of tuning fork longer than you can
       ii. Proprioception (position sense) — ask patient to report whether his finger or toe is being moved up or down
   f. Cortical/discriminatory sensation — receptors, sensory pathways, and primary receptive cortical area must be intact for accurate interpretation of following tests. Ability to perform tests accurately thus assesses association portions (parietal lobe) of cortex
       i. Stereognosis — ask patient, without aid of vision, to identify familiar objects placed in his hand

    ii.   Topognosia – ask patient to identify which finger the examiner is touching, and whether it is on right or left side

    iii. Graphognosia – ask patient to identify numbers or letters traced on skin of palm or fingers

    iv. Tactile inattention – determine if patient can identify that he has been touched on both sides of his body simultaneously

EXAMINATION OF THE PATIENT WITH AN ALTERED STATE OF CONSCIOUSNESS

1. **Consciousness:** an awareness of self and environment
   a. Disturbances in consciousness can result from extensive, bilateral cerebral lesions or from injury to diencephalon or pontomesencephalic (pons/midbrain) reticular formation
   b. Unilateral lesions of cerebrum and lesions of medulla or spinal cord do not cause coma

2. **Assessment:** the following all assist in determining location and extent of CNS damage, and provide an index by which progress or deterioration of patient can be measured
   a. Level of consciousness
      i. Determine stimuli necessary to arouse patient. Does he respond when his name is called? Does he have to be touched or shaken? Are painful stimuli necessary? Does he have no response at all?
      ii. Describe patient's behavior once aroused. Is he oriented or confused to person, place, time, environment? Is he restless, irritable, combative? Does he follow verbal commands?
      iii. Describe patient's verbal response. Is his speech clear, garbled, or confused? Does he use inappropriate words? Does he make incomprehensible sounds? Does he have any verbal response?
      iv. Determine patient's best motor response. Does he obey verbal commands? Does he localize or withdraw from noxious stimuli? Does he exhibit abnormal flexor or extensor posturing? Is there no response at all to stimuli? i.e., is he flaccid?
   b. Pupillary responses
      i. Describe size of pupils either in number of millimeters or in comparison to one another (e.g., right larger or smaller than left)
      ii. Describe direct light reflex of pupil as brisk, sluggish, or nonreactive (i.e., fixed)

      iii. Consensual light reflex — when one eye is stimulated with light, the other should respond. This tests integrity of optic (afferent limb) and oculomotor (efferent limb) of pupillary light reflex

c. Motor ability

      i.   If patient is able to follow verbal commands, assess strength and tone of extremities as described previously

      ii. If patient is unable to follow verbal commands, assess motor ability by observing which extremities he moves spontaneously or in response to noxious stimuli

      iii. Hemiparesis or hemiplegia may also be detected by lifting both arms off bed and releasing them simultaneously. Hemiparetic side will fall faster and more limply than normal side. Repeat maneuver with legs

      iv. Paratonia is increased muscular resistance of any part of body to passive movement. It usually accompanies diffuse forebrain dysfunction, but when seen unilaterally is associated with lesions of frontal lobe and increased ICP

      v.   Flexor posturing (decorticate rigidity) consists of flexion and adduction of upper extremity with extension, internal rotation, and plantar flexion in lower extremity. Associated with lesions of internal capsule (a compact band of afferent and efferent fibers near upper part of brain stem) or cerebral hemispheres

      vi. Extensor posturing (decerebrate rigidity) is characterized by extension, adduction, and hyperpronation of upper extremities and extension and plantar flexion of lower extremities. Results from lesions at the pontomesencephelic level

      vii. Unilateral, bilateral, or mixed responses may occur

d. Cranial nerves

      i.   Optic (II) is indirectly tested by pupillary light reflexes, since II is afferent limb of this arc. Oculomotor (III) is efferent limb of arc

      ii. Trigeminal (V) is tested by touching corneal with a wisp of cotton and observing for blink reflex. Efferent limb of corneal reflex is facial nerve (VII). An alternate method for testing V–VII arc is to apply pressure to supraorbital ridge and observe facial grimacing, which will be decreased or absent on same side as hemiplegia

      iii. Vestibular portion of cranial nerve VIII and its connections with nerves III and VI provides information regarding integrity of brain stem. Can be tested by

          (a) Caloric irrigation test (also called oculovestibular reflex) — see previous description. A normal coma response, i.e., one showing the connections between VIII and III and VI to be intact, consists of deviation and nystagmus toward irrigated ear

(b)   Doll's eye test (oculocephalic reflex). In a comatose patient who has intact connections between cranial nerves VIII and III and VI, brisk turning of patient's head will cause his eyes to move in opposite direction. CAUTION: before doing this maneuver, be sure that patient does not have a cervical spine injury

iv.   Cranial nerves IX and X are tested by the gag reflex

e.   Vital signs

  i.   Temperature

(a)   Hyperthermia increases metabolic needs of an already compromised CNS

(b)   Hypothermia, if extreme, can lead to cardiac dysrhythmias, and has not been consistently proved to be of therapeutic value in preventing or treating secondary effects of cerebral insult

  ii.   Respirations

(a)   Hypercapnia or hypoxia lead to vasodilatation, increased CBF, and, in patient with compromised intracranial dynamics, increased ICP

(b)   Respiratory dysrhythmias often correlate with lesions at various levels, although effects are variable and influenced by other factors

(1)   Posthyperventilation apnea – patient with metabolic or structural forebrain disease will have a period of apnea after taking deep breaths sufficient to lower $PaCO_2$ below normal. This response is abolished in sleep or obtundation

(2)   Cheyne-Stokes respiration – a pattern that alternately crescendos to hyperpnea and decrescendos to apnea. Associated with bilateral lesions of cerebral hemispheres, basal ganglia, or metabolic lesions.

(3)   Central neurogenic hyperventilation – sustained, regular, rapid, and deep hyperpnea. Seen in patients with lesions of midbrain, often secondary to transtentorial herniation, and midpontine lesions

(4)   Apneustic breathing – an end-inspiratory pause, often followed with expiratory pauses. Indicates injury to respiratory mechanisms at mid- or caudal-pontine level

(5)   Ataxic breathing (Biot's) – completely irregular pattern with both deep and shallow breaths occurring randomly. Represents disruption of medullary inspiratory and expiratory neurons, and thus occurs with lesions of posterior fossa

(6)   Cluster breathing – disorganized sequence of breaths with irregular periods of apnea. Seen in patients with lesions of caudal pons or rostral medulla

iii. Pulse and blood pressure
    (a) Although of vital importance in overall assessment and care of critically ill patients, pulse and BP are notoriously unreliable parameters in CNS disease. When changes do occur, they are seen late in course of increasing ICP, and are thus of little clinical use
    (b) Cushing's reflex is a rise in systolic pressure greater than rise in diastolic pressure. This leads to widening pulse pressure, and occasionally to reflex slowing of pulse

DIAGNOSTIC STUDIES

1. **Laboratory**
  a. Blood
    i. CBC, differential, sedimentation rate
    ii. Chemistries
    iii. Electrolytes
    iv. Clotting profile
    v. Arterial blood gases
    vi. Toxicology – alcohol, drugs
  b. Urinalysis
  c. CSF
    i. Gross description of appearance
    ii. Cell count
    iii. Protein – identify site specimen drawn
    iv. Wassermann test
    v. Culture and sensitivity
    vi. Glucose – compare with serum levels
    vii. Specific gravity
    viii. pH

2. **Radiologic**
  a. Skull series – used to diagnose skull fractures and illustrate status of cranial sutures. May also aid in diagnosis of other abnormalities such as tumors, degenerative processes, and increased ICP by presence of calcifications, erosion or exostosis of bone
  b. Spine series – used to diagnose fractures, dislocations, or degenerative processes of vertebrae
  c. Computerized axial tomography (CT, CAT, or CTT scan)
    i. Principle: a computerized composite of 180 views of selected sections of brain tissue, printed out as a digital picture. Digital composite may also be converted to a black-and-white picture and displayed on an oscilliscope or Polaroid picture. Scan may be repeated after patient has received an IV injection of a contrast solution that enhances some abnormal tissue
    ii. Clinical use: invaluable in diagnosis of almost all intracranial pathology, and of particular value in head trauma, tumors, hydrocephalus, cerebral edema, and infectious

processes. Of more limited value at present in diagnosing vascular lesions such as aneurysms or arteriovenous malformations

d. Cerebral angiography

   i. Principle: a contrast material, e.g., Conray, is injected into one or more arteries in order to obtain radiographic visualization of intracranial or extracranial circulation

   ii. Clinical use: particularly useful in diagnosis of vascular abnormalities such as aneurysms, arteriovenous malformations, vasospasm, or vascular tumors. Also aids diagnosis of other intracranial abnormalities that cause stretching/displacement of vessels or change in their diameter

e. Air encephalography

   i. Principle: injection of air into ventricles and subarachnoid space. Air is radiolucent as compared to soft tissue or bone, and thus appears dark on x-ray film. CSF is replaced with air injected either directly into ventricles through burr-hole made in skull (ventriculogram), or into subarachnoid space via lumbar or cisternal puncture (pneumoencephalogram)

   ii. Clinical use: diagnosis of lesions in and near ventricles or subarachnoid spaces

f. Radioisotope brain scanning

   i. Principle: a radioactive substance is introduced into blood, and brain is scanned to determine areas that have accumulated the substance. In some disorders, radioisotope accumulates in abnormal areas of brain in quantities sufficient to allow detection, probably owing to breakdown in bloodbrain barrier or increased vascularity of lesion

   ii. Clinical use: in screening patients for presence of brain tumors, and evaluating cerebrovascular disease and some infectious processes. Often used in conjunction with other diagnostic procedures

g. Myelography

   i. Principle: x-ray examination of spinal canal after injection of a radiopaque substance into subarachnoid space, usually in lumbar area

   ii. Clinical use: diagnosis of intervertebral disc disease, spinal cord tumors, and other diseases of or injuries to spinal cord

3. **Special**

   a. Electroencephalography (EEG)

      i. Principle: recording of electrical activity of brain by electrodes attached to scalp. Voltage fluctuations have rhythmicity depending on area of cerebrum being recorded, and age and level of alertness of patient

      ii.   Clinical use: most helpful in diagnosing epilepsy, space-occupying lesions, and (on occasion) coma. Used in many institutions to aid diagnosis of cerebral death

  b. Echoencephalography (Echo)

      i.   Principle: an ultrasonographic beam is reflected off surfaces of skull and midline structures of brain (i.e., third ventricle, calcified pineal gland). A transducer converts ultrasonic beam into an electrical impulse, which is displayed on an oscilloscope and in Polaroid pictures

      ii.   Clinical use: primarily to diagnose a shift of midline structures of cerebrum (shift of more than 2 mm is considered abnormal), particularly in patients with head trauma or coma of unknown etiology

  c. Electromyography (EMG)

      i.   Principle: needle electrodes are used to record electrical potentials from contracting muscle fibers. These are displayed on an oscilloscope

      ii.   Clinical use: to aid diagnosis of lower motoneuron disease or muscle disorders due to denervation or myopathy

  d. Nerve conduction velocity

      i.   Principle: a large motor nerve trunk is stimulated with an electrode and a response is recorded in one of its muscles. Velocity of impulse conduction can be calculated from distance and time elapsed between stimulus and response

      ii.   Clinical use: diagnosis of peripheral neuropathies and nerve compression. In myasthenia gravis, repetitive stimulation gives objective evidence of decreasing muscular strength

  e. Lumbar puncture, cisternal puncture

      i.   Principle: a needle is placed into subarachnoid space, usually at L_{4-5} interspace (or cisterna magna with a cisternal puncture)

      ii.   Clinical use: to obtain CSF for laboratory examination, measure/reduce CSF pressure, as a route for administration of medications, or in preparation for other diagnostic studies (e.g., myelography)

GENERAL PATIENT CARE MANAGEMENT

RECOGNIZE CLINICAL SIGNS OF INCREASED INTRACRANIAL PRESSURE (ICP)

1. **Definitive signs:** decreases in level of consciousness, motor ability, cranial nerve function (particularly oculomotor function), or changes in vital signs from one assessment to another indicate a change in patient's neurologic status, and possibly increasing ICP. Papilledema (edema of optic disc) is a positive sign of increased ICP, but is not seen in acute intracranial hypertension

2. **Other signs and symptoms:** those that indicate a change in patient's neurologic status or increased ICP must be evaluated in light of history and clinical presentation
   a. Increasing headache
   b. Blurred vision, diplopia, photophobia
   c. Seizure activity — may be due to head trauma, anoxia, tumors, or electrolyte disorders in acutely ill patient without history of seizure disorders
   d. Vomiting — lesions that produce vomiting are those that involve vestibular nuclei, impinge on floor of fourth ventricle, or (less often) produce brain stem compression secondary to increased ICP
   e. Nuchal rigidity — inability to flex patient's head indicates irritation of meninges, most commonly due to meningitis or subarachnoid hemorrhage

3. **Pathophysiology**
   a. Nondistensible intracranial cavity is filled to capacity with essentially noncompressible contents — CSF, intravascular blood, brain tissue water (interstitial fluid)
   b. Monro-Kellie hypothesis states that, if volume of one of constituents of intracranial cavity increases, a reciprocal decrease in volume of one or both of the others must occur, or an overall increase in ICP will result
   c. Principal spatial buffers that resist increases in ICP are displacement of CSF from cranial vault, and compression of low pressure venous system. Increased CSF absorption may also contribute to spatial compensation
      i. Volume of fluid that can be displaced is finite, and increase in ICP will ultimately occur if volume of intracranial mass exceeds volume of fluid displaced
      ii. Relationship between intracranial volume and pressure has been plotted and an elastance curve (inverse of compliance) constructed. See Figure 3–1. A flat portion of curve in which little change in pressure occurs with increases in volume (low elastance or high compliance), and a steep portion of curve in which large pressure changes occur with small increases in volume (high elastance or decreased compliance), have been described. Patient's response to changes in ICP therefore depend, in part, on where he is on volume/ pressure curve. Rate of volume change also influences magnitude of ICP change
   d. CBF varies with changes in cerebral perfusion pressure (CPP) and diameter of cerebrovascular bed

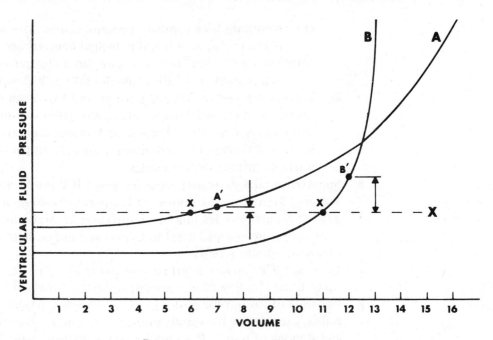

Figure 3-1. Two theoretical volume/pressure curves in two different patients. At the same resting pressure (*X*) addition of 1 unit produces a greater pressure increase on the *B* curve than on the *A* curve (B' > A'). (From Mauss, N.K., and Mitchell, P.H.: Increased intracranial pressure: an update. Heart Lung 5: 919, 1976.)

   i.   CPP is difference between mean systemic arterial pressure (SAP) and the mean intracranial pressure (ICP). Therefore, changes in either SAP or ICP will affect CPP

$$CPP = SAP - ICP$$

   ii.   CPP may change, but CBF is not affected over a wide range of arterial pressures owing to autoregulation, an alteration in diameter of resistance vessels that maintains constant blood flow over a range of perfusion pressures

  iii.   Increased ICP can increase CBF indirectly by producing cortical vascular dilatation, and appears to be principal mechanism responsible for maintenance of CBF in face of rising ICP

  iv.   When ICP approaches SAP, CPP decreases to point where autoregulation is impaired and CBF decreases

     (a)   When autoregulation is impaired, arterioles passively dilate with increases in arterial blood pressure, causing increase in CBF; however, pressure in venous system (capacitance system) also rises, cerebral blood volume increases, and ICP rises further

       (b)   Resultant high capillary pressure causes oozing of plasma from vessels and petechial hemorrhage

       (c)   Eventually, perfusion pressure can no longer be maintained, and CBF gradually falls as ICP increases

   v.   Increases in carbon dioxide tension, and to a lesser extent decreases in oxygen tension, also cause arteriolar dilatation and increases in CBF. Hypoxia and hypercapnia thus can lead to intracranial hypertension, especially in patients with unstable intracranial dynamics

e.   Supratentorial lesions that cause increased ICP can cause tentorial herniation (i.e., uncus of temporal lobe herniates over edge of tentorium), leading to compression or stretching of oculomotor nerve (ipsilateral to lesion) and impairment of its parasympathetic activity

f.   Increased ICP can also exert pressure on motor and sensory nerve tracts, leading to impairment or loss of function

g.   Ischemia of vasomotor center in brain stem may trigger Cushing's reflex, causing rise in systolic pressure, widening pulse pressure, and slowing of pulse. Respiratory rate or pattern may also change

4. **Etiology or precipitating factors**

a.   Any intracranial condition, e.g., hematomas, tumors, hydrocephalus, that leads to alteration in total intracranial volume beyond compensatory capacity will cause intracranial hypertension

b.   Extracerebral conditions, usually metabolic, can cause alterations in CNS functioning and may lead to changes in intracranial dynamics. This is often result of cerebral edema

   i.   Vasogenic cerebral edema is characterized by increased permeability of brain capillary endothelial cells. Commonest type of cerebral edema — can be caused by tumors, abscesses, hemorrhage, infarction or contusion of brain

   ii.   Cytotoxic cerebral edema causes all cellular elements of brain (neurons, glia, endothelial cells) to undergo swelling, with concomitant reduction of the ECF space. Occurs within seconds of hypoxia. Also with acute hypo-osmolality (i.e., water intoxication)

MONITOR AND CONTROL INCREASED ICP

1. **Intracerebral pressure:** because brain is deformed and displaced easily by mass lesions (i.e., is plastic), it is felt that persistent differences in pressure do not develop within its substance

2. **CSF pressure:** CSF is contained within a closed system, and since pressure is transmitted equally in all directions in fluid, CSF is most accessible indicator of overall ICP. Choroid plexus pulsations

are transmitted to CSF throughout ventricular system and subarachnoid space, and produce a wave form with same characteristics as an arterial wave form, although of lower amplitude. Variations coincident with respiratory cycle also occur

3. **Indications for ICP monitoring:** patients who benefit are those with head trauma (particularly closed head trauma), ruptured intracerebral aneurysms, known or suspected hydrocephalus, posterior fossa lesions, Reye's syndrome, or tumors

4. **Techniques:** the three most common are
   a. Intraventricular. Cannula is inserted into anterior horn of lateral ventricle (sometimes posterior horn), usually in nondominant hemisphere, via a twist drill hole through skull. Cannula is connected via a stopcock and/or fluid-filled pressure tubing to a transducer that is positioned at level of foramen of Monro (middle of ear may be used as reference)
      i. Advantages — ability to measure CSF pressure directly, drain CSF therapeutically, and withdraw CSF for analysis
      ii. Disadvantages — risks of infection, inadvertent loss of CSF (usually due to disconnection), and difficulty in placement of cannula if ventricles are small or displaced
   b. Subarachnoid screw. Hollow screw is placed into subarachnoid space through a twist drill hole in skull. Fluid-filled tubing connects screw to transducer
      i. Advantages — ability to measure CSF pressure directly, and also to remove CSF for examination or control of increased ICP, although occlusion of screw occurs frequently
      ii. Disadvantages — risks of infection and inadvertent loss of CSF
   c. Epidural. Device (e.g., fiberoptic transducer or balloon radio transmitter) is placed between skull and dura, with pressure-sensitive membrane toward dura. Transducer continually balances air pressure in transducer with pressure being applied to dura; it may also be placed subdurally
      i. Advantage — ability to monitor ICP while leaving dura intact. An intact dura should protect patient from intracerebral infection although wound, bone or epidural infections may still occur
      ii. Disadvantages — epidural pressure is higher than intraventricular pressure and may not always reflect true ICP. Once in place, fiberoptic transducer cannot be zero-balanced or calibrated, further contributing to possibility of inaccurate readings. Progress is being made in eliminating these problems. CSF sampling and drainage also are not possible with this system

5. **Nursing responsibilities:** these vary with monitoring technique used, but for intraventricular and subarachnoid screw techniques include
   a. Ensuring a closed system to prevent infection or inadvertent loss of CSF. All openings on stopcocks must be covered to prevent contamination, and Luer-Lok connections should be used whenever possible. Because system must be opened to obtain CSF specimens and to zero balance, great care must be taken to prevent contamination
   b. Maintaining transducer at level of foramen of Monro
      i. Zero balance and calibrate whenever bed or patient's position is changed, every 4 hours, or if erroneous readings are suspected
      ii. Keep transducer and tubing free of air bubbles to avoid dampening of wave form and inaccurate readings
   c. Reporting and recording changes in wave form, elevations in pressure, and therapy instituted
      i. Normal ventricular pressure is under 15 mm Hg — pressures above 20 mm Hg are regarded as elevated
      ii. Transient increases may occur with suctioning, coughing, Valsalva maneuvers, inappropriate positioning, or other nursing interventions
      iii. Three types of ICP wave forms have been described
         (a) A waves (also called plateau or Lundenberg waves)
            (1) Elevations of intracranial pressure between 50 and 100 mm Hg, lasting 5–20 minutes
            (2) May or may not be associated with clinical manifestations of increased ICP
            (3) Associated with advanced stages of intracranial hypertension
         (b) B and C waves are variations in pressure that correspond to respiratory and arterial pressure changes, respectively, but generally are not considered clinically significant

6. **Methods used to control increased ICP**
   a. Facilitate venous return
      i. Elevate head of bed 15–30°
      ii. Prevent hyperextension, flexion, or rotation of head
      iii. If patient has a tracheotomy, make sure ties are not too tight
   b. Limit suctioning to 15 seconds to minimize blood gas alterations. Some patients may also require hyperventilation/hyperoxygenation before/after suctioning
   c. Assist patient when moving in bed to avoid Valsalva maneuvers
   d. Therapy may be aimed at reducing volume of 1 of the 3 components of ICP: cerebral blood volume, CSF volume, and brain tissue water

     i.   Hyperventilation (usually to $PaCO_2$ of 25–30 mm Hg) causes vasoconstriction, and thus reduces cerebral blood volume

     ii.   Diuretics, including mannitol, urea, glycerol (osmotic diuretics) furosemide, or ethacrinic acid, aim at reduction of brain tissue water

     iii.   CSF may be drained in patients with enlarged ventricles via intraventricular cannulas or subarachnoid screws

  e. High potency glucocorticoids — e.g., dexamethasone or methylprednisolone — may help control cerebral edema from some causes, although mechanism is unclear

  f. Barbiturate coma (administration of pentobarbital or phenobarbital in doses and at intervals sufficient to produce complete unresponsiveness) has been employed alone and in conjunction with other methods. Barbiturates reduce metabolic activity and may have direct effect on ICP; exact mechanism not known. Patient must be intubated and on a ventilator; arterial blood pressure must be monitored continuously

  g. Hypothermia causes decrease in metabolic requirements. It has been used alone and in conjunction with other methods to control ICP

  h. Paralyzing agents — e.g., pancuronium or curare — also decrease body's metabolic requirements, and may be used alone or in conjunction with other therapy

PROVIDE PRE- AND POSTPROCEDURE CARE APPROPRIATE TO THE DIAGNOSTIC PROCEDURE

1. **Patient education:** all procedures and equipment should be explained to patient, and postprocedure assessment compared to preprocedure condition

2. **CT scan:** no specific preprocedure care is necessary. If contrast enhancement is done, quantity and specific gravity of urine will be increased for approximately 8 hours postscan

3. **Cerebral angiography:** patient may be premedicated and a consent should be signed. Postprocedure, check injection site for bleeding or hematoma formation. Pressure dressings/ice may be applied. A major complication is cerebrovascular accident (CVA) caused by dislodging of an atherosclerotic plaque from wall of artery or clot that has formed at end of catheter or needle

4. **Pneumoencephalography:** patient should be NPO prior to procedure and written consent should be obtained. Premedication may be necessary. If complications occur, they usually do so during proce-

dure — may include hypotension, cardiopulmonary arrest, brain herniation. Patient is usually on bed rest for 24–48 hours. Medication may be needed to relieve postprocedure headache. Nausea and vomiting may occur

5. **Radioisotope brain scanning:** radioisotope is injected at varying time intervals prior to scanning. No specific postprocedure care or complications

6. **Myelography:** written consent should be obtained. Patient may complain of headache postprocedure, and usually is required to lie flat for 4–24 hours

7. **EEG:** preprocedure care varies depending on institution and type of EEG (e.g., sleep EEG). Postprocedure care includes washing conductive paste from hair. No risks in this procedure

8. **Echoencephalography:** no pre- or postprocedure care and no risks involved

9. **Electromyography and nerve conduction velocity studies:** no risk to patient, although needle electrodes are uncomfortable

10. **Lumbar puncture:** written consent may be obtained. Contraindicated in patients with increased ICP as it may lead to herniation of brain stem. Infection, headache, or backache may occur as complications. Patient is usually required to lay flat for a few hours postprocedure

11. **Cisternal puncture:** written consent may be obtained. Injury to brain stem could occur and lead to changes in vital signs, shock. Hemorrhage or infection may also occur. Patient is usually kept flat for 4–6 hours.

PROVIDE POSTOPERATIVE CRANIOTOMY CARE: Craniotomy is done for intracranial lesions or pathologic conditions including hematomas, abscesses, tumors, aneurysms, arteriovenous malformations (AVMs), hydrocephalus. Although postoperative care includes aspects specific to the condition, there are general principles that apply to most patients.

1. **Assess neurologic status**
   a. Compare with preoperative status
   b. Use as baseline for determining progress or deterioration

2. **Monitor cardiovascular and renal status:** preoperative and intraoperative diuretic therapy and limited fluids postoperatively may lead to hypovolemia, hypotension, and inadequate renal perfusion. Intra-arterial, CVP or pulmonary artery catheters may be necessary to monitor fluid status accurately

3. **Alleviate headache:** avoid morphine as it may mask neurologic signs

4. **Use glucocorticoids:** appropriate for most patients with above disorders for prevention/treatment of increased ICP
   a. Antacids or cimetidine are recommended to diminish gastric irritation that may accompany steroid therapy
   b. Hyperglycemia may occur, particularly in patients receiving large doses. Frequent testing of urine or serum glucose levels should be done. Rarely necessary to treat; dissipates when dosage of steroids is decreased
   c. Dosage of steroids is tapered when discontinuing therapy to avoid iatrogenic adrenal insufficiency

5. **Elevate head of bed:** 15–30°: unless otherwise ordered (exceptions might include those with posterior fossa surgery)

6. **Check head dressings frequently for signs of drainage:** clear drainage indicates CSF leak and must be reported promptly

7. **Check subgaleal or subdural wound drains (e.g., Hemovac or Jackson-Pratt drains):** often in place for first 24–48 hours after surgery — note amount and kind of drainage

8. **Provide care appropriate to pre-existing medical problems**

9. **Recognize potential complications**
   a. Increased ICP may result from rebleed, cerebral edema, or hydrocephalus (see sections on prevention of increased ICP and monitoring and control of ICP)
   b. Seizures may be precipitated postoperatively by hypoxia, cerebral ischemia, hypoglycemia, fluid or electrolyte imbalances, or hyperthermia. Of particular concern in early postoperative period owing to possibility of elevated ICP and increased metabolic demand placed on brain (for further details see sections on seizures and status epilepticus)
   c. Fever causes an increase in rate of metabolism and, therefore, oxygen consumption
   d. Fibrinolysis and disseminated intravascular coagulation (DIC) may occur with extensive cerebral injury and may be related to release of large amounts of thromboplastin from injured brain tissue. Best treatment is elimination of causative factor. Replacement of lost blood components is often necessary
   e. Cushing's ulcers, one type of stress ulcer, are associated with severe brain lesions and seem to be characterized by high gastric acid output, possibly mediated by vagal stimulation. Both antacids and cimetidine have been recommended in prevention of gastric ulcerations

    f.   Electrolyte disorders, e.g., hypernatremia, hyperglycemia, or acute hyponatremia may occur as result of injury, surgery, or therapy. Diabetes insipidus or syndrome of inappropriate ADH may precipitate or aggravate sodium imbalances

    g.   Infection may result from an open wound, e.g., in compound depressed skull fracture, during surgery, or through monitoring devices, artificial ventilation, or Foley catheters

MAINTAIN ADEQUATE VENTILATION AND OXYGENATION: Respiratory patterns that cause hypoventilation or hypoxia can lead to increased ICP and further cerebral injury. Consult with physician before instituting postural drainage or clapping as this may also result in increased ICP.

MAINTAIN FLUID AND ELECTROLYTE BALANCE

1. **Hypovolemia and hypotension:** can occur through use of fluid restriction, diuretics, and glucocorticoids. Monitor arterial pressure, PAP, PCWP, and urine output for signs

2. **Hyperglycemia:** may occur as result of high dose steroid therapy and stress response. Monitor urine sugar and acetone and serum glucose levels frequently. Usually a transient finding and rarely needs treatment

3. **Hypernatremia:** may occur as result of osmotic diuretic therapy, sodium therapy, diabetes insipidus, hypothalamic disorders, or high-protein tube feedings. Represents hyperosmolality, and causes cellular dehydration and further neurologic deterioration

4. **Hyponatremia:** caused by either solute (Na^+ or K^+) loss or water retention. May occur as result of syndrome of inappropriate ADH (SIADH) as complication of diuretic therapy, or as result of gastrointestinal losses in which electrolyte replacement has been inadequate. Hypo-osmolar state thus produced may result in cerebral edema

5. **Other conditions:** since these patients are critically ill they may have other fluid and electrolyte problems that are iatrogenically produced or due to coexisting conditions

PROVIDE FOR BOWEL AND BLADDER FUNCTION: Intermittent catheterizations have been advocated in recent years to reduce the incidence of urinary tract infections that occur with indwelling catheters. Condom external catheter should replace indwelling catheters as soon as possible in male patients. Bowel function may be maintained (once the patient has begun feedings again) by stool softeners or suppositories.

MAINTAIN SKIN INTEGRITY AND PREVENT DEFORMITY: Proper positioning, the use of special mattresses, frequent turning, and passive/active range of motion (ROM) all aid in preventing skin breakdown and deformity. Patients with decerebrate rigidity are particularly prone to both breakdown and deformity.

MAINTAIN NORMOTHERMIA: Hyperthermia may be treated with antipyretic drugs, a cooling mattress, or an alcohol/ice sponge bath. Shivering may be controlled with medications (e.g., chlorpromazine) or by wrapping the extremities in towels. A warming mattress may be used if the patient is hypothermic.

PREVENT INFECTION: Careful handling of invasive monitoring equipment is essential. Dressings and patient care equipment should be changed every 24–48 hours.

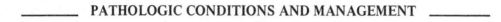

PATHOLOGIC CONDITIONS AND MANAGEMENT

CEREBROVASCULAR ACCIDENT (CVA): Patients with CVA are not routinely admitted to critical care units unless they are unstable, have multiple system failure, or definitive therapy is planned.

1. **Pathophysiology**
   a. Occlusive vascular disease – thrombosis or embolus
      i. Decreased oxygen to cerebral tissue leads to anaerobic glycolysis and loss of function
      ii. Cerebral ischemia, infarction, and edema may follow
   b. Intracerebral hemorrhage
      i. Causes pressure on and irritation of cerebral tissues and nerves, leading to loss of function and death of neurons
      ii. Cerebral vascular spasm often occurs secondary to hemorrhage, and contributes to ischemia or infarction

2. **Etiology or precipitating factors**
   a. Vascular occlusion
      i. Mural thrombi may embolize to cerebral vasculature
      ii. Atherosclerotic plaque
      iii. Cardiovascular disease may be a contributing factor in pathogenesis of emboli formation. May include
         (a) Coronary artery disease
         (b) Mitral stenosis
         (c) Dysrhythmias, e.g., atrial fibrillation
         (d) Endocarditis
      iv. Oral contraceptives have been correlated with an increased incidence of embolus formation and CVA

  b. Hemorrhage
      i.   Ruptured cerebral aneurysm or arteriovenous malformation
      ii. Hypertensive bleed
      iii. Bleeding of a vascular tumor

3. **Clinical presentation**
    a. Main presenting feature in hemorrhage or embolization is sudden onset of signs and symptoms
    b. Clinical presentation varies depending on area of brain involved and extent of injury
    c. Patients with injury to right cerebral hemisphere may exhibit some or all of following dysfunctions
        i.   Left homonymous hemianopia — blindness in left half of both visual fields
        ii. Left hemiparesis or hemiplegia
        iii. Sensory agnosia
             (a) Astereognosis — inability to recognize objects placed in hand without aid of visual clues
             (b) Astatoagnosia — inability to determine position of body parts
             (c) Tactile inattention — lack of attention to simultaneous stimuli
             (d) Anosognosia — unawareness of neurologic deficit, e.g., hemiplegia
             (e) Constructional apraxia — patient does not complete left half of figures he is drawing
             (f) Dressing apraxia — inability to dress oneself properly
        iv. Inattention to objects in left visual field and to left auditory stimuli
        v.   Deviation of head and eyes to right
    d. Patients with injury to left cerebral hemisphere may exhibit some or all of following dysfunctions
        i.   Right homonymous hemianopia — blindness in right half of both visual fields
        ii. Right hemiparesis or hemiplegia
        iii. Sensory agnosia
             (a) Astereognosis — see above
             (b) Astatoagnosia — see above
             (c) Finger agnosia — inability to identify the finger touched
             (d) Right-left disorientation
        iv. Aphasia
             (a) Expressive — inability to speak or write language, or name familiar objects
             (b) Receptive — inability to understand spoken (auditory aphasia) or written (visual aphasia-dyslexia) words
             (c) Mixed or global — both expressive and receptive language difficulties
        v.   Deviation of head and eyes to left

4. **Diagnostic findings**
   a. History
      i. Transient ischemic attacks (TIA) or reversible ischemic neurologic deficits (RIND) may precede vascular occlusion. TIAs resolve within minutes to hours, but RINDs may result in mild, residual neurologic deficits.
      ii. Hypertension — often associated with hemorrhage but not a uniform finding
      iii. Family history of vascular disease may be present
      iv. Arteriosclerosis
      v. Other cardiovascular disease
      vi. Diabetes mellitus
   b. Physical examination — signs vary depending on area of brain involved, on whether dominant or nondominant hemisphere affected, and on extent of injury (see Clinical presentation)
   c. Diagnostic findings
      i. Laboratory
         (a) CSF — may reveal RBCs and increased protein after hemorrhage
         (b) Serum glucose — should be checked to rule out hypoglycemic coma, diabetes mellitus
         (c) Clotting profile — check adequacy of clotting
      ii. Radiologic
         (a) Skull series — normal
         (b) Brain scan — may identify area of increased uptake
         (c) CT scan
            (1) Ischemia and infarctions are revealed as areas of decreased absorption or density
            (2) Hemorrhage appears as an area of increased absorption or density
         (d) Cerebral angiography — may reveal vessels in spasm, areas of hemorrhage, aneurysms, AVMs, or vessels displaced or stretched
      iii. Special — EEG may reveal focal abnormalities, slowing

5. **Complications**
   a. Depend on neurologic deficits in addition to age, general health, and severity of disease process
   b. Because CVA is a disorder of upper motoneurons, patient will have spastic paralysis that may lead to contractures
   c. Progression of stroke may occur as result of rebleed or further embolotic occlusion
   d. Seizures may occur

6. **Specific patient care**
   a. Communicate with patient in most effective way possible, e.g., writing, sign language

    b. Observe for signs of progression of stroke, i.e., further neurologic deterioration. Treat any cardiovascular abnormalities that may be contributing factors

    c. Surgical procedures, e.g., endarterectomy (removal of plaque formation from wall of artery) or bypass grafts (anastomosis of extracranial vessel with intracranial vessel), may be done in patients with signs of hemodynamic insufficiency

        i. In both types of patients, BP must be monitored closely postoperatively to ensure adequate cerebral perfusion

        ii. In patients who have undergone bypass surgery, the scalp area that the extracranial vessel supplied must be checked for ischemia. Assess neurologic function for effectiveness of bypass perfusion postoperatively

INTRACRANIAL HEMATOMAS

1. **Pathophysiology**

    a. Subdural hematoma (SDH) — usually caused by venous bleeding; accumulates below dura mater

        i. Acute SDH — signs and symptoms occur within 48 hours after injury

        ii. Subacute SDH — signs and symptoms occur within 2 weeks after injury

        iii. Chronic SDH — clot has organized and a membrane forms around it; may not be readily attributable to trauma and signs and symptoms may not occur for weeks to months after trauma

    b. Epidural hematoma (EDH) — usually caused by arterial bleeding; accumulation of blood above the dura mater

    c. Intracerebral hematoma (ICH) — hemorrhage into brain substance itself

2. **Etiology or precipitating factors**

    a. Any of the 3 types of hematomas may be caused by trauma to head, and are often associated with scalp lacerations, skull fractures, cerebral contusion, or penetrating head injuries (gunshot wound, stab wound)

    b. SDH may occur spontaneously, particularly if patient has a coagulation disorder or is taking anticoagulation medication

    c. EDH is often associated with linear skull fractures that cross major vascular channels, e.g., middle meningeal artery, transverse or superior sagittal sinus

    d. ICH may also occur as result of rupture of intracranial aneurysm, arteriovenous malformation, vascular tumor, or rupture of a vessel due to hypertension

3. **Clinical presentation**
   a. SDH
      i. Usually present with signs of increasing ICP e.g., decreasing level of consciousness, ipsilateral oculomotor paralysis with contralateral hemiparesis/hemiplegia. May cause ipsilateral hemiparesis
      ii. Acute and subacute SDH may present with an alteration in sensorium, and progress to unconsciousness shortly after injury
      iii. Chronic SDH may present with history of slowly progressing change in behavior that may lead to decrease in consciousness, with or without history of trauma. Often associated with acute or subacute subdural hematoma
   b. EDH
      i. Classically presents with short period of unconsciousness followed by lucid interval of varying duration. Rapid deterioration follows
      ii. Signs of increasing ICP develop rapidly owing to arterial bleeding, e.g., decreasing level of consciousness, ipsilateral oculomotor paralysis with contralateral hemiparesis/hemiplegia
   c. ICH
      i. Signs and symptoms vary with area of brain involved, size of hematoma, and rate at which blood accumulates
      ii. May or may not exhibit signs of increased ICP in addition to above neurologic deficits

4. **Diagnostic findings**
   a. History
      i. Trauma to head
      ii. Loss of consciousness, with or without return to consciousness
      iii. SDH or ICH may present varying history (see Etiology)
   b. Physical examination – findings vary with area of brain involved, rate of bleeding, and size of hematoma
      i. Signs of trauma to head, e.g., hematomas of scalp, areas of tenderness
      ii. Signs of increased ICP
      iii. Focal neurologic signs generally lateralize to one cerebral hemisphere. Exception is hematomas in posterior fossa
   c. Diagnostic studies
      i. Laboratory
         (a) Lumbar puncture (LP) is contraindicated by increased ICP, and is rarely indicated in diagnosis of head trauma

(b) ABG's may reveal respiratory alkalosis due to spontaneous hyperventilation or metabolic acidosis if patient is in shock, is hypoxic, or has high level of physical activity, e.g., seizures, combative behavior, or decerebrate posturing all causing lactic acidosis

  ii. Radiologic

(a) CT scan will show an area of increased density that indicates presence, location, and extent of intracranial hematomas

(b) Skull films

    (1) May reveal associated skull fractures

    (2) In presence of increased ICP, calcified pineal gland or choroid plexus may be shifted from midline

(c) Cerebral angiogram may reveal avascular mantle with displacement or stretching of vessels

(d) Cervical spine x-rays — may show associated injury

(e) Brain scan may reveal increased uptake of isotope in area of hematoma

  iii. Special — echoencephalogram may reveal a shift of midline structures

5. **Complications**

a. Respiratory insufficiency — hypoxia and hypercapnia cause increased CBF and increased ICP and may cause further neurologic deterioration

b. Hydrocephalus can occur as result of trauma or subarachnoid hemorrhage

c. Infection — wound infection, osteomyelitis, abscess, or meningitis can result from improperly cared for scalp lacerations

d. Diabetes insipidus may develop owing to injury to hypothalamus or pituitary

e. Cerebral edema can develop as result of hypoxia or contusion

f. Seizures may result from injury or complications, e.g., hypoxia, electrolyte imbalance

g. Residual neurologic deficits may be present

6. **Specific patient care:** see sections on Increased ICP and Intracranial Monitoring

a. Trauma sufficient to cause intracranial bleeding may also result in scalp lacerations that can lead to significant blood loss, sometimes enough to lead to shock. Direct pressure is usually sufficient, although suturing may be necessary, to control bleeding. Careful cleansing and debridement must be done to avoid extracranial or intracranial infection

b. If patient shows signs of shock, check for abdominal, chest, or retroperitoneal trauma; fractures; scalp laceration; or other injuries that could cause blood loss. Intracranial bleeding in adults is never sufficient to cause shock

   c.   Treat patient as for cervical fracture until spine films rule out fracture. Do not flex or hyperextend head; nasotracheal intubation may be used if respiratory function is compromised

   d.   Monitor and assess neurologic status closely postoperatively for signs of rebleed

   e.   Control pain, e.g., headache, with mild analgesics or codeine if necessary

   f.   Provide seizure precautions. Prophylactic anticonvulsant drugs are usually given

   g.   Burr-holes or craniotomy is usually performed to remove hematoma and associated damaged brain tissue (see section on Postoperative Craniotomy Care)

CLOSED HEAD INJURIES

1. **Pathophysiology**
   a. Cerebral concussion — a transient state of partial or complete paralysis of cerebral functioning. Recovery complete within 12 hours (usually much sooner) with no detectable residual effects other than transient post-traumatic amnesia. Diagnosis is clinically based
   b. Cerebral contusion — partial or complete dysfunction of CNS functioning that persists longer than 12 hours. Contused area may act as intracranial mass owing to cerebral edema and petechial hemorrhages

2. **Etiology or precipitating factors**
   a. Cerebral concussion — neurologic deficit or unconsciousness caused by blunt head trauma. Mechanism of unconsciousness unknown
   b. Cerebral contusion — cerebral dysfunction caused by head trauma with resultant bruising and small petechial hemorrhages. Cerebral edema may occur

3. **Clinical presentation**
   a. Concussion
      i.   May present with gross neurologic deficit or alteration in consciousness that clears spontaneously within 6–12 hours or less
      ii. Post-traumatic amnesia of varying periods is usually present
   b. Contusion
      i.   Signs vary depending on severity of trauma and area of brain involved
      ii. May present in coma with little or no response to noxious stimuli
      iii. Cerebral edema may result and is maximal at about 72 hours. May cause increased ICP

4. **Diagnostic findings**
   a. History
      i. Head trauma
      ii. Neurologic deficits or loss of consciousness
   b. Physical examination
      i. Signs of trauma to head may be present
      ii. There may be mild-to-severe alterations in neurologic status
      iii. Other systems are usually intact, except as altered by severe involvement of brain stem, e.g., vasomotor instability, or multiple trauma
   c. Diagnostic studies
      i. Laboratory — no specific findings
      ii. Radiologic
         (a) Skull, brain scan, angiogram essentially normal
         (b) CT scan may reveal cerebral edema or areas of petechial hemorrhages with severe contusions. Hydrocephalus may be present
      iii. Special — echoencephalogram is usually midline, except with severe cerebral edema involving only one hemisphere

5. **Complications**
   a. Cerebral edema
   b. Residual neurologic deficits as result of contusion. Persistent coma may result from severe contusion
   c. Seizures — approximately 5% incidence with contusion
   d. Respiratory failure/infection

6. **Specific patient care:** see section on Increased ICP and Intracranial Monitoring. Care is supportive as there is no specific surgical intervention commonly employed. If patient exhibits intractable increased ICP, craniectomy and temporal lobectomy may be done to relieve pressure

SKULL FRACTURES

1. **Pathophysiology**
   a. Linear — no displacement of bone. Of significance if fracture interrupts major vascular channel, e.g., middle meningeal artery or superior sagittal sinus
   b. Depressed
      i. Fracture that depresses outer table of skull so that it lies beneath inner table of adjacent skull
      ii. If associated with scalp laceration (i.e., open fracture), is considered a surgical emergency
      iii. Bone fragments may lacerate brain tissue and lead to ICH or other intracranial pathology

   c.   Basal: fracture of base of skull that may extend into ear, orbit, nasal cavity, or walls of paranasal cavities. Difficult to confirm radiologically – diagnosis usually made on basis of clinical signs

2. **Etiology or precipitating factors**
   a. Caused by trauma to head, or penetrating injuries (stab wounds, gunshot wounds)
   b. Depressed fractures may lead to laceration of brain tissue by bone fragments, or lodging of fragments or debris in brain tissue
   c. Basal skull fractures may cause injury to one or more cranial nerves or tearing of dura, with resultant CSF leak

3. **Clinical presentation**
   a. Linear – may have swollen, ecchymotic, tender area of scalp or scalp laceration
   b. Depressed
      i. Significant contusion and edema of scalp without laceration, i.e., closed fracture
      ii. May have scalp laceration, i.e., open fracture
      iii. May present in altered state of consciousness, depending on associated injuries and amount of brain damage
   c. Basal
      i. Anterior fossa
         (a) May result in CSF rhinorrhea if dura is torn
         (b) May also result in bilateral ecchymotic eyes owing to bleeding into sinuses – sometimes referred to as "owl's eyes" or "raccoon's eyes"
         (c) Injury to olfactory nerve (I) is not uncommon
      ii. Middle fossa
         (a) Bleeding, with resultant ecchymosis over mastoid bone – commonly referred to as "battle's sign"
         (b) CSF otorrhea occurs if dura is torn and tympanic membrane ruptured. CSF seeks exits via eustachian tube, and CSF rhinorrhea results if tympanic membrane is intact – in this case, tympanic membrane will bulge and patient may complain of difficulty in hearing
         (c) May also result in cranial nerve injuries

4. **Diagnostic findings**
   a. History
      i. Head trauma
      ii. Patient may have been unconscious
   b. Physical examination
      i. Linear – may have swollen, ecchymotic, tender area of scalp
      ii. Depressed
         (a) Closed – contusion with significant edema of scalp; bone edge may be palpable

    (b) Open – scalp laceration with palpable or visible bone fragments

    (c) Altered state of consciousness

    (d) Other signs depend on severity and other associated injuries

  iii. Basal

    (a) Bilateral, periorbital ecchymosis or bruising over mastoid

    (b) CSF rhinorrhea/otorrhea

    (c) Signs of head trauma

    (d) Altered state of consciousness

    (e) Cranial nerve injury

 c. Diagnostic studies

  i. Laboratory

    (a) Linear or depressed – nothing specific to injury

    (b) Basal – CSF drainage from nose/ear positive for glucose (controversial as to whether this is a positive sign for CSF)

  ii. Radiologic

    (a) Skull series

      (1) Linear or depressed – may be seen on plain films

      (2) Basal – frequently difficult to see on x-ray film; diagnosis usually based on clinical signs

    (b) CT scan – done if other intracranial pathology suspected

    (c) Cervical spine – may be an associated cervical spine fracture

    (d) Other diagnostic studies unnecessary unless associated injuries/complications known or suspected

5. Complications

 a. Linear – if fracture crosses major vascular channel, particularly middle meningeal artery in temporoparietal area, or superior sagittal or transverse sinuses, could cause vessel injury with resultant intracranial hemorrhage (usually EDH)

 b. Depressed

  i. Laceration of brain tissue by bone fragments

  ii. Intracranial hemorrhage or contusion

  iii. CNS infection

 c. Basal

  i. Intracranial hemorrhage

  ii. Meningitis, intracerebral abscess

  iii. Cranial nerve injury

  iv. Carotid-cavernous fistula

6. Specific patient care: see sections on Increased ICP

 a. Linear – if fracture crosses major vascular channel, be alert for signs of increased ICP from intracranial hemorrhage

b. Depressed
  i. Meticulous cleansing and debridement of associated scalp laceration necessary
  ii. Surgical intervention includes removal of bone fragments and necrotic brain tissue, repair of dural defects, and smoothing edges of bony defect; bone is not replaced at this time. Protect brain under cranial defect from post-operative injury
d. Basal
  i. Avert further tearing of dura by preventing transient increases in ICP
    (a) Instruct patient not to blow nose
    (b) Prevent Valsava maneuvers
    (c) Prevent vigorous coughing
    (d) Instruct patient not to inhibit sneezes
  ii. Prevent infection — because there is communication with CSF due to dura tear, meningitis/abscess is possible
    (a) Do not put anything into nose or ears. This includes tissue, dressings, cotton, suction catheters, nasogastric tubes
    (b) Instruct patient to allow fluid to drain freely (although a mustache dressing may be used if rhinorrhea is significant)
    (c) Patient is usually placed on prophylactic antibiotics. CSF leak normally stops spontaneously. Rarely, surgery may be done to repair dura

ACUTE SPINAL CORD INJURY

1. **Pathophysiology**
   a. Compression, contusion, or transection of spinal cord can be caused by bony dislocation; fracture fragments; rupture of ligaments, vessels, or intravertebral discs; interruption of blood supply; or overstretching of neural tissue
   b. Subsequent histopathologic changes may be result of decreased spinal cord blood flow mediated by loss of autoregulation; progressive edema causing small vessel compression; decreased tissue oxygen levels; or release of vasoactive substances such as dopamine, serotonin, or norepinephrine

2. **Etiology or precipitating factors**
   a. Most spinal cord injuries are caused by trauma including falls, motor vehicle accidents, sports injuries, gunshot wounds, or stab wounds
   b. Mechanisms include flexion, hyperextension, and rotational injuries leading to fracture, dislocation, or vascular injury

      c. Disease processes, e.g., tumors, ruptured arteriovenous malformations, infectious processes, or hematomas may also precipitate acute loss of function

3. **Clinical presentation**
    a. Signs and symptoms depend on
      i. Type and extent of lesion
        (a) Complete transection – total loss of sensory and motor function below level of lesion; irreversible
        (b) Incomplete lesion – varying degree of motor and sensory loss below level of lesion; represents sparing of some tracts
          (1) Central cord syndrome – greater motor loss in upper extremities than in lower; varying sensory loss
          (2) Brown-Séquard syndrome (hemisection of cord) – ipsilateral loss of motor, position, and vibratory sense; contralateral loss of pain and temperature sensation
          (3) Anterior cord syndrome – complete motor loss, and loss of pain and temperature below level of lesion, with sparing of proprioception, vibratory sense, and touch
          (4) Other incomplete lesions cause partial dysfunction of some or all spinal cord tracts
      ii. Level of lesion
        (a) C_{1-4} – quadriplegia with total loss of respiratory function
        (b) C_{4-5} – quadriplegia with possible phrenic nerve involvement due to edema that results in loss of respiratory function
        (c) C_{5-6} – quadriplegia with gross arm movements; sparing of diaphragm leads to diaphragmatic breathing
        (d) C_{6-7} – quadriplegia with biceps muscles intact; diaphragmatic breathing
        (e) C_{7-8} – quadriplegia with triceps and biceps intact, but no function of intrinsic hand muscles; diaphragmatic breathing
        (f) T_1 to L_2 – paraplegia with loss of varying amounts of intercostal and abdominal muscle function
        (g) Below L_2 – cauda equina injury; mixed picture of motor-sensory loss, bowel and bladder dysfunction
    b. Patients are areflexic with flaccid paralysis immediately after injury – "spinal shock"
    c. Respiratory failure is seen with complete cervical lesions at C_4 or above owing to loss of innervation to diaphragm, intercostal and abdominal muscles. Diaphragmatic breathing is seen with lesions below C_4

   d. May be associated injury to head or other systems

   e. Assessment of other systems is difficult owing to lack of motor-sensory function, e.g., patient does not complain of abdominal pain, and guarding is not present

   f. Patient may complain of neck pain/tenderness

4. **Diagnostic findings**
   a. History
      i. Trauma resulting in acute decrease or loss of function
      ii. Acute loss of function without history of trauma, e.g., rupture of AVM
   b. Physical examination
      i. Motor-sensory loss — extent and location varies with pathologic condition and level of injury
      ii. Decrease or loss of deep tendon and cutaneous reflexes
      iii. Bladder/bowel disturbance
      iv. Signs of trauma
   c. Diagnostic studies
      i. Laboratory — CSF analysis if pathology other than trauma. Usually done at time of myelogram
      ii. Radiologic
         (a) Spinal series — fractures, dislocation, degeneration will be visualized
         (b) Tomography identifies bony lesion that is difficult to visualize on plain films
         (c) Myelogram may be done if occlusion of spinal subarachnoid space suspected or pathology unclear

5. **Complications**
   a. In first 7–10 days after injury can generally be related to stage of spinal shock, and can affect all systems of body. Many are life-threatening if not prevented or treated promptly. More profound in patients with cervical injuries
   b. Cardiovascular
      i. Hypotension — due to loss of sympathetic outflow caused by spinal cord transection above T_5. Vasodilatation, decreased venous return, and hypotension results. May be further complicated by hemorrhage from associated injuries
      ii. Bradycardia — probably due to sympathetic blockade. May lead to junctional escape beats or rhythm, rarely to ventricular beats. Aggravated by hypothermia or hypoxia
      iii. Vasovagal reflex — cardiac arrest induced by suctioning that leads to hypoxia and vagal stimulation
      iv. Poikilothermism — results from interruption of sympathetic pathways to temperature-regulating centers in hypothalamus. Patients tend toward ambient temperature and become hypo- or hyperthermic, depending on room temperature

      v. Venous thrombosis — decreased rate of blood flow and flaccid paralysis contribute to venous stasis in legs and pelvis

  c. Respiratory

      i. Hypoventilation — injury below C_4 results in diaphragmatic breathing, decreased tidal volume and vital capacity. Paralysis of abdominal and intercostal muscles leads to ineffective cough and retention of secretions. Abdominal distention may restrict diaphragmatic excursions

      ii. Pneumonia — collection of secretions in dependent segments of lung caused by immobility, ineffective cough, and decreased vital capacity. Artificial airways offer easy access for infection. Aspiration is a common complication

      iii. Pulmonary edema — usually attributable to overtransfusion of fluids. There have been case reports of apparent neurogenic pulmonary edema with cervical spinal cord injuries, but mechanism is unclear

      iv. Pulmonary embolus — may result from venous thrombosis of pelvis or legs

  d. Gastrointestinal

      i. Gastric dilatation and ileus — probably due to loss of central control. Can subsequently interfere with diaphragmatic functioning, causing hypoventilation/ hypoxia. Vomiting and pulmonary aspiration may occur

      ii. Cushing's ulcer — a type of stress ulcer seen with CNS injuries. Probably the result of vagal-stimulated gastric acid production and/or ACTH release

      iii. Hemorrhage secondary to abdominal trauma — difficult to diagnose because of loss of usual clinical indicators, e.g., pain. May progress rapidly owing to loss of sympathetic compensatory mechanisms

  e. Urinary

      i. Urinary retention — due to bladder atony. May lead to urinary reflux, stone formation, upper urinary tract back pressure, and renal deterioration

      ii. Urinary tract infection — may result from urinary retention or catheterization

  f. Musculoskeletal

      i. Skin breakdown — denervated areas break down faster and heal slower than those with normal nerve supply. Poor circulation may be contributory

      ii. Muscle atony and wasting — occurs during flaccid paralysis that characterizes spinal shock

      iii. Contractures — may occur owing to spastic paralysis that occurs as spinal shock dissipates

  g. Metabolic

      i. Acidosis due to hypoperfusion

      ii. Alkalosis due to gastric suctioning

      iii. Hypokalemia due to gastric suctioning and trauma

      iv. Extracellular volume excess due to overtransfusion

h. Psychologic (see Psychosocial section)
    i.   Grief and loss
    ii. Body image changes
    iii. Dependency

6. **Specific patient care**
    a. Assess motor function of all major muscle groups and evaluate
        their relative strength (see Assessment section). This tests
        integrity of corticospinal (pyramidal) tracts
    b. Assess sensory ability
        i.   Assess spinothalamic tract function (pain and temperature)
             by having patient identify areas stimulated by pinprick with
             his eyes closed
             (a) Use a clean pin; do not scratch or puncture skin
             (b) Starting at toes, gently tap skin and ask patient to
                  identify at what point he can feel taps. Do this both
                  sides of body, including arms and legs
             (c) Record sensory level by describing distance from
                  anatomic landmarks, i.e., iliac crest, umbilicus, nipple
                  line, clavicle
             (d) Test temperature sense with test tubes of hot and cold
                  water in manner previously described (assessment of
                  pain is usually a sufficient indicator of spinothalamic
                  function, however)
        ii. Assess functioning of posterior columns (proprioception and
             vibratory sense), i.e., fasciculus gracilis and fasciculus
             cuneatus, by again testing either vibratory or position sense
             (a) Position sense is tested by asking patient to close his
                  eyes and identify if a finger or toe is moved away from
                  or toward head
             (b) Vibratory sense is assessed by applying tuning fork to
                  bony prominences and soft tissue, and asking patient
                  to identify if he feels vibration
        iii. Touch is mediated by both the spinothalamic tracts and
             posterior columns
    c. Prevent further damage to spinal cord
        i.   Injured area may be immobilized by traction, casts, braces,
             or surgery. Maintenance of continuous immobilization is
             essential
        ii. Special bed (e.g., Stryker or Circ-O-Electric) may be used to
             assist with turning. Log roll if special bed is not being
             utilized
    d. Treat/prevent complications
        i.   Cardiovascular
             (a) Hypotension — usually self-limiting, but judicious
                  fluid replacement may be necessary — colloid as well as
                  crystalloid may be required
                  If hypotension is severe, as with multiple trauma,
                  hemodynamic monitoring may be instituted

(b) Bradycardia — treat with atropine if symptomatic or other dysrhythmias occur. Treat contributing factors, e.g., hypothermia/hypoxia

(c) Vasovagal reflex — oxygenate prior to suctioning; monitor cardiac rate and rhythm

(d) Poikilothermism — ensure cool environment to avoid hyperthermia. Treat with warming mattress if hypothermic

(e) Venous thrombosis — prophylactic anticoagulation (normal and low dose) has been recommended. Effects of antiembolic stockings and alternating pressure devices for legs are being studied. Recent research has revealed that clinical observation for usual signs of venous thrombosis is often inadequate for lower extremities and of no value in pelvic thrombi. [125] I-fibrinogen test is recommended for diagnosis

ii. Respiratory

(a) Hypoventilation — measure vital capacity and tidal volume at regular intervals to assess deterioration. Monitor arterial blood gases. Nasotracheal intubation, using a fiberoptic bronchoscope, and mechanical ventilation may become necessary to facilitate respiratory care

(b) Pneumonia — assist patient with deep breathing and diaphragmatic coughing (physical therapist can teach this). Provide adequate humidification for airway to prevent tracheobronchitis. Use sterile suctioning technique. Change respiratory equipment at least daily. Monitor sputum with cultures

(c) Pulmonary edema — use hemodynamic monitoring to guide fluid therapy. Chest auscultation will detect presence of rales. Monitor oxygenation status and chest x-ray films

(d) Pulmonary embolus — prevention and early detection of venous thrombosis is best means of prevention. Should be suspected in patients who exhibit sudden change in respiratory status. Remember that pain and hemoptysis will not be clinical indicators in quadriplegic patients

iii. Gastrointestinal

(a) Gastric dilatation and ileus — inspect abdomen for distention. Insert NG tube and attach to intermittent suction. Monitor amount and quality of output

(b) Cushing's ulcer — antacids and cimetidine have been recommended in prevention and treatment. Gastric bleeding has been treated with both warm and cold saline lavage. Check for coagulation defects. Intra-arterial infusion of vasopression has been used.

Surgery — vagotomy and pyloroplasty or gastrectomy — may become necessary

    (c) Hemorrhage — intraperitoneal lavage may be used to detect presence of intra-abdominal hemorrhage

  iv. Urinary

    (a) Urinary retention — intermittent or indwelling catheterization is necessary in initial stages

    (b) Urinary tract infections — intermittent catheterization is recommended to decrease incidence. Early detection is essential, as infection can prolong period of spinal shock and may lead to sepsis

  v. Musculoskeletal

    (a) Skin breakdown — frequent turning (every 1–2 hours) and meticulous skin care are essential. Protect bony prominences

    (b) Muscle contractures — ROM keeps joints mobile. Position properly, employing orthopedic appliances as necessary

  vi. Metabolic — secondary complications to those of other body systems. Correction of cause or replacement of lost electrolytes usually eliminate problems

  vii. Psychologic (see Psychosocial section) — deal honestly with patient and his family while maintaining positive attitude. Allow patient to participate in his care and make decisions when possible. Define and set appropriate limits of behavior, and provide consistency of care

e. Treatment, other than reduction and immobilization, is still in experimental stages, mostly involving laboratory animals. Treatment is directed at preventing or reversing histopathologic changes thought to take place after injury (see Pathophysiology)

  i. Immediate immobilization and reduction is accepted therapy. Early surgical repair of fracture is controversial except to remove bony fragments or intraspinous discs

  ii. Glucocorticoids have been widely advocated and used in early treatment of spinal cord injuries, but no substantial data have emerged to indicate their efficacy

  iii. Induced hypothermia of the spinal cord, with or without durotomy (opening of the dura mater) and/or tissue perfusion, remains controversial — infrequently used in humans

  iv. A variety of pharmacologic agents, including dextran, phenobarbital, methyldopa, phenoxybenzamine, and vasopressors, have been used with nonconclusive results in experimental animals

  v. Generally agreed that effective treatment requires immediate immobilization and institution of definitive therapy within 4 hours of injury

MENINGITIS

1. **Pathophysiology**
   a. Pathologic organisms gain access to subarachnoid space and meninges via blood stream, sinuses, middle ear — directly through penetrating injuries or ventriculostomy catheters, or indirectly as result of cerebral abscess or encephalitis
   b. Exudate forms in subarachnoid space, and inflammation of meninges occurs. There is congestion of tissues and blood vessels
   c. This leads to cortical irritation, and increased ICP may result from hydrocephalus/cerebral edema
   d. Progressive involvement leads to
      i. Vasculitis with necrosis of cortical parenchyma
      ii. Ependymitis or pyrocephalus
      iii. Petechial hemorrhage within brain
      iv. Hydrocephalus or subdural hygroma
      v. Cranial nerve neuritis

2. **Etiology or precipitating factors**
   a. Infecting organisms
      i. Virus
      ii. Bacteria — infecting organisms most often seen include
         (a) Meningococcus — most common
         (b) Streptococcus
         (c) Pneumococcus
         (d) *Haemophilus influenzae* — most common in young children
   b. Penetrating head injury
   c. Basal skull fracture
   d. Middle ear infection
   e. Intracranial surgery
   f. ICP monitoring
   g. Septicemia, septic embolus

3. **Clinical presentation**
   a. Severe, persistent headache
   b. Meningismus
   c. Hyperthermia
   d. Convulsions
   e. Cranial nerve involvement (see Physical examination)
   f. Decreased sensorium — irritability, confusion, lethargy
   g. Nausea and vomiting
   h. Clinical signs of increased ICP
   i. Skin rash common in meningococcal meningitis

4. **Diagnostic findings**
   a. History
      i. A highly suspect injury, procedure, or pathologic condition

  ii. Headache that has grown progressively worse, fever, nausea and vomiting, irritability, confusion, seizures
b. Physical examination
  i. Decreased level of consciousness
  ii. Hyperthermia
  iii. Meningismus
      (a) Nuchal rigidity — resistance to flexion of neck
      (b) Brudzinski's sign — adduction and flexion of legs as attempts are made to flex neck
      (c) Kernig's sign — after flexing thigh on abdomen, attempts at extending it are met with resistance
  iv. Cranial nerve irritation
      (a) II — papilledema may be present; blindness can occur
      (b) III, IV, VI — impairment of ocular movement, ptosis and unequal pupils, and diplopia are common findings
      (c) V — photophobia
      (d) VII — facial paresis
      (e) VIII — tinnitus, vertigo, deafness
  v. Tendon and superficial reflexes may be decreased
  vi. Petechiae or purpura common in meningococcal meningitis
c. Diagnostic studies
  i. Laboratory
      (a) CSF — findings depend on type of organism
          (1) Elevated protein seen in most cases, higher in bacterial meningitis than in viral meningitis
          (2) Low sugar content seen in most bacterial meningitis — may be normal in viral form
          (3) Purulent — turbid. May be clear with some viruses
          (4) Cells — predominantly polymorphonuclear leukocytes
      (b) Blood cultures — culture CSF, drainage from sinuses or wounds to identify organism
      (c) Nasopharyngeal smear — causative bacteria may be present
      (d) Electrolytes — either hypo- or hypernatremia may be seen
  ii. Radiologic
      (a) CT scan — usually normal in acute uncomplicated meningitis, but may show diffuse enhancement in some types or reveal evidence of increased ICP
      (b) Skull — infected sinuses may be seen
  iii. Special — EEG may show generalized slow-wave activity

5. **Complications**
  a. Seizures
  b. Waterhouse-Friderichsen syndrome (adrenal hemorrhage) with resulting hemorrhage and shock. May be seen in fulminating meningococcal meningitis

      c. DIC

      d. Brain abscess, subdural effusions, encephalitis

      e. Hydrocephalus

      f. Cerebral edema

      g. Hyperthermia

      h. Persistent neurologic deficits, e.g., deafness, blindness, hemiparesis

6. **Specific patient care**: see sections on Increased ICP and Intracranial Monitoring

      a. Treat infective organism with large doses of appropriate antibiotics if bacterial in origin. Take isolation precautions

      b. Control body temperature with hypothermia mattress, tepid water bath, antipyretic medications

      c. Provide quiet environment with little stimulation – darken room if photophobia present

      d. Control seizure activity with anticonvulsant medications. Protect from injury, and observe and describe seizure activity carefully

      e. Control headache with analgesics

      f. Control increased ICP (see section on Control of Increased ICP)

GUILLAIN-BARRÉ SYNDROME: Also called Landry-Guillain-Barré-Strohl syndrome, polyneuritis, polyradiculoneuritis, infectious polyneuritis.

1. **Pathophysiology**

      a. Edema and inflammation of spinal nerve roots, with subsequent demyelination

      b. Focal perivascular lymphocytic infiltration occurs within nerve roots, peripheral nerves, and CNS

      c. Schwann cells deposit myelin around axon. Myelin insulates axon and is interrupted at 1–2-mm intervals by nodes of Ranvier. Impulse of myelinated fibers is conducted from node to node (i.e., saltatory conduction) instead of continuously along axon, and thus allows for more rapid impulse conduction. When demyelination occurs, this ability is lost, and nerve impulses are conducted more slowly or not at all. In addition, anterior horn cells in spinal cord may then undergo chromatolysis, i.e., degeneration. This resolves as edema and inflammation of nerves resolves, and remyelination occurs

      d. Demyelination classically begins in distal nerves and ascends symmetrically, resulting in ascending paralysis. This process may halt at any point, or may progress to quadriplegia and involvement of cranial nerves

      e. When demyelination ceases, remyelination occurs slowly, resulting in return of transmission of nerve impulses and restoration of function. Return of function first occurs proximally

and proceeds distally, with complete recovery in an overwhelming majority of cases

2. **Etiology or precipitating factors**
    a. Etiology unknown, but an autoimmune disease theory is popular
        as it explains a mechanism common to a variety of etiologies
    b. A viral infection, such as upper respiratory tract infection or
        gastroenteritis, may precede onset of symptoms by 2–3 weeks.
        Vaccination for smallpox, flu, tetanus, or measles has also been
        associated with syndrome
    c. Previous surgery and pre-existing illnesses, e.g., Hodgkin's
        disease or SLE, have also been associated with syndrome
    d. Many patients have no history of any of these

3. **Clinical presentation**
    a. Paresthesias usually precede paresis/paralysis in extremities
    b. Progressive, symmetric ascending weakness
    c. Dysphagia
    d. Muscle tenderness
    e. Decreased or absent reflexes (areflexia is the rule)
    f. Vital capacity decreased
    g. Objective, minimal, transient sensory loss, hyperesthesia,
        hypalgesia
    h. Cranial nerve involvement – VII most frequently involved,
        followed by VI, III, XII, V, and X. Order of involvement may
        be varied

4. **Diagnostic findings**
    a. History of viral infection 2–3 weeks prior to onset of symptoms
        and progressive ascending weakness
    b. Physical examination
        i.   Muscle weakness – symmetric involvement (distal muscles
              most severely affected)
        ii.   Cranial nerve involvement – most commonly dysphagia and
              facial weakness
        iii. Depressed or absent reflexes
        iv.   Decreased vital capacity due to weakness of respiratory
              muscles
        v.   Paresthesias, hyperesthesia, hypalgesia
    c. Diagnostic studies
        i.   CSF – elevated protein with normal cell count, referred to
              as "albuminocytologic dissociation" (a classical finding)
        ii.   Radiologic – all normal
        iii. Special – electromyography not generally used during acute
              stages, but may be done during rehabilitation to document
              nerve regeneration

5. Complications
   a. Respiratory failure, infection
   b. Gastric dilatation, ileus
   c. Venous thrombosis, pulmonary embolus
   d. Immobilization problems
   e. Autonomic dysfunction — most frequently manifested by wide fluctuations in BP and pulse rate
   f. ADH secretion dysfunction

6. Specific patient care
   a. Monitor vital capacity frequently to assess need for assisted ventilation. Know predicted norm for patient
   b. Prevent and control respiratory and urinary tract infections, as these can greatly prolong rehabilitation period. If catheterization becomes necessary, intermittent catheterization is preferable
   c. Some physicians advocate steroids to decrease symptoms and/or promote regeneration — efficacy controversial, and of no apparent benefit in acute stages
   d. Observe for signs of phlebitis. Antiembolic stockings have been advocated for prevention, but efficacy is controversial. Anticoagulation therapy may become necessary
   e. Handle extremities gently to prevent discomfort. There may be paresthesias as regeneration of nerves occurs
   f. Observe for and treat autonomic dysfunction — BP and cardiac rate and rhythm most seriously affected. These patients are more sensitive to drugs, so dosage may need to be modified. Vasoactive drugs not advised
   g. Monitor fluid and electrolyte balance carefully to detect abnormalities of ADH secretion early
   h. Maintain adequate nutrition, initially with tube feedings

MYASTHENIA GRAVIS

1. Pathophysiology
   a. Chronic disorder of neuromuscular transmission characterized by abnormal muscular fatigability brought on by activity; improves with rest
   b. Normally, each nerve impulse liberates ACh from nerve terminal causing depolarization, i.e., end-plate potential. Subsequent AP in turn, initiates events that result in muscular contraction
   c. Physiologic defect is thought to be at neuromuscular junction, although exact mechanism has been controversial. Presynaptic defects, e.g., impairment of ACh synthesis, packaging or ' release; and decreased amplitude and/or frequency of miniature end-plate potentials, have been proposed as possible mechanisms
   d. Recent research implicates a postsynaptic defect as cause. This theory suggests reduction of available ACh receptors at neuro-

muscular junction, brought about by an autoimmune process, i.e., antibodies directed against skeletal muscles

e. Decrease in number of ACh receptor sites leads to reduced amplitude of end-plate potentials and impairment of impulse transmission, and therefore of muscular contraction

2. **Etiology or precipitating factors**
   a. Etiology unknown — most accepted theory is that it is an autoimmune disorder affecting postsynaptic receptor sites. Significant incidence of thymoma and thymic hyperplasia associated with myasthenia gravis lends support to this theory
   b. Precipitating factors of crisis
      i. Inadequate anticholinesterase drug levels (myasthenic crisis)
      ii. Overdosage of anticholinesterase drugs (cholinergic crisis)
      iii. Influenza
      iv. Menstrual cycle or pregnancy (especially first trimester)
      v. Certain drugs — quinidine, -mycin antibiotics, procainamide, quinine, phenothiazines, barbiturates, tranquilizers, narcotics
      vi. Emotional stress
      vii. Fatigue
      viii. Alcohol

3. **Clinical presentation**
   a. Easy fatigability of voluntary muscle groups with repeated use
   b. Ptosis
   c. Diplopia
   d. Dysphagia
   e. Jaw weakness, especially with chewing and speaking (dysarthria)
   f. Hoarseness after talking a few minutes
   g. Limb weakness, usually symmetric in terms of involvement, although not necessarily in terms of severity
   h. Respiratory difficulty -- decreased vital capacity

4. **Diagnostic findings**
   a. History
      i. Complaints of feeling tired and weak, especially after sustained activity or late in day
      ii. Improvement in strength and recovery from fatigue after rest
      iii. Complaints of weakness of specific muscle groups with repetitive use
      iv. Deviation from medication regime
   b. Physical Examination
      i. Includes asking patient to perform repetitive actions using involved muscle groups, to assess for fatigability
      ii. Other physical signs vary depending on type and number of muscles involved, and severity

   c. Diagnostic studies
- i. Laboratory — serum antibody tests
  - (a) Radioimmunoassay studies — positive (increased) serum antibody titers
  - (b) Mouse transfer assay leads to myasthenic symptoms in mice
  - (c) Receptor-blocking assay — positive result
  - (d) Negative T_3 and T_4 to rule out thyroid etiology
- ii. Radiologic
  - (a) Thymus scan may reveal thymoma or thymic hyperplasia
  - (b) Chest x-ray film, occasionally with tomograms, may reveal thymic abnormality
- iii. Special
  - (a) Repetitive nerve stimulation studies — electrical stimulation of nerves at various frequencies leads to progressive decrement of muscle APs
  - (b) Anticholinesterase tests
    - (1) Tensilon (edrophonium chloride) — injection of 2 mg is given IV and patient is assessed for improvement in muscle strength. If no reaction within 45 seconds, repeated doses of 2–5 mg may be given at 2-minute intervals until response is obtained or a total of 10 mg has been given. Duration of Tensilon is about 5 minutes
    - (2) Neostigmine, 0.5–1.0 mg IV, may be used if Tensilon test not conclusive
  - (c) Curare test — Administration of small doses (nonparalytic doses in normal individuals) leads to clinically documented increase in weakness
    Note: Not commonly used for diagnosis owing to risk of respiratory collapse. Be prepared to support ventilation.

5. **Complications**
   - a. Respiratory failure
   - b. Aspiration
   - c. Myasthenic crisis
   - d. Cholinergic crisis

6. **Specific patient care**
   - a. Control symptoms
     - i. Improve neuromuscular transmission
       - (a) Administer anticholinesterase agents — neostigmine, pyridostigmine, Mytelase (ambenonium chloride)
         - (1) Very important to administer on schedule
         - (2) Carefully note all muscular responses to medications. Atropine may control side effects (e.g.,

excessive oral secretions or diarrhea), but may
mask cholinergic crisis — use with caution

    (b)   Administer adrenal corticosteroids

        (1)   Although controversial, steroids are generally
indicated in patients not satisfactorily controlled
by anticholinesterase medication or thymectomy.
Mechanism of action not precisely known, but is
thought to interrupt autoimmune response

        (2)   To circumvent producing an increase in weakness
upon initiation of steroid therapy, patient may
be started on small daily doses (e.g., 25 mg
prednisone) that are gradually increased

        (3)   When adequate improvement has occurred,
alternate-day therapy may be instituted. When
maximal improvement is reached, prednisone is
gradually decreased over period of 1 year to a
maintenance dose

        (4)   Anticholinesterase drugs are regulated as neces-
sary. When patient begins to respond to prednisone, dosage of anticholinesterase drugs can be
decreased as tolerated

        (5)   Alternate-day therapy may minimize some side
effects of prednisone, but side effects of prolonged steroid therapy do occur and must be
promptly dealt with

    (c)   Although controversial in patients without thymoma,
thymectomy has been shown to produce improvement
in or remission of symptoms in high percentage of
myasthenic patients. Improvement may occur gradually
and may not be maximal for as long as 1–10 years.
Many patients continue to require steroids and/or
anticholinesterase medications after thymectomy,
although often in smaller amounts

  ii.   Anticipate problems of inability to ventilate adequately.
Observe for weak cough, difficulty in swallowing, and
ineffective response of muscles to medications. Measure
vital capacity every 2–4 hours

 iii.   Avoid certain drugs that might precipitate problems (see
Precipitating factors)

  iv.   Prevent aspiration. Patient may have difficulty chewing or
swallowing. Semisoft foods are generally tolerated best.
NG tube feedings may become necessary during crisis

   v.   Develop method of communication with patient if he is
unable to talk. Explain care and procedures to him

b. Treat myasthenic crisis (inadequate dosage of or tolerance to
anticholinesterase drugs)

   i.   Tensilon test may be used to differentiate between myasthenic crisis and cholinergic crisis. If patient's symptoms

              improve after receiving Tensilon, crisis is myasthenic; if they get worse, it is cholinergic

  ii. Monitor patient's ability to ventilate

    (a) Observe for restlessness, dyspnea. Measure vital capacity every 2 hours, and know predicted norm for patient

    (b) Monitor arterial blood gases as necessary — generally a late indicator of respiratory distress in these patients

    (c) Endotracheal intubation or tracheostomy and assisted ventilation may become necessary

    (d) Chest physical therapy should be done often

  iii. Improve neuromuscular transmission by administering anticholinesterase drugs, repeating as necessary. Steroids are usually avoided in crisis

  iv. Maintain communication with patient — often very frightened of weakened condition and dependency on ventilator

  v. Monitor and assess muscle strength frequently

  vi. Treat any underlying condition that may have precipitated crisis or may be perpetuating it

c. Treat cholinergic crisis (overdosage of anticholinesterase drugs)

  i. Improve neuromuscular transmission by withholding anticholinesterase drugs, usually for 72 hours while supporting patient

  ii. Anticholinesterase drugs are then reinstituted slowly

  iii. Cholinergic symptoms may be controlled with medications such as atropine (which again carries danger of masking important signs of anticholinesterase overdosage)

d. Care for patient post-thymectomy

  i. Anticholinesterase drugs may be discontinued prior to surgery. Patient will need ventilator support and frequent suctioning to handle secretions

  ii. A transcervical or sternal approach may be used. Institute appropriate care after chest surgery, e.g., chest tubes

  iii. Anticholinesterase medications and/or steroids will be reinstituted slowly postoperatively, starting with low doses. Assess response carefully

  iv. Monitor respiratory status

  v. Remind patient that full effects of thymectomy may not be apparent for some time

e. Care for patient undergoing plasma exchange — often referred to as "plasmapheresis," this is process of separating blood into component parts for purpose of removing one or more components (in this case, the autoantibodies believed to be cause of myasthenia gravis). Used infrequently — see literature for further details of procedure and nursing care

  i. Patients who do not respond to traditional therapy may be candidates for plasma exchange. Its use is very limited at this time, and studies are still being conducted

      ii.   Course of plasma exchange usually involves 3 exchanges per week for 2–4 weeks. It is not a cure for myasthenia, and may or may not result in clinical improvement. Degree and duration of response cannot be predicted, nor can the need for or efficacy of future exchanges. Concomitant immuno-suppression is necessary.

     iii.   Muscle strength is monitored closely before, during, and after procedure. Particular attention is given to vital capacity, swallowing ability, ptosis, and diplopia

     iv.   Complications

        (a)   Medications contained in plasma are removed during procedure. When possible, they should be given after exchange procedure, or dosage modified accordingly

        (b)   Venous trauma may occur with repeated punctures and action of machine

        (c)   Electrolyte imbalances are not uncommon during plasma exchange. In particular, calcium and potassium must be monitored closely

SEIZURES

1. **Pathophysiology**
   a. Paroxysmal high frequency or synchronous low frequency, high voltage electrical discharge in neurons of cerebral cortex, and possibly neurons of the brain stem
   b. Properties of epileptogenic neurons
      i. Generation of autonomous paroxysmal discharges is influenced by synaptic activity
      ii. Increased electrical excitability is present
      iii. Cortical surface is electrically negative to surrounding normal cortex
      iv. Initiation of volleys of high frequency impulses is caused by depolarization of RMP
      v. They are able to induce secondary epileptogenic foci in synaptically related areas

2. **Etiology or precipitating factors**
   a. Genetic
   b. Perinatal injury
   c. Craniocerebral trauma
   d. Cerebrovascular disease
   e. Infections, particularly of CNS
   f. Cerebral tumors
   g. Metabolic or toxic disorders
   h. A–V malformations of the brain
   i. Abrupt withdrawal of anticonvulsant medications or chronically used sedatives

3. **Clinical presentation**
    a. Generalized
        i. Grand mal
            (a) Tonic-clonic symmetric movements involving whole body
            (b) No focal onset but may have high-pitched epileptic cry at beginning of seizure
            (c) Loss of consciousness
            (d) Profuse salivation during seizure
            (e) Apnea and cyanosis may develop, clearing as seizure terminates
            (f) Incontinence is common
            (g) Usually lasts 1–5 minutes
        ii. Petit mal
            (a) Brief loss of contact with environment, i.e., absence
            (b) Patient may exhibit minor motor movements such as drooping or twitching of lips, rolling or turning up of eyes
            (c) Lasts 2–10 seconds; ends abruptly. Patient (usually a child) is generally unaware that anything has happened
            (d) Not usually seen in patients over 12 years of age
        iii. Myoclonic – sudden, brief, muscular contractions that may occur singly or repetitively; usually involve arms
        iv. Akinetic – sudden, brief loss of muscle tone that may be manifest as "drop attacks"
    b. Partial
        i. Partial seizures with elemental symptomatology
            (a) Motor
                (1) Focal motor seizures that are confined to specific body parts but may progress and become generalized (commonly called "jacksonian")
                (2) May be associated with "aura" – a sensory phenomena preceding seizure activity
            (b) Sensory
                (1) Somatic sensory seizures that patient usually describes as numbness or tingling, may generalize
                (2) Special sensory seizures may include visual, auditory, or vertiginous symptoms
        ii. Partial seizures with complex symptomatology
            (a) Automatisms or temporal lobe seizures (psychomotor)
                (1) May present as simple or elaborate behavioral or sensory alterations
                (2) Although behavior appears intentional, patient has amnesia regarding the event
                (3) Usually lasts 1–5 minutes
            (b) Visceral or autonomic symptoms

4. **Diagnostic findings**
   a. History
      i. Ask for details of subjective and objective events occurring at onset of attack
      ii. Ask those observing seizure about postictal events
      iii. Ask patient and his family about frequency and duration of seizure disorder
      iv. Inquire into genetic history for possible etiology
   b. Physical examination
      i. Neurologic examination may reveal possible causative factor, e.g., abnormality that suggests intracranial pathology
      ii. If seizures are idiopathic, examination will be normal unless patient is in postictal state
      iii. Examination of other body systems may reveal possible causative factors, e.g., signs of electrolyte imbalances, blood gas abnormalities, or other serious illness
   c. Diagnostic studies
      i. Laboratory – dependent on cause or related pathology
      ii. Radiologic – dependent on intracranial pathology, if any – e.g., tumors, abscesses, hematomas, aneurysm or AVM
      iii. Special – EEG
         (a) May be done under variety of conditions, e.g., sleeping, hyperventilation, photostimulation
         (b) May be repeated at different times of day or under different conditions
         (c) Abnormal results vary depending on causative pathology, but generally reveal localized or diffuse slowing of the pattern when patient is not having a seizure, and localized or diffuse increase in EEG activity during seizures. Certain seizures, e.g., petit mal, have characteristic EEG patterns

5. **Complications**
   a. Status epilepticus
   b. Injury during seizure activity
   c. Aspiration
   d. Respiratory embarassment

6. **Specific patient care**
   a. Observe seizure activity, record and report observations
      i. Note time and signs of impending attack
      ii. Observe parts of body involved, order of involvement, and character of movements
      iii. Check for deviation of eyes, nystagmus; note change in pupillary size

      iv.   Assess respiratory pattern
      v.   Note tonic and clonic stages
      vi.   During postictal stage
         (a)   Insure adequate airway and check for apparent injury
         (b)   Evaluate patient's neurologic status, particularly motor weakness and speech

b. Prevent injuries during convulsive seizure activity
    i.   Never force anything into mouth
    ii.   Do not attempt to restrain patient's movements
    iii.   Remove objects from vicinity that could cause injury
    iv.   Protect head from injury
    v.   Remove restraining or constricting clothing

c. Improve control of seizure activity
    i.   Monitor and maintain therapeutic plasma levels of anticonvulsant medications — more than one drug may be used at a time
       (a)   Phenytoin (Dilantin) — generalized or partial seizures. Therapeutic range 9–20 μg/ml
       (b)   Phenobarbital — generalized or partial seizures. Therapeutic range 20–40 μg/ml
       (c)   Primidone (Mysoline) — generalized and complex partial seizures. Therapeutic range 7–15 μg/ml
       (d)   Carbamazepine (Tegretol) — generalized and simple or complex seizures. Therapeutic range 4–10 μg/ml
       (e)   Ethosuximide (Zarontin) — petit mal and complex partial seizures. Therapeutic range 40–90 μg/ml
       (f)   Clonazepam (Clonopin) — myoclonic and akinetic seizures. Therapeutic range 40–100 μg/ml
    ii.   Diagnose and treat causative factors, e.g., metabolic disorders, cerebral tumors, or infections
    iii.   Eliminate precipitating factors
       (a)   Alcohol abuse
       (b)   Emotional stress
       (c)   Lack of proper nutrition or sleep
       (d)   Inadequate or inappropriate anticonvulsant medication
       (e)   Nonadherence to drug regime

d. Combat toxic side effects of drugs
    i.   Draw serum levels and maintain at therapeutic levels
    ii.   CNS dysfunction is most common result of toxicity
    iii.   Encourage good oral hygiene to prevent gingival hypertrophy, which commonly occurs with phenytoin
    iv.   Many drugs increase or decrease plasma concentration of certain anticonvulsant drugs, particularly phenytoin. Phenytoin may also decrease plasma concentrations of other drugs. Consult a pharmacist for patient on multiple medications

e. Care for patient postoperatively (see also section on Postoperative craniotomy care, most of which applies here too)

    i.   Cerebral lobectomy or hemispherectomy may be done if patient suffers from intractable seizures that significantly interfere with life

    ii.   Specific epileptic focus must be identified by physician prior to surgery. Dominant hemisphere must also be identified to avoid producing aphasia if seizure focus is in the dominant hemisphere

    iii. Carefully observe for seizure activity in postoperative period — may continue for some time after surgery

STATUS EPILEPTICUS

1. **Pathophysiology**
   a. Same as for seizures, except that seizures persist
   b. Prolonged grand mal seizure activity leads to hypoxia, hypoglycemia, and hyperthermia as result of increased metabolic activity. These conditions may perpetuate seizure activity, causing metabolic and physical exhaustion

2. **Etiology or precipitating factors**
   a. Acute alcohol withdrawal
   b. Withdrawal from anticonvulsant medications
   c. Electroshock therapy
   d. CNS infections, e.g., meningitis, encephalitis, abscesses
   e. Brain tumors, particularly in frontal lobe
   f. Acute withdrawal from chronically used drugs that have sedative or depressant effects
   g. Metabolic disorders, e.g., uremia, hypoglycemia, hyponatremia
   h. Craniocerebral trauma
   i. Cerebral edema

3. **Clinical presentation**
   a. Petit mal status — 200–300 absences in 24 hours
   b. Epilepsia partialis continua — partial or focal seizures that occur regularly or are continuous. Not usually accompanied by loss of consciousness. May generalize
   c. Grand mal status — grand mal seizures that recur. with incomplete recovery between seizures. As seizures repeat, postictal interval becomes progressively shorter. Seizures may become continuous. Life-threatening owing to metabolic and physical exhaustion that occurs
   d. Electrical status — little or no clinical evidence of seizure activity, although EEG shows continuous spike discharges

4. **Diagnostic findings**
   a. History
      i. Presence of one or more precipitating factors
      ii. Seizure activity
   b. Physical examination — see Clinical presentation

    c. Diagnostic studies
        i. Laboratory
            (a) Electrolyte abnormalities may be precipitating cause of seizure activity or may result from prolonged seizures. Pay particular attention to Na^+ and K^+ levels
            (b) Blood sugar should be monitored. Again, may be precipitating cause or may result from prolonged seizure activity. Glucose consumption is increased during seizures and may lead to hypoglycemia
            (c) Arterial blood gases — hypoxia may precipitate or result from seizures. Hypoxia and CO_2 retention may result in acidosis due to increased lactic acid production
            (d) Serum enzymes, particularly CPK, will be elevated after seizure activity
            (e) Myoglobinuria is not uncommon after seizures
       ii. Radiologic — after seizures are controlled, diagnostic studies may be done to find precipitating or complicating cause
      iii. Special — EEG will show seizure activity

5. **Complications**
    a. Respiratory and metabolic acidosis
    b. Hypoxemia
    c. Hypoglycemia
    d. Hyperthermia
    e. Electrolyte imbalances
    f. Renal failure

6. **Specific patient care**
    a. Establish or maintain patent airway and adequate ventilation
        i. Endotracheal intubation and controlled ventilation with volume-cycled ventilator may become necessary if seizures cannot be controlled rapidly
       ii. Monitor arterial blood gases frequently and combat respiratory or metabolic acidosis
      iii. Maintain adequate oxygenation — seizure activity increases oxygen consumption
    b. Stop seizure activity — following drugs may be used
        i. Diazepam — 5–10 mg IV over 2 minutes, repeated as necessary. Do not dilute. Monitor BP and respiratory status
       ii. Phenobarbital — 5–8 mg/kg IV slowly. Watch for respiratory depression and hypotension. Not recommended for use in conjunction with diazepam
      iii. Phenytoin — 13 mg/kg given IV no faster than 50 mg per minute. Do not dilute. Monitor ECG for dysrhythmias

      iv. Paraldehyde – 0.1 – 0.15 ml/kg IM or IV rectally.
          Caution should be used in IV administration – a 1:10
          dilution should be given slowly

  c. Monitor and assess condition closely to prevent complications
      i.   Insert NG tube and attach to gastric suction to prevent
          vomiting and aspiration
      ii. Establish IV route for medications
      iii. Monitor cardiac rate and rhythm
      iv. Cardiovascular drugs should be readily available
      v.   Assess neurologic status frequently
      vi. Treat hyperthermia

  d. Maintain fluid and electrolyte balance
      i.   Maintain accurate intake and output
      ii. Administer glucose solutions IV based on blood glucose
          levels
      iii. Assess electrolytes, calcium and magnesium levels, renal and
          liver function
      iv. Myoglobinuria may result from prolonged seizure activity
          and can lead to renal failure. Treat with fluid and diuretics

  e. Maintain seizure-free state
      i.   If diazepam is used to stop seizures, anticonvulsant drugs,
          preferably phenytoin, must be given simultaneously to
          prevent recurrent seizures
      ii. Phenytoin is often preferred as it does not mask neurologic
          signs
      iii. Phenobarbital may be used if sedation is not a concern
      iv. General anesthesia may be indicated to control seizures if
          they cannot be stopped in 2–4 hours

  f. Investigate and treat underlying pathology

INTRACRANIAL ANEURYSMS

1. **Pathophysiology**
  a. Dilatation of an artery resulting from weakness in media layer
      and internal elastic laminar layer of arterial wall
  b. Aneurysms most commonly occur at bifurcations of arteries
  c. Most cerebral aneurysms occur in vessels of anterior portion of
      circle of Willis
  d. High arterial pressures and continuous arterial pulsations lead to
      ballooning of weakened arterial wall
  e. Rupture of aneurysm can cause intracerebral hematoma and
      subarachnoid hemorrhage
  f. Clot forms in and around rupture site and inhibits continuing
      hemorrhage

2. **Etiology or precipitating factors**
  a. May include congenital defects of walls of artery, complicated by
      degenerative changes

    b. No specific precipitating causes present in all patients

    c. Hypertension not present in all patients, but may be contributing factor to rupture of aneurysm in hypertensive patients

3. **Clinical presentation**

    a. Patient is usually well until rupture of aneurysm

    b. Sudden, severe headache

    c. Patient may be nauseated or may have vomited

    d. Seizures may have occurred

    e. Meningismus — nuchal rigidity, headache, photophobia, diplopia, Kernig's or Brudzinski's sign may be present

    f. Neurologic deficit — motor, sensory, speech

    g. Altered sensorium

4. **Diagnostic findings**

    a. History

        i.   Headache — onset usually sudden and severe

        ii. Seizures

        iii. Change in sensorium

        iv. Hypertension may or may not be present

    b. Physical examination — neurologic examination reveals varying signs and symptoms depending on severity and location of hemorrhage. Aneurysms may be categorized as follows

        i.   Grade I

           (a) Patient alert, no neurologic deficit

           (b) Minimal headache

           (c) Slight nuchal rigidity

        ii. Grade II

           (a) Patient awake, minimal neurologic deficit — e.g., cranial nerve III palsy

           (b) Mild-to-severe headache

           (c) Nuchal rigidity

           (d) No vasospasm

        iii. Grade III

           (a) Drowsiness, confusion, mild focal neurologic deficit

           (b) Nuchal rigidity

        iv. Grade IV

           (a) Patient unresponsive, hemiplegic

           (b) Nuchal rigidity

           (c) Patient may or may not have vasospasm

        v.   Grade V

           (a) Patient comatose — moribund

           (b) Decerebrate posturing

           (c) Patient may have vasospasm

    c. Diagnostic studies

        i.   Laboratory

           (a) Lumbar puncture — not done if signs of increased ICP are present. If done, will reveal bloody CSF, elevated

CSF protein and cell count. CSF pressure may be
elevated
  ii. Radiologic
      (a) Cerebral angiogram will usually illustrate size, shape,
           and location of aneurysm. May also show spasm of
           involved vessels. May detect ICH or hydrocephalus
      (b) CT scan will reveal ICH and intraventricular blood.
           Hydrocephalus will be evident if present. Vasospasm
           may be detected
      (c) Radioisotope brain scan may reveal area of increased
           uptake — not a routine study

5. **Complications**
   a. Rebleeding — most common cause of death. Greatest incidence
       is 7–11 days after initial bleed, owing to lysis of clot
   b. Vasospasm — seen by about 3rd day postbleed. Vasospasm
       increases cerebral ischemia
   c. Neurologic deficits
   d. Cerebral edema
   e. Hydrocephalus

6. **Specific patient care**: see sections on Increased ICP, Intracranial
   Monitoring, and Postoperative Craniotomy Care
   a. Minimize potential for rebleed and promote stabilization of
       patient
       i.   Complete bed rest — surgery is usually delayed until
             patient's condition has improved to Grades I or II
       ii.   Elevate head of bed 15–30° to promote venous drainage
       iii. Limit fluids but avoid dehydration. Vasospasm may be
             treated with hypervolemia
       iv.   Ensure quiet, dark environment, especially if patient has
             photophobia
       v.   Keep patient quiet. Sedatives, e.g., phenobarbital, may be
             necessary. Avoid restraints
       vi.   Take axillary temperatures
       vii. Avoid letting patient strain
       viii. If patient hypertensive, drugs may be used to control BP,
             although not necessarily to bring it to normal levels
       ix.   Epsilonaminocaproic acid (Amicar), an antifibrinolytic
             agent, may be used to delay spontaneous lysis of aneurysmal
             clot (high incidence of rebleed at 7–11 days)
             (a) If given orally, administer every 2 hours to maintain
                  adequate blood levels of about 130 mg/ml
             (b) If given IV, administer as continuous infusion to
                  maintain above levels
             (c) Efficacy of this drug in reducing morbidity and
                  mortality is controversial
             (d) Complications of therapy include thrombus formation

b. Monitor patient's postoperative condition closely (see section on Postoperative Craniotomy Care)

    i.   Frequency of neurologic assessments depends on type of procedure done and status of patient

        (a) Carotid ligation — neurologic assessments may be needed as often as every 5 minutes while clamp on artery is being tightened

        (b) If a clip is applied to neck of aneurysm, routine post-craniotomy care is required

        (c) Wrapping of aneurysm with muslin or other material, or embolization of aneurysm, may be done if aneurysm cannot be clipped. Postoperative craniotomy care is required

    ii. Prevent seizure activity. Ensure adequate oxygenation and electrolyte balance. Give prophylactic anticonvulsant medications routinely

    iii. Prevent increased ICP

    iv. Amicar may be given for a few days postoperatively

REFERENCES

Adams, M., et al.: Psychological responses in critical care units. Am. J. Nurs. *78*:1504, 1978.

Albin, M.S.: Resuscitation of the spinal cord. Crit. Care Med. *6*:270, 1978.

Bader, D.C.H.: Microsurgical treatment of intracranial aneurysms. J. Neurosurg. Nurs. *7*:25, 1975.

Barr, M.L.: The Human Nervous System. Harper and Row, New York, 1974.

Bartol, G.: Psychological needs of the spinal cord injured person. J. Neurosurg. Nurs. *10*:171, 1978.

Bates, B.: A Guide to Physical Examination, 2nd ed. J.B. Lippincott Co., Philadelphia, 1979.

Behrends, E.: Superficial temporal artery anastomosis to middle cerebral artery. J. Neurosurg. Nurs. *10*:113, 1976.

Bellamy, R., Pitts, F.W., and Stauffer, E.S.: Respiratory complications in traumatic quadriplegia. J. Neurosurg. *39*:596, 1973.

Berk, J.L., and Levy, M.N.: Profound reflex bradycardia produced by transient hypoxia or hypercapnia in man. Eur. Surg. Res. *9*:75, 1977.

Blount, M., Kinney, A.B., and Stone, M.: Plasma exchange in the management of myasthenia gravis. Nurs. Clin. North Am. *14*:173, 1979.

Blount, M., et al.: Obtaining and analyzing cerebrospinal fluid. Nurs. Clin. North Am. *9*:593, 1974.

Bouvett, J.M.: Preoperative and postoperative care of patients with cerebral aneurysms. Nurs. Clin. North Am. *9*:655, 1974.

Bruce, D.A., Gennarelli, T.A., and Langfitt, T.W.: Resuscitation from coma due to head trauma. Crit. Care Med. *6*:254, 1978.

Burke, D.E., and Murray, D.D.: Handbook of Spinal Cord Medicine. Raven Press, New York, 1975.

Calvin, R.P.: Continuous ventricular or lumbar subarachnoid drainage of cerebrospinal fluid. J. Neurosurg. Nurs. *9*:12, 1977.

Carpenter, M.B.: Core Text of Neuroanatomy. Williams and Wilkins Co., Baltimore, 1978.

Casas, E.R., et al.: Prophylaxis of venous thrombosis and pulmonary embolism in patients with acute traumatic spinal core lesions. Paraplegia *15*:209, 1977.

Chusid, J.: Correlative neuroanatomy and functional neurology. Lange Medical Publications, Los Altos, California, 1979.

Clark, R.G.: Manter and Gatz's Essentials of Clinical Neuroanatomy and Neurophysiology. F.A. Davis Co., Philadelphia, 1975.

Conway, B.L.: Carini and Owens' Neurological and Neurosurgical Nursing. C.V. Mosby Co., St. Louis, 1978.

Cooper, P.R., Moody, S., Clark, W.K., et al.: Dexamethasone and severe head injury. J. Neurosurg. *51*:307, 1979.

Dahl, D.S.: The management of myasthenia gravis. Drug Ther. *1*:21, 1976.

Davis, A.G.: Inappropriate secretion of antidiuretic hormone in Guillain-Barré syndrome. Postgrad. Med. J. *47*:651, 1971.

DeArmond, S.J., Fusco, M.M., and Dewey, M.M.: Structure of the Human Brain. Oxford University Press, Inc., New York, 1976.

DeMyer, W.: Technique of the Neurological Examination. McGraw-Hill Book Co., New York, 1980.

Dodd, M.J.: Assessing mental status. Am. J. Nurs. *78*:1501, 1978.

Donohoe, K.M., et al.: Cerebral circulation and cerebral angiography. Nurs. Clin. North Am. *9*:623, 1974.

Dorsch, N.W.C., and Symon, L.: A practical technique for monitoring extradural pressure. J. Neurosurg. *42*:249, 1975.

Drachman, D.B.: Myasthenia gravis: part I. N. Engl. J. Med. *298*:136, 1978.

Drachman, D.B.: Myasthenia gravis: part II. N. Engl. J. Med. *298*:186, 1978.

Edmonds, V.E., et al.: The role of laboratory research in the clinical treatment of acute spinal cord injuries. J. Neurosurg. Nurs. *8*:18, 1976.

Elias, S.B., and Appel, S.H.: Recent advances in myasthenia gravis. Life Sci. *18*:1031, 1976.

Engel, W.K., et al.: Myasthenia gravis. Ann. Intern. Med. *81*:225, 1974.

Feig, P.U., and McCurdy, D.K.: The hypertonic state. N. Engl. J. Med. *297*:1444, 1977.

Ferris, G.S.: Treatment of Epilepsy. Medical Economics Co., Oradell, N.J., 1978.

Feustel, D.: Autonomic hyperreflexia. Am. J. Nurs. *76*:228, 1976.

Fincham, R.W., and Davenport, S.S.: Occlusive cerebrovascular disease. Am. Fam. Physician *7*:69, 1973.

Fischer, K.C., and Schwartzman, R.J.: Oral corticosteroids in the treatment of ocular myasthenia gravis. Neurology *24*:795, 1974.

Fischman, R.A.: Brain edema. N. Engl. J. Med. *293*:706, 1975.

Foldes, F.F., and Glaser, G.H.: Diagnostic tests in myasthenia gravis and significance of clinical classification. Ann. N.Y. Acad. Sci. *183*:275, 1971.

Fowler, R., and Fordyce, W.: Adapting care for the brain injured patient. Am. J. Nurs. *72*:1832, 2056, 1972.

Ganong, W.F.: The Nervous System. Lange Medical Publications, Los Altos, CA, 1977.

Gifford, R.M., and Plaut, M.R.: Abnormal respiratory patterns in the comatose patient caused by intracranial dysfunction. J. Neurosurg. Nurs. *7*:57, 1975.

Groteber, J.: Stroke, carotid endarterectomy, and the neurosurgeon. J. Neurosurg. Nurs. *10*:52, 1978.

Gudeman, S.K., Miller, J.D., and Becker, D.P.: Failure of high-dose steroid therapy to influence intracranial pressure in patients with severe head injury. J. Neurosurg. *51*:301, 1979.

Guttmann, L.: Spinal Cord Injuries: Comprehensive Management and Research. Blackwell Scientific Publications, Oxford, England, 1976.

Hanlon, K.: Description and uses of intracranial pressure monitoring. Heart Lung *5*:277, 1976.

Harper, M., et al.: Blood flow and metabolism in the brain. Churchill Livingstone, London, 1975.

Hodges, L.C.: Human sexuality and the spinal cord injured: role of the clinical specialist. J. Neurosurg. Nurs. *10*:125, 1978.

Howe, J.R.: Patient care in neurosurgery. Little, Brown & Co., Boston, 1977.

Jacobansky, A.M.: Stroke. Am. J. Nurs. *72*:1260, 1972.

Jacobs, G.B., et al.: The treatment of intracranial aneurysms. J. Neurosurg. Nurs. *8*:149, 1976.

Jimm, L.: Nursing assessment of patients for increased intracranial pressure. J. Neurosurg. Nurs. *6*:27, 1974.

Johnson, J.H. and Cryan, M.: Homonymous hemianopsia: assessment and nursing management. Am. J. Nurs. *79*:2131, 1979.

Johnson, M., and Quinn, J.: The subarachnoid screw. Am. J. Nurs. *77*:448, 1977.

Josephson, D.A.: Status epilepticus. Am. Fam. Physician *10*:168, 1974.

Kealy, S.L.: Respiratory care in Guillain-Barré syndrome. Am. J. Nurs. *77*:58, 1977.

Kinash, R.G.: Experiences and nursing needs of spinal cord injured patients. J. Neurosurg. Nurs. *10*:29, 1978.

Langfitt, T.W.: Increased intracranial pressure. Clin. Neurosurg. *16*:436, 1969.

Langfitt, T.W.: Pathophysiology of increased intracranial pressure. *In* Brock, M., and Dietz, H. (eds.): Intracranial Pressure. Springer-Verlag, New York, 1972.

Levin, A.B., Duff, T.A., and Javid, M.J.: Treatment of increased intracranial pressure: a comparison of different hyperosmolar agents and the use of thiopental. Neurosurgery *5*:570, 1979.

Lichtenfeld, P.: Autonomic dysfunction in the Guillain-Barré syndrome. Am. J. Med. *50*:772, 1971.

Lorenz, R.: The Cushing response. *In* Beks, J.W.F., and Bosch, D.A. (eds.): Intracranial Pressure III. Springer-Verlag, New York, 1976.

Lundberg, N.: Continuous recording and control of ventricular fluid pressure in neurosurgical practice. Acta Psychiatr. Scand. Suppl. *149*:1, 1960.

Madeja, C.: Computerized tomography: an introduction. J. Neurosurg. Nurs. *9*:87, 1977.

Mandrillo, M.P.: Brain scanning. Nurs. Clin. North Am. *9*:633, 1974.

Marshall, L.F., King, J., and Langfitt, T.W.: The complications of highdose corticosteroid therapy in neurosurgical patients: A prospective study. Ann. Neurol. *1*:201, 1977.

Marshall, L.F., Smith, R.W., Raucher, L.A., and Shapiro, H.M.: Mannitol dose requirements in brain-injured patients. J. Neurosurg. *48*:169, 1978.

Matthews, W.B., and Miller, H.: Diseases of the nervous system. Blackwell Scientific Publications, Oxford, England, 1975.

Mauss, N.K., and Mitchell, P.H.: Increased intracranial pressure: an update. Heart Lung *5*:919, 1976.

McGraw, C.P.: Continuous intracranial pressure monitoring: review of techniques and presentation of method. Surg. Neurol. *6*:149, 1976.

McKibbin, B., and Brotherton, B.J.: The early management of cervical spine injuries. Resuscitation *2*:241, 1973.

McLaurin, R.L., and King, L.R.: Metabolic effects in head injury. *In* Vinken, P.J., and Bruyn, G.W. (eds): Handbook of Clinical Neurology — Injuries of the brain and skull, Part I. American Elvesier Publishing Co., Inc., New York, 1975, pp. 109–131.

Mechner, F.: Patient assessment: examination of the eye, part II. Am. J. Nurs. *75*:1, 1975.

Mechner, F.: Patient assessment: neurological examination, parts I, II and III. Am. J. Nurs. *75*:1511, 2037, 1975; *76*:609, 1976.

Merritt, H.H.: A Textbook of Neurology. Lea and Febiger, Philadelphia, 1973.

Meyd, C.J.: Acute brain trauma. Am. J. Nurs. *78*:40, 1978.

Miller, J.D., and Leech, P.: Effects of mannitol and steroid therapy on intracranial volume-pressure relationships in patients. J. Neurosurg *42*:274, 1975.

Mitchell, P.H., and Irvin, N.J.: Neurological examination: nursing assessment for nursing purposes. J. Neurosurg. Nurs. 9:23, 1977.

Mitchell, P.H., and Mauss, N.K.: The relationship of patient and nurse activity to intracranial pressure variations. Nurs. Res. 27:4, 1978.

Moody, R.A., and Poppen, J.L.: Arteriovenous malformations. J. Neurosurg. 32:503, 1971.

Mulder, D.G.: Effects of thymectomy in patients with myasthenia gravis. Am. J. Surg. 128:202, 1974.

Namba, T., el al.: Corticotropin therapy in myasthenia gravis: effects, indications and limitations. Neurology 21:1008, 1971.

National Institute of Health: Diagnostic criterion for Guillain-Barré. J.A.M.A. 240:1709, 1978.

New, P.F.J.: Computed tomography: a major diagnostic advance. Hosp. Prac. 2:55, 1975.

Nicol, C.F.: Status epilepticus. J.A.M.A. 234:419. 1975.

Nikas, D.L., and Konkoly, R.: Nursing responsibilities in arterial and intracranial pressure monitoring. J. Neurosurg. Nurs. 7:116, 1975.

Noback, C.R., and Demarest, R.J.: The nervous system: introduction and review. McGraw-Hill Book Co., New York, 1972.

Norman, S.: Diagnostic categories for the patient with a right hemisphere lesion. Am. J. Nurs. 79:2126, 1979.

Norman, S., and Baratz, R.: Understanding aphasia. Am. J. Nurs. 79:2135, 1979.

Odachowski, S.: Cerebrospinal fluid in acid-base balance: importance in neurosurgical nursing. J. Neurosurg. Nurs. 6:117, 1974.

O'Flynn, J.D. : Early management of neuropathic bladder in spinal cord injuries. Paraplegia 12:83, 1974.

Okawara, S.H.: Warning signs prior to rupture of an intracranial aneurysm. J. Neurosurg. 38:575, 1973.

Overgaard, J., and Tweed, W.A.: Cerebral circulation after head injury: part 2: The effects of traumatic brain edema. J. Neurosurg. 45:292, 1976.

Ozdemir, C., and Young, R.R.: Electrical testing in myasthenia gravis: an overview. Ann. N.Y. Acad. Sci. 183:287, 1971.

Patton, H.D., et al.: Introduction to Basic Neurology. W. B. Saunders Co., Philadelphia, 1976.

Papatestas, A.E., et al.: Studies in myasthenia gravis: effects of thymectomy. Am. J. Med. 50:465, 1971.

Penny, M.D., Walters, G., and Wilkins, D.G.: Hyponatremia in patients with head injury. Inten. Care Med. 5:23, 1979.

Pepper, G.A.: A person with a spinal cord injury: psychological care. Am. J. Nurs. 77:1330, 1977.

Plum, F., and Posner, J.B.: Diagnosis of stupor and coma. F.A. Davis Co., Philadelphia, 1980.

Poe, R.H., Reisman, J.L., and Rodenhouse, T.G.: Pulmonary edema in cervical spinal cord injury. J. Trauma 18:71, 1978.

Polk, B.V.: Cardiopulmonary complications of Guillain-Barré syndrome. Heart Lung 5:967, 1976.

Ramon, R.K., et al.: Pulmonary embolism in Laundry-Guillain-Barré-Strohl syndrome. Chest 60:555, 1971.

Redelman, K.: The management of acutely ill patients with ruptured intracranial aneurysms. J. Neurosurg. Nurs. 5:69, 1973.

Reid, M.: The berry aneurysm patient: the surgical management — from hemorrhage to follow-up. J. Neurosurg. Nurs. 6:78, 1974.

Ricci, M.M.: Water and electrolyte metabolism in patients with intracranial lesions. J. Neurosurg. Nurs. 9:165, 1977.

Roberts, J.R.: Pathophysiology, diagnosis and treatment of head trauma. Top. Em. Med. 1:41, 1979.

Rose, B.D.: Clinical physiology of acid-base and electrolyte disorders. McGraw-Hill Book Co., New York, 1977.

Rosenberg, R.N., and Mendoza, G.: Idiopathic, acute, symmetrical polyradiculoneuritis. West. J. Med. *120*:124, 1974.

Rosenberg, R.N., et al.: The Treatment of Neurological Diseases. SP Medical and Scientific Books, New York, 1979.

Ross, A.J., et al.: Neuromuscular diagnostic procedures. Nurs. Clin. North Am. *14*:107, 1979.

Ross, G.S., and Klassen, A.: The stroke syndrome: part I — clinical and diagnostic aspects. Hosp. Med. *9*:8, 1973.

Ross, G.S., and Klassen, A.: The stroke syndrome: part II — clinical and diagnostic aspects. Hosp. Med. *9*:55, 1973.

Safar, P.: Cerebral edema. *In* Weil, M.H., and Shubin, H. (eds.): Critical Care Medicine Handbook. John H. Kolen, Inc., New York, 1974.

Saito, I., et al.: Vasospasm assessed by angiography and computerized tomography. J. Neurosurg. *51*:466, 1979.

Schmidt, R.P., and Wilder, B.J.: Epilepsy. F.A. Davis Co., Philadelphia, 1968.

Seybold, M.E., and Drachman, D.B.: Gradually increasing doses of prednisone in myasthenia gravis. N. Engl. J. Med. *299*:81, 1974.

Shalit, M.N., and Umanshy, F.: Effect of routine bedside procedures on intracranial pressure. Isr. J. Med. Sci. *13*:881, 1977.

Shapiro, H.M.: Intracranial hypertension: therapeutic and anesthetic considerations. Anesthesiology *43*:443, 1975.

Silver, J.R.: The prophylactic use of anticoagulant therapy in the prevention of pulmonary emboli in one hundred consecutive spinal cord injury patients. Paraplegia *12*:188, 1974.

Sodaro, E., and Perlick, N.: Gullain-Barré: the syndrome, patient care and some case findings. J. Neurosurg. Nurs. *6*:97, 1974.

Solomon, G., and Plum, F.: Clinical Management of Seizures. W. B. Saunders Co., Philadelphia, 1976.

Stackhouse, J.: Myasthenia gravis. Am. J. Nurs. *73*:1544, 1973.

Steinbok, P., and Thompson, G.B.: Metabolic disturbances after head injury: abnormalities of sodium and water balance with special reference to the effects of alcohol intoxication. Neurosurgery *3*:9, 1978.

Steinbok, P., and Thompson, G.B.: Serum cortisol abnormalities after craniocerebral trauma. Neurosurgery *5*:559, 1979.

Toole, J.F.: Special Techniques for Neurological Diagnosis. F.A. Davis Co., Philadelphia, 1969.

Trockman, G.: Caring for the confused or delirious patient. Am. J. Nurs. *78*:1495, 1978.

Trubuhovick, R.V.: Management of acute intracranial disasters. International Anesthesiology Clinics. Vol. I-II. Little, Brown and Co., Boston, 1979.

Tyson, G.W., et al.: Acute care of the head-injured patient. Crit. Care. Q. *2*:23, 1979.

Vassilouthis, J., and Richardson, A.E.: Ventricular dilatation and communicating hydrocephalus following spontaneous subarachnoid hemorrhage. J. Neurosurg. *51*:341, 1979.

Vinken, P.J., and Bruyn, G.W.: Handbook of Clinical Neurology: Infections of the Nervous System, Part I. American Elsevier Publishing Co., Inc., New York, 1976.

Vinken, P.J., and Bruyn, G.W.: Handbook of Clinical Neurology: Injuries of the Spine and Spinal Cord, Part II. American Elsevier Publishing Co., Inc., New York, 1976.

Vries, J.K., Becker, D.P., and Young, H.F.: A subarachnoid screw for monitoring intracranial pressure. J. Neurosurg. *39*:416, 1973.

Walleck, C.: Pulmonary complications in the neurosurgical patient. J. Neurosurg. Nurs. *9*:102, 1977.

Wallhagen, M.I.: The split brain: implications for care and rehabilitation. Am. J. Nurs. *79*:2118, 1979.

Walton, J.N. Brain's Diseases of the Nervous System, 8th ed. Oxford University Press, New York, 1977.

Warmolts, J.B., and Engel, W.K.: Benefit from alternate day prednisone therapy in myasthenia gravis. N. Engl. J. Med. *286*:17, 1972.

Watson, N.: Anticoagulant therapy in the treatment of venous thrombosis and pulmonary embolism in acute spinal injury. Paraplegia *12*:197, 1974.

Weiss, M.H.: Axioms on the management of head injury. Hosp. Med. *11*:94, 1975.

Wille, R.L., et al.: Anatomy of the brain and skull. J. Neurosurg. Nurs. *9*:99, 1977.

Williams, A.: Classification and diagnosis of epilepsy. Nurs. Clin. North Am. *9*:747, 1974.

Youmans, J.R.: Neurological Surgery. W. B. Saunders Co., Philadelphia, 1973.

THE
RENAL
SYSTEM

prepared by
JUNE STARK, R.N.

BEHAVIORAL OBJECTIVES

Functional Anatomy

1. Describe the anatomic relationship of the nephron to the cortex and medulla of the kidney.

2. List the two functional segments of the nephron.

3. Identify the sequence of blood flow from the renal artery to the renal vein.

Physiology

1. Relate alterations of renal circulation to glomerular filtration rate.

2. Explain the neurohypophyseal–ADH mechanism in terms of plasma osmolality.

3. Discuss the role of the renin–aldosterone system in the regulation of blood pressure.

4. Differentiate between renal and respiratory regulations of acid-base balance.

Assessment

1. Identify four sources of data collection used to assess the renal system.

2. Relate pertinent parts of the nursing history to assessment of the renal system.

3. Describe three components of the physical examination of the renal system.

4. Discuss the interpretation of laboratory results with respect to pathophysiology of the renal system.

General Patient Care Management

1. Formulate a general plan of care for the management of a patient with renal dysfunction.

2. Differentiate between peritoneal dialysis and hemodialysis as modes of therapy.

3. Discuss the psychosocial implications of renal disease.

Pathologic Conditions and Management

1. Contrast prerenal, renal, and postrenal failure with respect to the pathophysiology of each category.

2. Identify the systemic effects of acute renal failure.

3. Discuss the implications of the nursing management of acute renal failure.

4. Describe selected electrolyte imbalances with particular reference to etiology, pathophysiology, and management.

THE RENAL SYSTEM

EXTERNAL STRUCTURES

1. **Renal capsule**
   a. Thin, tough structure that covers each kidney
   b. Prevents kidney swelling, thereby affecting renal interstitial pressure since it resists expansion

2. **Perirenal fat**: cushions kidneys against trauma

INTERNAL STRUCTURES

1. **Cortex**
   a. Outermost layer of kidney — the metabolically active portion where aerobic metabolism occurs and NH_3 is formed
   b. Site of glomerulus, and proximal and distal tubules of nephron

2. **Medulla**
   a. Middle layer of kidney is region of anaerobic and glycolytic metabolism that supplies energy for active transport
   b. Composed of 6 to 10 renal pyramids, formed by collecting tubules and ducts
   c. Also site of deepest part of Henle's loop in nephron

3. **Renal sinus and pelvis**
   a. Papillae are rounded projections of renal tissue located at tips of renal pyramids
   b. Calyx (calyces)
      i. Minor calyx wraps around papilla and collects urine flow from collecting duct
      ii. Major calyx channels urine from renal sinus to renal pelvis
      iii. Urine flows from renal pelvis to ureter

4. **Nephron**: microscopic structure
   a. Structural and functional unit of kidney
   b. Approximately 1 million in each kidney
   c. Able to compensate for significant degree of nephron destruction by
      i. Filtering a higher solute load
      ii. Hypertrophy of remaining functional nephrons
   d. Types of nephrons, based on position and function in cortex
      i. Cortical nephrons are located in outer region of cortex and are characterized by short, sodium-losing loops of Henle

ii. Juxtamedullary nephrons are located in inner cortex adjacent to medulla. They have long loops of Henle that penetrate deep into medulla, and a greater capacity for concentration of urine because they are sodium-retaining nephrons

e. Functional segments of nephron
   i. Renal corpuscle
      (a) Bowman's capsule — a specialized portion of proximal tubule that supports glomerulus
      (b) Glomerulus — a capillary bed
         (1) Semipermeable membrane, normally permeable to water, electrolytes, nutrients, wastes; relatively impermeable to large protein molecules and cells
         (2) Albumin and RBCs, composed of 3 cellular layers — endothelial, basement membrane, and epithelial cells
   ii. Renal tubules
      (a) Segmentally divided into proximal convoluted tubule, descending loop of Henle, ascending loop of Henle, distal convoluted tubule, and collecting duct
      (b) Each segment has a specific cellular structure and function

5. **Renal vasculature**
   a. Kidneys receive 20–25% of cardiac output
   b. Specialized arrangement of renal blood vessels reflects interdependence of blood supply with kidney function
   c. Pathway of blood supply
      i. Kidney: Aorta → renal artery → interlobar artery → arcuate artery → interlobular artery → (nephron) interlobular vein → arcuate vein → interlobar vein → renal vein → inferior vena cava
      ii. Nephron: Afferent arteriole → glomerular capillary → efferent arteriole → peritubular capillary → vasa recta adjacent to tubules → interlobular vein → renal vein → inferior vena cava
   d. Juxtaglomerular apparatus
      i. A complex of specialized cells composed of juxtaglomerular cells and macula densa
         (a) Juxtaglomerular cells—enlarged, smooth muscle cells containing granules of inactive renin
         (b) Macula densa—portion of distal tubule making contact with afferent arterioles of its respective glomerulus. These epithelial cells are characteristically "denser" in comparison to other distal tubule cells
      ii. Monitors arterial blood pressure in afferent and efferent arteriole in addition to amount of sodium in distal tubule

    iii. Factors that trigger juxtaglomerular cells to release renin reflect diminished glomerular filtration rate (GFR)

        (a) Decreased arterial BP in afferent and efferent arteriole

        (b) Reduced sodium content or concentration at distal tubule

        (c) Increased sympathetic stimulation of kidneys

6. **Lymphatics**: abundant supply that drains into venous circulation via thoracic duct

7. **Route of nerve supply**: along renal blood vessels, maintaining vasoactive tone of arteriole

---

PHYSIOLOGY

FORMATION OF URINE: This involves 4 processes—filtration, absorption, secretion, and excretion.

1. **Glomerular ultrafiltration**: first step in formation of urine
   a. Characteristics of filtrate
      i. Normal — protein-free, plasma-like substance with specific gravity of 1.010
      ii. Abnormal — increased permeability of glomerular membrane allows large amounts of RBCs and protein to be filtered into urine. Specific gravity of urine may artifactually increase owing to presence of protein or glucose
   b. Filtration determined by pressure
      i. Glomerular hydrostatic pressure is 50 mm Hg and favors filtration. This capillary hydrostatic pressure is reflective of cardiac output
      ii. Colloid osmotic pressures of 25 mm Hg and Bowman's capsule pressure of 10 mm Hg opposes hydrostatic pressure and thereby opposes filtration
         (a) Colloid osmotic pressure results from oncotic pressure of plasma protein in glomerular blood supply
         (b) Bowman's capsule pressure is reflective of renal interstitial pressure
      iii. Net filtration pressure

Glomerular hydrostatic pressure	+50mm Hg
Colloid osmotic pressure (opposes)	−25mm Hg
Bowman's capsule pressure (opposes)	−10mm Hg
Net pressure favoring filtration	+15mm Hg

   c. Glomerular filtration rate (GFR)
      i. A clinical assessment tool to determine renal function

    ii.   Definition — volume of plasma cleared of a given substance per minute (may be determined using endogenous creatinine)

   iii.   GFR equation:

$$GFR = \frac{(Ux \cdot V)}{Px}$$

Where:

        x = a substance freely filtered through glomerulus and not secreted or absorbed by tubules
        P = plasma concentration of x
        V = urine flow rate
        U = urine concentration of x

   iv.   Normal GFR is 125 ml per minute or 180 liters per day
    v.   Normal urine volume is approximately 1 liter per day; this indicates greater than 99% reabsorption of filtrate
   vi.   Factors affecting GFR
       (a)   Changes in glomerular hydrostatic pressure
          (1)   Secondary to changes in systemic blood pressure
          (2)   Variation in afferent or efferent arteriolar tone
       (b)   Alterations in oncotic pressure
          (1)   Dehydration
          (2)   Hypoproteinemia or hyperproteinemia
       (c)   Alterations in Bowman's capsule pressure
          (1)   Urinary tract obstruction
          (2)   Nephron destruction
          (3)   Interstitial edema of kidney
          (4)   Disease processes, i.e., changes in GFR

2. Tubular functions of absorption, secretion, and excretion
   a.   Conversion of 180 liters of plasma filtered per day to 1 liter of excreted urine
   b.   Absorption and secretion by two processes
      i.   Passive — diffusion following concentration gradients
     ii.   Active — ion transport requiring energy
    iii.   Both processes influenced by hormones, electrochemical gradients, and Starling's law
   c.   Proximal convoluted tubule
      i.   Reabsorbs 60–80% of filtrate which remains isotonic to plasma
     ii.   Major function is active reabsorption of NaCl with passive reabsorption of water
    iii.   Other nutrients reabsorbed are glucose, amino acids, phosphates, uric acid, potassium
    iv.   Regulates acid-base balance through reabsorption of HCO_3^- and secretion of H^+

v.   Secretes organic acids and foreign substances such as drugs
d. Loop of Henle
  i.   Variations in length depending on type of nephron
    (a) Juxtamedullary with long loops
    (b) Cortical with short loops
  ii. Two distinct segments
    (a) Descending segment, the thin limb, permeable to water only
    (b) Ascending segment, the thick limb, which has active Na^+ or Cl^- pump and is impermeable to water
  iii. Major function is concentration or dilution of urine, accomplished by countercurrent mechanism that maintains hyperosmolar concentration in renal medulla
e. Distal convoluted tubule
  i.   Receives hyposmotic or hypotonic urine from ascending loop of Henle
  ii. Major functions are reabsorption of water, sodium chloride, and sodium bicarbonate, and secretion of potassium, ammonia, and hydrogen ions
  iii. Water permeability at this site is controlled by antidiuretic hormone (ADH), and sodium reabsorption is determined by aldosterone
f. Collecting duct
  i.   Receives urine isosmotic with plasma from distal convoluted tubule
  ii. Functions with distal convoluted tubule and is influenced by presence or absence of ADH and aldosterone
  iii. Final adjustments of urine are made in this segment before urine enters renal pelvis and progresses to ureter and bladder

BODY WATER REGULATION: Maintenance of volume and concentration of body water content via thirst-neurohypophyseal-renal axis.

1. **Thirst:** regulator of water intake
  a. Thirst center is located in anterior hypothalamus
  b. Neuronal cells of this center are stimulated by intracellular dehydration, causing sensation of thirst
  c. Role is maintenance of satiety state, i.e., drinking exact amount of fluid to return body to normal hydration state

2. **Antidiuretic hormone (ADH):** osmosodium receptor mechanism for control of extracellular fluid (ECF) osmolality and sodium concentration
  a. Synthesized in supraoptic nuclei of hypothalamus. It then travels along axons of supraopticohypophyseal tract to be stored or released from posterior pituitary. Supraoptic area of hypothalamus may overlap with thirst center, thus leading to an

integration of thirst mechanism, osmolality detection, and ADH release.

b. Release of ADH occurs during

    i.   An increased serum osmolality that stimulates osmoreceptor cells in hypothalamus (*Note:* Normal serum osmolality is 280–300 mOsm/liter). These cells transmit a message along neurohypophyseal tracts, causing ADH release from posterior pituitary

    ii. Volume contraction states, leading to reversal of inhibitory effect on ADH release controlled by stretch receptors in left atrium, thus allowing activation of ADH mechanism

c. In presence of ADH, water reabsorption occurs in distal tubule and collecting ducts, resulting in

    i.   Production of hypertonic urine

    ii. A hypotonic medullary interstitium

    iii. Eventual correction of concentrated ECF

d. Inhibition of ADH secretion occurs when serum osmolality is decreased (as seen during water intoxication)

e. When ADH secretion is inhibited (as above), distal tubule and collecting duct are relatively impermeable to water

    i.   Large volumes of hypotonic filtrate will be delivered to collecting duct, resulting in dilute urine

    ii. Final results are excess water loss in comparison to extracellular solute concentration, returning serum osmolality toward normal limits

3. **Countercurrent mechanism of kidney**: mechanism for concentration and dilution of urine, able to adjust urine osmolality from 200 to 1400 mOsm/liter

a. Occurs in juxtamedullary nephrons' long loop of Henle and peritubular capillary of vasa recta. Both anatomic structures are necessary for existence of this mechanism

    i.   Loop of Henle acts as countercurrent multiplier, since it "multiplies" concentration of medullary interstitium

    ii. Peritubular capillaries act as countercurrent exchangers. This means that any shift in water or sodium from tubular lumen is taken up by peritubular capillaries, enabling medullary interstitium osmotic pressure to remain fairly constant

b. A continuous process

    i.   Isotonic glomerular filtrate leaves proximal tubule and enters loop of Henle at 300 mOsm/liter

    ii. Descending loop of Henle is permeable to water only. This water is gradually drawn into hypertonic medullary interstitium, resulting in

        (a) Gradual increase in osmolality of glomerular filtrate as it becomes dehydrated. At hairpin turn of the loop, osmolality is dramatically increased secondary to

removal of water. Osmolality can reach 1200–1400 mOsm/liter
    (b) Medullary interstitium becoming hypotonic
  iii. Thick ascending limb of loop of Henle is permeable to sodium chloride and impermeable to water. Medullary interstitium becomes more hypertonic as sodium concentration is increased by pumping action at ascending limb
  iv. A dilute filtrate reaches distal tubule
    (a) In absence of ADH, dilute filtrate is excreted unchanged, resulting in dilute urine with water excretion in excess of solute
    (b) In presence of ADH, water is reabsorbed from dilute filtrate in collecting duct (via mechanism described in section above on ADH), resulting in excretion of concentrated urine

ELECTROLYTE REGULATION

1. **Sodium regulation**: normal serum concentration is 136–143 mEq/L
  a. Sodium is the major extracellular cation and osmotically active solute. Since variations in body sodium can be associated with an exchange of water between intracellular and extracellular compartments, sodium affects ECF volume
  b. Renal reabsorption sites
    i.   Proximal tubule – 65% of filtered sodium
    ii. Loop of Henle   – 25% of filtered sodium
    iii. Distal tubule   – 6% of filtered sodium
    iv. Collecting duct – 3–4% of filtered sodium
  c. Three major factors influence sodium excretion
    i.   GFR
    ii. Aldosterone
    iii. Third factor
  d. Sodium reabsorption increases at renal tubules during
    i. Decreased GFR secondary to renal hypoperfusion (e.g., shock, myocardial infarction) – less sodium is delivered to renal tubules and less is excreted
    ii. Aldosterone secretion
      (a) Aldosterone is a steroid, a mineralocorticoid secreted from zona glomerulosa of adrenal cortex
      (b) Its major effect is to increase renal tubular reabsorption of sodium, and selective renal excretion of potassium
      (c) Result of aldosterone secretion is an increased quantity of sodium in ECF, which in turn promotes water reabsorption. At same time, potassium ions are secreted into distal tubule and collecting duct to be passed out into urine

        (d)   Regulating factors for aldosterone secretion are potassium concentration in ECF renin-angiotensin-aldosterone mechanism, total amount of body sodium, and adrenocorticotropic hormone (ACTH).

    iii. Suppression of third factor — function of third factor appears to be promotion of sodium excretion by inhibition of sodium reabsorption along nephron. Therefore, suppression of this factor assures sodium reabsorption

    iv. Sodium reabsorption decreases at renal tubules during

        (a)   Increased glomerular filtration rate (e.g., excess ECF volume) — effect is increased perfusion to kidneys, and therefore increased GFR. More sodium is delivered into renal tubules and more sodium is excreted into urine

        (b)   Inhibition of aldosterone secretion, which causes renal sodium excretion.

        (c)   Third factor secretion (see above)

        (d)   Secretion of ADH — in addition to its role in water balance, ADH has a secondary effect that enhances sodium excretion

        (e)   Action of diuretics, especially loop-affecting diuretics

2. **Potassium regulation:** normal serum concentration is 3.5–5.0 mEq/L
   a. Potassium is the major intracellular cation necessary for maintenance of osmolarity and electroneutrality of cell
   b. Renal transport sites — potassium is actively reabsorbed in proximal tubule, and actively and passively secreted in distal tubule to maintain electroneutrality of urine. This electrical gradient is determined primarily by reabsorption of sodium from urine
   c. Factors enhancing potassium excretion
      i. Increase in cellular potassium
        (a)   Elevated levels of available potassium increase incidence of exchange between sodium and potassium ions. Potassium ions are excreted into urine and sodium ions are reabsorbed
        (b)   A clinical situation is acute metabolic or respiratory alkalosis that results in movement of potassium ions into cells
     ii. High volume flow rates in distal portion of nephron, which increase number of available potassium ions, and thus increase excretion. This situation can be created by effect of osmotic and other diuretics
    iii. Aldosterone, which provides a feedback mechanism for maintenance of ECF potassium ion concentration. It functions as follows

(a) Elevation of serum potassium stimulates zona glomerulosa cells of adrenal cortex to secrete aldosterone

(b) Aldosterone acts on distal nephron and collecting ducts, enhancing retention of sodium and excretion of potassium

(c) Excretion of excess potassium eventually returns patient to a normal potassium ion concentration

3. **Calcium regulation:** normal serum concentration is 8.5–10.5 mg/dl
  a. The calcium ion has several functions and is required for
    i. Transmission of nerve impulses and muscular contraction
    ii. Blood coagulation
    iii. Formation of bones and teeth
    iv. Maintenance of cellular permeability
  b. Renal transport sites – 98% of filtered calcium is reabsorbed
    i. Reabsorptive pathways are similar to those utilized for sodium transport
    ii. Most active reabsorption occurs in proximal tubule
    iii. Other sites include loop (20–25%) and distal tubule (10%)
  c. Factors influencing calcium reabsorption
    i. Parathyroid hormone (PTH) – decrease in serum calcium stimulates secretion of PTH; PTH stimulates tubular reabsorption of calcium at a distal portion of nephron, and increased phosphate excretion. PTH also mobilizes calcium from bone, all in an effort to elevate serum calcium levels
    ii. Vitamin D – calcium absorption from small intestine is dependent on presence of activated vitamin D (1, 25-dihydroxycholecalciferol)
      (a) Activation process – ingestion of ultraviolet light converts 7-dihydrocholesterol in skin to cholecalciferol
        (1) Liver further hydroxylates vitamin D to form 25-hydroxycholecalciferol
        (2) Kidney further hydroxylates to final activated form of vitamin D (1, 25 – dihydroxycholecalciferol)
      (b) PTH stimulates this activation process
      (c) Reduction in serum calcium results in decreased urinary calcium excretion. Therefore, activated vitamin D must be available to absorb calcium from small intestine to maintain adequate serum calcium levels
    iii. Corticosteroids' effect
      (a) Large doses decrease calcium absorption in intestines
      (b) Suspected of interfering with activation of vitamin D in liver

      iv. Diuretic effect:
- (a) These drugs can cause sodium and calcium excretion. Ultimate effect of reduced serum calcium concentration is decreased excretion
- (b) Volume loss – decrease in total body volume, leading to diminished GFR, reduces calcium excretion

4. **Phosphate:** normal serum concentration is 3.0–4.5 mg/dl
   a. The phosphate ion
      i. Is located in bone as is calcium
      ii. Plays a significant role in intracellular energy-producing reactions
      iii. May also be connected with DNA and RNA, i.e., genetic code information
      iv. Is a component of phosphoproteins and phospholipids, which are important constituents of intracellular molecules
   b. Renal transport sites – reabsorption of phosphate is an active process that occurs in proximal tubule and is dependent on presence of sodium
   c. Factors influencing phosphate excretion at renal tubule
      i. PTH secretion inhibits proximal tubular reabsorption of phosphates
      ii. Alterations in GFR
         (a) Increased GFR results in decreased reabsorption of plasma phosphates
         (b) Decreased GFR results in increased reabsorption of plasma phosphates

5. **Magnesium:** normal serum concentration is 1.5–2.5 mEq/L
   a. Magnesium ion is the second major intracellular ion, and is a significant factor in cellular enzyme systems and biochemical reactions
   b. Renal transport site: reabsorptive process is similar to calcium, thereby requiring sodium reabsorption in proximal tubule
   c. Factors influencing magnesium reabsorption along renal tubules
      i. Availability of sodium – presence of sodium ion is necessary for this reabsorptive process
      ii. PTH, although this has a minimal effect on magnesium reabsorption. Mechanisms that stimulate this reabsorptive process are believed to be similar to those utilized in calcium reabsorption

6. **Chloride:** normal serum concentration is 98–100mg/dl
   a. Renal transport sites – reabsorbed with sodium at all sodium absorptive sites in nephron
   b. Factors influencing excretion
      i. Acidosis – bicarbonate reabsorbed while chloride is excreted to maintain electrochemical balance

    ii.   Alkalosis – bicarbonate excreted while chloride is
        reabsorbed to maintain electrochemical balance

EXCRETION OF METABOLIC WASTE PRODUCTS: A primary role of
renal function. It is presently postulated that the kidney excretes over 200
metabolic waste products. The two measured for interpretation of renal
function are blood urea nitrogen (BUN) and serum creatinine.

1. **Urea:** a nitrogen waste product of protein metabolism that is
   filtered and reabsorbed along entire nephron
   a. Unreliable measurement of GFR since urea excretion is
      influenced by
      i. Urine flow (decrease in urine flow rate, such as with volume
         depletion, may allow for backleak and reabsorption of
         BUN)
      ii. Extrarenal factors such as hypoperfusion states
      iii. Catabolic rate as seen with fever, infections, and trauma
         conditions
      iv. Changes in protein metabolism
      v. Drugs
      vi. Diet
   b. Elevation in BUN *without* an associated rise in creatinine is
      indicative of
      i. Volume depletion
      ii. Low renal perfusion pressure states
      iii. Increased catabolic process
   c. Elevations of *both* BUN and creatinine (10:1 ratio) are indicative
      of renal disease

2. **Creatinine:** a waste product of muscle metabolism
   a. Amount produced each day is proportional to body's muscle
      mass, and occurs at a constant rate
   b. Normal kidney excretes creatinine at a rate equal to the kidney's
      blood flow or GFR
   c. Creatinine is freely filtered, i.e., neither reabsorbed nor secreted
      at nephron
   d. Combination of equal creatinine production and excretion makes
      it a reliable assessment for determination of kidney function
   e. Elevation in serum creatinine can be directly related to a change
      or deterioration in kidney function

RENAL REGULATION OF ACID-BASE BALANCE: The kidneys regulate
acid-base balance by minimizing wide variations in body fluid balance, in
conjunction with the appropriate retention or excretion of hydrogen ions.
Normal acid-base balance is also regulated by the lungs and the body buffers
(serum bicarbonate, blood, and plasma proteins).

1. **Bicarbonate reabsorption**
   a. Most bicarbonate (HCO_3) is reabsorbed in proximal tubule, and this process is completed in distal tubule
   b. Bicarbonate is reabsorbed with sodium ions
   c. Bicarbonate reabsorption occurs when filtrate contains more than 28 mEq/L (T max). This may increase in acidemia

2. **Hydrogen ion secretion**
   a. Passive secretion occurs in proximal tubule, and active secretion occurs distally in exchange for sodium (Na^+) ions
   b. Acid is buffered by ammonia (NH_3) or phosphate (HPO_4) before excretion, providing for hydrogen (H^+) excretion without lowering pH
   c. Hydrogen secretion increases during acidemia and decreases during alkalemia

3. **Renal buffers of hydrogen ions**
   a. Buffers that are filtered by glomerulus
      i.   Bicarbonate is completely reabsorbed (up to 28 mEq/L)
      ii. Phosphate (HPO_4) is secreted, then reacts with hydrogen:

$$H^+ + HPO_4^{-2} \rightarrow H_2PO_4^{-1}$$

   b. Buffers produced by kidney tubule
      i.   Bicarbonate can be synthesized in distal tubule. It involves excretion of hydrogen into urine at same time that bicarbonate is delivered to ECF with sodium. Hydrogen and bicarbonate both come from distal tubule cell as result of ionization of carbonic acid (H_2CO_3), thus:

$$H_2CO_3 \overset{CA}{\rightleftharpoons} H^+ + HCO_3^-$$

      ii. Carbonic acid (H_2CO_3) comes from hydration of carbon dioxide (CO_2) via carbonic anhydrase (CA):

$$H_2O + CO_2 \overset{CA}{\rightleftharpoons} H_2CO_3$$

      iii. Carbon dioxide (CO_2) is derived from either cellular metabolism or dissolved carbon dioxide in venous blood; thus *new* bicarbonate can be made in distal tubule from extraurinary sources.
      iv. Complete equation:

$$H_2O + CO_2 \overset{CA}{\rightleftharpoons} H_2CO_3 \overset{CA}{\rightleftharpoons} H^+ + HCO_3^-$$

4. **Renal response to acidosis:** a summary
   a. Increased hydrogen ion secretion at distal nephron with an increased excretion of titratable acids (HPO_4^{-2})
   b. All bicarbonate (HCO_3^-) is reabsorbed in proximal nephron
   c. Production of ammonia to accommodate hydrogen ion excretion

$$NH_3 + H^+ \leftrightharpoons NH_4^+$$

   d. Urinary pH is as low as 4.4 owing to excretion of a more acid urine

5. **Renal response to alkalosis:** a summary
   a. Decreased hydrogen ion secretion in distal nephron
   b. Excess bicarbonate (HCO_3^-) excretion
   c. Decreased production of ammonia
   d. Urine is alkaline with a pH over 7.0

RENAL ROLE IN REGULATION OF BLOOD PRESSURE: This involves four mechanisms.

1. **Maintenance of volume and composition of ECF**
   a. Normal plasma volume is essential for control of BP
   b. Alterations in plasma volume eventually affect BP
      i. Contraction of plasma volume lowers arterial BP, leading to compensation by vasoconstriction, thus impairing oxygen perfusion
      ii. Expansion of plasma volume results in increased cardiac preload affecting Starling curve, with ultimate rise in BP

2. **Aldosterone-body sodium balance determines ECF volume:** aldosterone is one of the substances that preserve sodium balance by stimulating renal tubular reabsorption of this ion (see p. 269)

3. **Renin-angiotensin-aldosterone system:** a regulatory mechanism to preserve BP and avoid serious volume contraction. System is stimulated in response to factors causing decreased GFR
   a. Renin is released from juxtaglomerular cells into afferent arteriole
   b. Upon entering circulation
      i. Renin acts on renin substrate to split away vasoactive peptide, angiotensin I
      ii. Angiotensin I is split to angiotensin II in presence of "converting enzyme" found in lung tissue

        iii. Angiotensin II is a potent vasoconstrictor, with potential to cause pronounced vasoconstriction throughout body

   c. Circulatory effect of angiotensin II on arterial BP
      i. Significant constriction of peripheral arterioles
      ii. Venous constriction, a moderate response resulting in reduction of vascular volume
      iii. Renal arteriolar constriction, which causes kidneys to retain sodium and water. This expands ECF volume, thereby increasing arterial BP

   d. Fluid volume response to angiotensin II is restoration of effective circulating volume by
      i. Angiotensin II stimulation of zona glomerulosa cells for release of aldosterone, which enhances renal sodium reabsorption
      ii. Vasoconstriction, to further decrease GFR, leading to sodium and water reabsorption
      iii. Stimulation of thirst mechanism

4. **Prostaglandins**: intrarenal autoregulation mechanism
   a. Lipid compounds present in most cells (especially kidney, brain, and gonads)
   b. Synthesized in collecting tubule and medullary interstitial cells
   c. Postulated role — vasodilatation of renal vascular bed, creating increase in renal blood flow and increase in sodium and water excretion. This mechanism may occur as physiologic response to renal artery constriction in an attempt to maintain renal perfusion

RED BLOOD CELL SYNTHESIS AND MATURATION

1. **Erythropoietin secretion**: stimulates production of RBCs in bone marrow and prolongs life of RBC

2. **Postulated methods for erythropoietin synthesis and stimulus for secretion**
   a. Synthesis process — kidneys either produce erythropoietin or they synthesize an enzyme that catalyzes its formation
   b. Stimulation for formation is believed to be decreased oxygen delivery to kidney

3. **Erythropoietin deficiency**: this is primary cause of anemia seen in chronic renal failure

_____ **ASSESSMENT** _____

HISTORY

1. **Family history**
   a. Hypertension
   b. Diabetes mellitus
   c. Gout
   d. Malignancy
   e. Polycystic kidney disease
   f. Hereditary nephritis
   g. Renal calculi
   h. Cardiovascular disease

2. **Previous history**
   a. Kidney disease
   b. Urinary tract disease
   c. Cardiovascular disease
      i. Hypertension
      ii. Congestive heart failure (CHF)
      iii. Atherosclerosis
   d. Diabetes mellitus
   e. Immunologic disorders and allergies
   f. Pulmonary disease
   g. Recent infections
   h. Other
      i. Toxemia of pregnancy
      ii. Renal transplant
      iii. Anemia
      iv. Recent surgery
      v. Dialysis
      vi. Drugs and toxins
      vii. Renal calculi
      viii. Infections
      ix. Azotemia

3. **Specific signs and symptoms:** history of present illness
   a. Urinary tract disorders
      i. Dysuria
      ii. Abnormal appearance of urine
         (a) Hematuria (grossly bloody)
         (b) Pyuria (cloudy)
         (c) Biliuria or bilirubinuria (orange)
         (d) Myoglobinuria (usually clear; hematest positive on dipstick)
      iii. Frequency or urgency of urination

iv. Nocturia (may be due to diabetes insipidus, diabetes mellitus, or CHF)
    v.   Polyuria, polydipsia
    vi. Incontinence
    vii. Oliguria, anuria
    viii. Fever
    ix. Pain in costovertebral angle, flank or groin pain
  b. Uremia
    i.   Nausea or vomiting
    ii. Itching (pruritus) and hiccoughing
    iii. Changes in sensorium
    iv. Weakness and fatigue
    v.   Weight loss with muscle wasting
    vi. Edema
    vii. Bleeding
    viii. Asterixis
    ix. Peripheral neuropathy
    x.   Uremic odor of breath
    xi. Uremic frost (skin)

4. **Medication history**
  a. Nephrotoxic agents
    i.   Antibiotic therapy (tetracyclines, aminoglycosides, and gentamicin)
    ii. Analgesic abuse (combination of aspirin and phenacetin)
  b. Diuretics
  c. Cardiac glycosides (digoxin)
  d. Antihypertensives and antiarrhythmic agents
  e. Electrolyte replacement therapy
  f. Immunosuppressives
    i.   Steroids
    ii. Imuran, cytoxan, antilymphocyte globulin (ALG)

5. **Other pertinent information**
  a. Exposure to chemicals or poisons (carbon tetrachloride, lead, mercury)
  b. Recent blood transfusions (history of incompatibility reactions)
  c. Results of past blood studies and x-rays

PHYSICAL EXAMINATION

1. **Inspection**
  a. Diminished level of consciousness (lethargy, coma)
  b. Skin
    i.   Abnormal color — grayish tinge if anemia, and yellowish tinge if retained carotenoids present
    ii. Skin capillary integrity is fragile, and as a result is easily bruised

      iii. Skin turgor is dependent on age and state of hydration
      iv. Purpura lesions — in some forms of renal failure
  c. Eye — cataracts, periorbital edema
  d. Ear — nerve deafness
  e. Edema
      i. Presence and significance of edema is dependent on amount of water retained
      ii. Form of presentation varies from localized edema to anasarca with ascites and pleural effusions
      iii. Edema of renal failure is often related to hypoalbuminemia and can be found in other than dependent areas, such as periorbital tissue
  f. Respiratory pattern — air hunger in severe acidosis similar to Kussmaul respiratory pattern of diabetes ketoacidosis
  g. Urine — volume and characteristics are indications
  h. Muscle tremors, weakness, and weight loss resulting from generalized debilitation seen with uremic syndrome
  i. Tetany
      i. Result of severe hypocalcemia or very rapid correction of acidosis (calcium moves into cell in exchange for potassium ions, and rapid calcium depletion ensues)
      ii. Positive Chvostek's and Trousseau's signs (see p. 306)
  j. Asterixis
      i. Indicative of progressive uremic state
      ii. Ask patient to face practitioner and raise upper extremities in a fixed hyperextensive position. Palms of hands should be visible to practitioner, with fingers separated. Positive sign occurs within 30 seconds — irregular movements of wrists and flapping movements of fingers

2. **Palpation:** generally performed to determine size and shape of kidney and to check presence of tenderness, cysts, and masses
  a. Right kidney is easier to palpate than left
  b. Palpate bladder for presence of urine: if grossly enlarged, suspect bladder neck obstruction
  c. In males, palpate prostate to check size, shape, and potential for infection or cause of obstruction

3. **Percussion**
  a. Performed at the costovertebral angles in attempt to elicit pain and tenderness, which is indicative of
      i. Pyelonephritis
      ii. Calculi
      iii. Renal abscess or tumor
      iv. Glomerulonephritis
      v. Intermittent hydronephrosis

    b. If a mass is present, suspect hydronephrosis, polycystic disease, perinephric abscess or tumor

    c. Percuss abdomen for presence of ascites

4. Auscultation

    a. Listen for aortic or renal artery bruits, heard in flanks or intercostal regions of anterior abdomen

    b. Presence of bruit can be a sign of hypertension, atherosclerosis, and aneurysm

5. Vital signs

DIAGNOSTIC STUDIES

1. Laboratory studies

    a. Blood

        i.   CBC

        ii. Serum creatinine and BUN

        iii. Electrolytes

        iv. Chemistries (calcium, phosphate, alkaline phosphatase, bilirubin, uric acid)

        v.   Baseline blood gases

        vi. Glucose, cholesterol, albumin

        vii. Clotting profile

    b. Urine

        i.   Visual examination for color and clarity

           (a) Clear and colorless with hyposthenuria

           (b) Cloudy when infection is present

           (c) Foamy when albumin is present

        ii. Osmolality (40–1200 mOsm/kg water)

        iii. Specific gravity (1.003–1.030) wide range of normal – this test provides reasonable estimate of urinary osmolality

           (a) Below normal (less than 1.010) – suspect diabetes insipidus or overhydration

           (b) Above normal (1.030) – suspect proteinuria, presence of x-ray contrast media, or severe dehydration

        iv. 24-hour urine collection – check creatinine clearance to assess renal function. In average-sized patients, satisfactory 24-hour collection, regardless of degree of renal function, always has 1 gm of creatinine

        v.   Culture and sensitivity – check for presence or absence of infection

        vi. pH (normal range 4.5–8.0)

           (a) Average value is 6.0

           (b) Alkaline urine frequently seen with infection; if infection is absent, consider renal tubular acidosis if both

               (1) Persistent alkaline urine

               (2) Systemic acidosis present

    vii. Glucose – appears in urine when renal threshold for glucose is exceeded

    viii. Acetone – seen in urine during starvation and diabetic ketoacidosis. A false-positive occurs when patient is taking salicylates

    ix. Protein

        (a) Expressed qualitatively as 1+ or 4+
Quantified accurately if more than a trace is present in urine over 30 mg/24 hrs

        (b) Diagnostic for presence of nephrotic syndrome or for detection of myeloma proteins causing renal failure

    x. Spot urine electrolytes

        (a) Screening test for tubular function

        (b) Measure sodium and potassium concentrations

    xi. Urinary sediment

        (a) Casts – precipitation of protein within kidney that takes on shape of tubule in which it originally formed

            (1) Hyaline casts – entirely protein, small amounts normal in urine. If present in large numbers, suspect significant proteinuria such as albumin or myeloma protein

            (2) RBC casts – diagnostic for active glomerulonephritis

            (3) WBC casts – indicative of infectious process

            (4) Granular casts – small number normal, possibly result of degenerating RBC or WBC casts

            (5) Fatty casts containing lipoid material – when seen in abundance, consider lipoid nephrosis or nephrotic syndrome

            (6) Renal tubular casts – seen in acute renal failure

        (b) Bacteria – Gram stain

        (c) Erythrocytes – small numbers normal. In abundance during active glomerular nephritis, interstitial nephritis, malignancies, infections

        (d) Leukocytes – small numbers normal. Present in infection, interstitial nephritis

        (e) Renal epithelial cells – rarely seen. Present in abundance during acute tubular necrosis, nephrotoxic injury of kidney, allergic reaction

        (f) Crystals – seen in diseases of stone formation or following certain intoxication, e.g., oxalate stones or ethylene glycol

        (g) Eosinophils – when present in urine, indication of allergic reaction in kidney

2. **Radiologic examination**

    a. Plain abdominal x-ray (KUB) determines position, shape and size of kidney and identifies calcification in urinary system

b.   Intravenous pyelography (IVP)
   i.   Visualizes urinary tract to diagnose partial obstruction, renovascular hypertension, tumor, cysts, congenital abnormalities
   ii.   Complications – allergic reaction to dye, dehydration
   iii.   Contraindicated in presence of
      (a)   Poor renal function – can further compromise function because of dehydrating effect and nephrotoxicity of IVP dye
      (b)   Multiple myeloma – IVP dye may potentiate precipitation of myeloma protein in kidney
      (c)   Pregnancy – abdominal irradiation should be avoided
      (d)   CHF – IVP dye has an acute osmotic effect that can further compromise heart failure
      (e)   Diabetes mellitus – rapid deterioration of renal function is commonly seen in these patients after IVP; mechanism is unknown
      (f)   Sickle cell anemia – elevation in renal tissue oncotic pressure from dye can promote sickling and infarction of renal tissue
c.   High excretion tomography – indicated when kidneys cannot be readily visualized on IVP
d.   Renal scan – determines renal perfusion and function, and can also provide information about obstructed renal mass
   i.   Radioactive dye is taken up by normal kidney tubule cells. Decrease in uptake indicates hypoperfusion due to any cause
   ii.   Commonly utilized to assess status of renal transplants
e.   Retrograde pyelography – provides information regarding upper region of urinary collecting system, i.e., obstruction
f.   Retrograde urethrography – provides information about status of urethra
g.   Cystoscopy – detects bladder or urethral pathology
h.   Renal arteriography
   i.   Identifies tumors and differentiates type of existing renal or renovascular disease (e.g., renal artery stenosis)
   ii.   Complications
      (a)   Dye utilized can be allergenic and cause same complications as IVP dye (see above)
      (b)   Puncturing of a peripheral artery, with consequential hematoma, embolism, or thrombosis formation, is greatest technical risk
i.   Diagnostic ultrasonography – identifies hydronephrosis, differentiates between solid and cystic tumors, localizes cysts or fluid collections
j.   Computerized axial tomography (CT scan) – identifies tumors and other pathologic conditions that create variations in body density (e.g., abscess lymphocele)

k. Voiding cystourethrography — identifies abnormalities of lower urinary tract, urethra, and bladder to determine presence of reflux and residual urine

l. Chest x-ray
   i. Standard procedure
   ii. Identifies presence of pulmonary disease, pulmonary edema, cardiomegaly, left ventricular hypertrophy, pericardial effusion, uremic lung, Goodpasture's disease, infections (e.g., tuberculosis or fungal infiltrates)

3. **Kidney biopsy**: most common invasive diagnostic tool
   a. Indicated for renal disease that cannot be definitively diagnosed by other methods
   b. Determines cause and extent of lesions — helpful when planning treatment regime
   c. Open and closed biopsies
      i. Open — perform if severe anatomic deformities, or "deep specimen" needed for diagnosis of polyarteritis nodosa or dense deposit disease
      ii. Closed — a simple procedure; no contraindications (see below)
   d. Contraindications — bleeding tendency, hydronephrosis, hypertension, cystic disease, neoplasms

--------- **GENERAL PATIENT CARE MANAGEMENT** ---------

MAINTENANCE OF FLUID BALANCE

1. **Determine state of hydration**
   a. Indications of overhydration
      i. Weight gain
      ii. Elevated BP
      iii. Edema, anasarca, ascites
      iv. Neck vein distention, elevated CVP measurements
      v. Dyspnea
      vi. Stupor (water intoxication)
   b. Indications of dehydration
      i. Weight loss
      ii. Poor skin turgor
      iii. Decreased BP
      iv. Little or no evidence of neck vein distention in supine position
      v. Decreased CVP (less than 5 cm H_2O)
      vi. Stupor (severe hypovolemia)

2. **Measure body weight**
   a. To assess fluid status and dietary adequacy

b. To determine accuracy of intake and output record (approximately 500 ml = 1 lb)

c. Provides guideline for regime of fluid replacement or restriction

3. **Documentation of intake and output record**
    a. Consider insensible losses — fluid losses via lungs, skin, and bowels (approximately 750–800 ml/day)
    b. Consider catabolic rate — result of fluid liberated from food ingested (carbohydrate metabolism: approximately 300–350 ml/day)

4. **Assess renal function**
    a. Urine volume and creatinine clearance
    b. Urinalysis
    c. Urine concentration — specific gravity, urine osmolality, spot electrolytes
    d. Urine protein content for 24 hours

5. **Fluid therapy**
    a. Administer fluids for dehydration, which can be associated with gastrointestinal losses, diuretic abuse, surgery, infection, or hypercatabolic states such as ketoacidosis
    b. Restrict fluids in overhydration, which can be associated with impaired renal function, impaired cardiac function (CHF), or syndrome of inappropriate ADH

MAINTENANCE OF ELECTROLYTE BALANCE

1. **Obtain knowledge of conditions that can precipitate imbalances**
    a. Nasogastric suction
    b. Vomiting and diarrhea
    c. Diuretic therapy
    d. Hyperglycemic (osmotic) diuresis
    e. Massive tissue destruction (in catabolic states with release of hydrogen, potassium, and increase in BUN)

2. **Determine dietary restrictions and provide electrolyte supplements**

3. **Ensure adequate hydration (essential)**

4. **Monitor serum and urine electrolyte values**

MAINTENANCE OF ADEQUATE NUTRITION

1. **Essential amino acids and adequate calories**

2. **Protein and electrolyte intake**: adjust to avoid uremic symptoms and electrolyte imbalances

MAINTENANCE OF ADEQUATE RENAL PERFUSION

1. **Control of hypertension**
   a. Monitor BP frequently
   b. Restrict salt and water intake
   c. Avoid drugs that can elevate BP (e.g., steroids and sympathomimetic-containing antihistamines)
   d. Assess need for diuretics or antihypertensives
   e. Monitor response to antihypertensive therapy. If hypertension is refractory to these medications, further evaluation is necessary — consider
      i. Assessment of renin-angiotensin-aldosterone mechanism (i.e., determine plasma renin activity)
      ii. Renal artery stenosis
      iii. Pheochromocytoma
      iv. Surgery — vascular repair of renal artery stenosis or nephrectomy

2. **Treatment of hypotension**
   a. Administer fluid challenges with volume expanders (normal saline, albumin, dextran) to increase BP
   b. If hypotension persists after correcting volume, vasopressors (e.g., dopamine) are indicated

3. **Treatment of renal hypoperfusion**
   a. Administer drugs to increase cardiac output (e.g., furosemide, digoxin, aminophylline, isoproterenol, dopamine)
   b. Since intratubular blockage can impair renal perfusion, consider agents that increase urine flow in responding nephrons, in order to improve renal function (e.g., furosemide, mannitol)

MAINTENANCE OF ACID-BASE BALANCE

1. **Obtain baseline blood gases** (for comparison)

2. **Assess degree of acidosis**
   a. Frequent concomitant of renal failure
   b. In emergency situations, administer sodium bicarbonate slowly by IV infusion to correct systemic pH
   c. Dialysis and oral sodium bicarbonate provide long-term control
   d. Electrolyte imbalances associated with acidosis are hyperkalemia, hyperchloremia, and increased free calcium ions

3. **Alkalosis**
   a. Rare in renal disease
   b. Presence can be associated with
      i. Excessive vomiting
      ii. Diuretic abuse
      iii. Hypokalemia

BLOOD COMPONENT THERAPY

1. **Give fresh blood whenever possible**
   a. Decreases risk of hyperkalemia
   b. Hypocalcemia can occur from anticoagulants (citrate) present in banked blood

2. **Hepatitis risk**
   a. Numerous blood transfusions increase risk of hepatitis-B to patient and staff
   b. Precautions include early recognition of HAA-positive individuals, followed by isolation measures

3. **Chronic anemia:** medication therapy includes
   a. Oral iron or Imferon IM, unless patient has excess body iron stores
   b. Folic acid and pyridoxine — important especially in dialysis patient since these are dialyzable vitamins. Also indicated in microcytic anemias of folate and B_6 deficiency.
   c. Vitamin B_{12}, for B_{12}-responsive anemia
   d. Anabolic steroids — stimulates RBC formation

PREVENTION OF UREMIC SYNDROME

1. **Prevent dehydration and restrict oral protein intake**

2. **Treat infection and other catabolic states**

3. **Remove blood if present in GI tract:** this is another protein source that will be metabolized to ammonia and urea, which cannot be handled by diseased kidneys

MAINTENANCE OF SKIN INTEGRITY: Insults to skin integrity may precipitate infection, which will further compromise renal function and increase severity of uremia (increase in BUN) — e.g., frequent and unnecessary venipunctures (see also section on shunt and fistula care).

PREVENTION AND TREATMENT OF INFECTIONS: Major cause of death in patients with acute renal failure. In order to minimize the possibility of further compromising existing renal disease, the following precautions are suggested.

1. **Obtain urine culture on admission:** urinary tract infection (UTI) may be asymptomatic

2. **Prevent introduction of microorganisms**
   a. Avoid indwelling urinary catheters
   b. Avoid unnecessary invasive monitoring techniques

3. **Provide aseptic technique for urinary and intravenous catheter care**

PREVENTION OF TOXIC OR SIDE EFFECTS OF DRUGS ADMINISTERED

1. **Drug metabolism:** kidneys play a major role

2. **Drug dosage:** essential to be well informed about drugs and dosages administered in relationship to degree of renal failure — mild, moderate, or severe
   a. Closely observe patient to prevent or recognize toxicity due to drug accumulation
   b. Question nephrotoxic agents ordered to prevent further renal damage
   c. Report any untoward signs, especially elevation in serum creatinine, so that drug can be reconsidered, reduced in dosage, or discontinued

DEVELOPMENT OF CARE PLAN: This should be compatible with the physical, cognitive, and behavioral status of the patient and his family, in order to support both in the adjustment process.

1. **Assessment of adaptation vs maladaptation to disease state**
   a. Gain information about patterns of adaptation and stress responses to previous failures, illnesses, and deaths
   b. Describe responses to changes in life style
   c. Determine degree of compliance to treatment regime (e.g., diet, fluid restriction)

2. **Nursing intervention**
   a. Orient patient to unit, and introduce him to personnel and procedures
   b. Explain alterations in daily activities
      i. Increased levels of fatigue
      ii. Restrictions created by shunt or fistula
      iii. Demands of dialysis schedule
      iv. Reversal in family roles
      v. Independence vs dependency conflict
      vi. Effects on sexual behavior
      vii. Question of maintenance or resumption of work

     c. Support incorporation of body image changes into individual self-concept

     d. Provide support systems, e.g., counseling sessions and visits with successfully adjusted patients

PATHOLOGIC CONDITIONS AND MANAGEMENT

ACUTE RENAL FAILURE: A syndrome of varying etiology, subclassified into prerenal, renal, and postrenal conditions, resulting in an acute deterioration of renal function. Oliguria can be associated with this disease process; anuria is an uncommon feature.

1. **Pathophysiology**
   a. Prerenal conditions
      i. Physiologic states leading to diminished perfusion to kidney without renal tubular damage
      ii. Effect of diminished kidney perfusion is
         (a) Decreased pressure to renal artery
         (b) Decreased afferent glomerular arterial pressure (below 100 mm Hg), which diminishes forces favoring filtration
         (c) After drop or cessation of GFR, ultimate result is oliguria or anuria
   b. Intrarenal conditions
      i. Cortical involvement of vascular, infectious, or immunologic processes
         (a) Causes renal capillary swelling and cellular proliferation, which eventually decreases GFR
         (b) Decreased GFR occurs secondary to obstruction of glomeruli by edema and cellular debris
         (c) Ultimate result is fall in urine output
      ii. Medullary involvement occurs after prolonged ischemia or nephrotoxic injury, specifically to tubular portion of nephron
         (a) Tubular necrosis produced is localized into a patchy pattern; extent of damage in nephrotoxic and ischemic injury differs
            (1) Nephrotoxic injury affects epithelial cellular layer; this layer can regenerate
            (2) Ischemic injury extends to basement membrane, sometimes involving other parts of nephron and peritubular capillaries. This pattern of damage is crucial, since tubular basement membrane cannot regenerate
         (b) Three phases

(1) Oliguric phase reflects pathophysiology of 2 processes
    (a) Obstruction of tubules by cellular debris, tubular casts, or tissue swelling
    (b) Total reabsorption or backleak of urine filtrate through damaged tubular epithelium and into circulation

(2) Diuretic phase signifies that tubular function is returning
    (a) Presents with large daily urine output sometimes exceeding 3 liters
    (b) This is due to osmotic-diuretic effect produced by elevated BUN and impaired ability of tubules to conserve sodium and water

(3) Recovery phase
    (a) Occurs after gradual improvement of kidney function extending over 3–12-month period
    (b) Permanent reduction in GFR may be the end result

c. Postrenal conditions – associated with obstruction of urinary collecting system
  i. Partial obstructions – can increase renal interstitial pressure, which increases opposing forces of glomerular filtration. End result is diminished urine output
  ii. Complete obstruction – impediment of urine flow accompanies bilateral kidney involvement

2. Etiology or precipitating factors

a. Prerenal failure
  i. Hypovolemia secondary to hemorrhage, gastrointestinal losses and third spacing phenomena, decreasing ECF volume
  ii. Excessive use of diuretics
  iii. Impaired cardiac function – myocardial infarction, CHF, acute pulmonary embolism, cardiac tamponade
  iv. Sepsis, progressing to gram-negative shock with vasodilatation
  v. Increased renal vascular resistance resulting from anesthesia or surgery
  vi. Bilateral renal vascular obstruction caused by embolism or thrombosis

b. Intrarenal failure (cortical involvement)
  i. Acute poststreptococcal glomerulonephritis
  ii. Acute cortical necrosis
  iii. Systemic lupus erythematosus (SLE)
  iv. Goodpasture's syndrome

        v.   Bilateral endocarditis

       vi. Pregnancy as seen with abruptio placentae and abortion

     vii. Malignant hypertension.

  c. Intrarenal failure (medullary involvement) — acute tubular necrosis (ATN) is most common type of acute renal failure. ATN, or "vasomotor nephropathy," is result of nephrotoxic or ischemic injury

        i. Nephrotoxic injury occurs after exposure to nephrotoxic agents, the effects of which are accentuated by dehydration, creating more extensive tubular damage. Examples include

           (a) Antibiotics — aminoglycosides, tetracyclines, penicillins

           (b) Carbon tetrachloride

           (c) Heavy metals — lead, arsenic, mercury, uranium

           (d) Pesticides and fungicides

           (e) X-ray contrast media

       ii. Ischemic injury - during this condition, mean arterial blood flow drops below 60 mm Hg for over 40 minutes. Specific disorders include

           (a) Massive hemorrhage

           (b) Transfusion reaction — tubules are obstructed with hemolyzed RBCs

           (c) Septic or cardiogenic shock

           (d) Major trauma or crush injuries

           (e) Postsurgical hypotension

           (f) Postpartum hemorrhage of pregnancy

  d. Postrenal failure — obstructive process can occur anywhere from kidney to urinary meatus

        i. Urethral obstruction

       ii. Prostatic hypertrophy

      iii. Bladder involvement — obstruction, carcinoma, infection, or neurogenic problems

      iv. Ureteral obstruction resulting from renal calculi and edema

       v. Extraureteral problems — e.g., abdominal tumor

3. **Clinical presentation:** during first few days of oliguria, clinical picture is dominated by primary disease process or underlying illness

  a. Acute onset of renal involvement

  b. Uremic manifestations

        i. Mental disturbances — confusion, lethargy, stupor

       ii. Gastrointestinal disturbances — nausea, vomiting, anorexia, sometimes constipation or diarrhea

      iii. Respiratory conditions — deep or rapid respirations due to metabolic acidosis and occasionally pulmonary edema

      iv. Cardiovascular problems — tachycardia, dysrhythmias, pericarditis; BP may be normal

v.   Genitourinary conditions – oliguria defined as less than 400 ml/24 hrs, urinalysis compatible with etiology for acute renal failure

vi.   Integument: dry skin; uremic frost may be present, and pruritus

vii.   Other – increased susceptibility to infection

4.   **Diagnostic findings**
   a.   History – collect data necessary to determine etiology of abrupt fall in renal function, elevated BUN and creatinine, or decrease in urine volume
      i.   Prerenal conditions
         (a)   History of dehydration
         (b)   History of cardiac failure
         (c)   History of venacaval obstruction
         (d)   Profound liver disease (hepatorenal)
      ii.   Intrarenal conditions
         (a)   Nephrotoxicity – history of exposure to nephrotoxic drugs, either environmental, occupational, or iatrogenic (including radiographic contrast media, e.g., IVP dye)
         (b)   Hypotensive-ischemic catastrophes causing ATN – history of recent surgery, cardiogenic or septic shock, trauma, anesthesia, aortic aneurysm, severe hemorrhage
         (c)   Bilateral emboli to both kidneys causing infarction
         (d)   Glomerular disease – cortical necrosis secondary to pregnancy or anaphylaxis, and acute glomerulonephritis occurring after streptococcal infections
         (e)   Tubular plugging – occurs with formation of abnormal proteins; seen in multiple myeloma, hemoglobin plugging following hemolysis, and myoglobin plugging as in rhabdomyolysis
      iii.   Postrenal conditions (bilateral obstruction)
         (a)   History of prostatic disease
         (b)   History of disease of cervix (e.g., malignancy)
         (c)   History of colonic disease
         (d)   Bladder malignancy
         (e)   History of renal calculi with bilateral flank pain and hematuria
         (f)   History of disease that causes bilateral renal calculi, e.g., leukemia (results in hyperuricemia and bilateral uric acid stones)
         (g)   Pregnancy
         (h)   Recent pelvic surgery (hysterectomy or ureteroligation)
         (i)   Bilateral retroperitoneal disease, e.g., lymphoma, sarcoma, retroperitoneal fibrosis

b. Physical examination
   i. Etiology most commonly determined from history and clinical setting or presentation. Severe systemic symptoms are not direct result of renal failure but of associated conditions (see Clinical presentation and History)
   ii. Neurologic – lethargy, confusion, neuromuscular twitching, and weakness related to development of metabolic acidosis
   iii. Gastrointestinal – loss of appetite, vomiting and possibly diarrhea, abdominal distention
   iv. Hematologic – bruising: if gastrointestinal bleeding is present, coffee ground emesis or melena stools can be observed
   v. Respiratory – rales indicative of pulmonary edema
   vi. Cardiovascular
     (a) Friction rub may be indicative of uremic pericarditis
     (b) BP may be normal, depending on fluid status and cardiac status
     (c) ECG may reveal dysrhythmias secondary to electrolyte imbalances or cardiac involvement (CHF)
   vii. Genitourinary – flank pain may be present
   viii. Integument – dry skin, uremic frost
   ix. Other – signs of infection (e.g., wound infection)
c. Diagnostic studies
   i. Laboratory
     (a) Prerenal
       (1) Urinary Na^+ less than 10 mEq/L
       (2) Specific gravity greater than 1.020
       (3) Serum BUN elevated in greater proportion than rise in creatinine (greater than the normal 10:1)
       (4) Minimal or no proteinuria
       (5) Normal urinary sediment
     (b) Intrarenal (cortical disease)
       (1) Urinary Na^+ less than 10 mEq/L
       (2) Specific gravity varies
       (3) Moderate-to-heavy proteinuria
       (4) Serum BUN and creatinine elevated
       (5) Hematuria
       (6) Urinary sediment with RBC casts and WBCs
     (c) Intrarenal (medullary disease)
       (1) Urinary Na^+ greater than 20 mEq/L
       (2) Specific gravity 1.010 to 1.015
       (3) Minimal-to-moderate proteinuria
       (4) Serum BUN and creatinine elevated
       (5) Urinary sediment with numerous renal tubular epithelial cells, tubular casts, and a rare RBC

(d) Postrenal
  (1) Serum BUN and creatinine elevated when complete obstruction present
  (2) Bacteriology report significant for a specific organism
  ii. Radiologic (see p. 281). Major reason for urographic studies is to rule out obstruction as cause of oliguria or anuria. Presence of obstruction must be determined, since its immediate treatment may reverse symptoms of renal failure
  iii. Special
    (a) Antistreptolysin-O (ASO) titer to diagnose recent streptococcal infection, which may cause poststrepto-coccal glomerulonephritis
    (b) Antiglomerular basement membrane titers to diagnose Goodpasture's syndrome, a devastating disease of pulmonary hemorrhage and renal failure
    (c) Serum studies for complement components — fall in complement levels is seen in active complement-mediated glomerulonephritis (e.g., lupus nephritis)
    (d) Serum electrophoresis for immunoglobulin levels — abnormal proteins, as seen in multiple myeloma, can irreversibly damage kidneys

5. Complications
  a. Cardiovascular — dysrhythmias, hypertension, pulmonary edema
  b. Neurologic — asterixis, coma, seizure
  c. Metabolic — electrolyte imbalances, e.g., hyponatremia, hyper-kalemia, hypermagnesemia. Acid-base, fluid, and electrolyte imbalances can become incompatible with life (especially in hyperkalemia)
  d. Hematologic — anemias, uremic coagulopathies
  e. Infection — increased susceptibility to pneumonias, septicemias, urinary tract and wound infections

6. Specific patient care: utilize all the objectives of care described in section on General Patient Care Management, in addition to the following
  a. Maintenance of patient during acute phase of illness is primary goal. Emphasis must be placed on
    i. Correction of fluid, electrolyte, and acid-base imbalances
    ii. Protection from infection
    iii. Establishment of a plan with patient care objectives that addresses underlying disease process and acute renal failure
  b. Peritoneal dialysis
    i. Principles utilized

    (a) Osmosis — movement of fluid across a permeable membrane from area of lesser to one of greater concentration

    (b) Diffusion — movement of molecules from area of higher concentration to one of lower concentration

    (c) Filtration — movement of particles through a permeable membrane by means of hydrostatic pressure

ii. Indications

    (a) Fluid overload

    (b) Electrolyte or acid-base balance

    (c) Acute or chronic renal failure

    (d) Intoxication from dialyzable drugs and poisons

    (e) Peritonitis

    (f) Unavailability of vascular access for hemodialysis (arteriovenous access crisis)

iii. Contraindications

    (a) Bleeding disorders

    (b) Abdominal adhesions

    (c) Recent peritoneal surgery

iv. Important nursing tasks

    (a) Explain procedure to patient (approach varies according to mental status) — duration, limited mobility, discomfort

    (b) Weigh patient before and after treatment

    (c) Prepare equipment utilizing aseptic technique

    (d) Dialysate solution — 1.5% or 4.25% of glucose; select concentration according to desired osmotic gradient necessary for water removal

    (e) Add medications to dialysate as prescribed

        (1) Heparin to prevent clotting in dialysis catheter

        (2) KCl — dosage varies according to serum potassium levels and state of digitalization

        (3) Antibiotics for treatment of peritonitis

        (4) Lidocaine for control of local discomfort (approximately 50 mg/2 L dialysis fluid)

    (f) Patient must void before procedure is begun, to eliminate bladder distention and thus decrease risk of bladder perforation during trocar insertion. If unable to void, patient must be catheterized

    (g) Assist physician during trocar insertion

    (h) First dialysate solution must be drained immediately to determine if catheter is patent — outflow should drain in a steady stream

    (i) Allow all other infusions to "pool" or "dwell" in abdomen (20–45 minutes) for optimal fluid and electrolyte exchange

    (j) Drain at end of dwell time and observe characteristics of dialysate outflow

   (1) Normal — clear, pale yellow

   (2) Cloudy — infection, peritonitis

   (3) Brownish — bowel perforation

   (4) Amber — bladder perforation

   (5) Bloody — common occurrence first to fourth exchange; if bleeding continues, may indicate abdominal bleeding or uremic coagulopathy

  (k) Obtain periodic culture and sensitivity of outflow fluid

  (l) Monitor total body intake and output, and maintain records

   (1) Follow established therapeutic goal for fluid and electrolyte removal

   (2) Measure amount of fluid removed for each exchange, and record positive and negative balance

  (m) Monitor vital signs during outflow phase

   (1) Anticipate changes in baseline BP and pulse rate/rhythm indicative of impending shock or over-hydration

   (2) When using hypertonic dialysate (4.25%) expect osmotic effect

   (3) In diabetic patients it is important to monitor glucose levels

c. Hemodialysis — extracorporeal technique for removing waste products or toxic substances from systemic circulation

 i. Principles are same as for peritoneal dialysis

 ii. Indications

  (a) Acute renal failure due to trauma or infection

  (b) Chronic renal failure when medications and diet no longer provide effective therapy

  (c) Rapid removal of toxic substances from blood stream (e.g., alcohol, aspirin, barbiturates, some antibiotics, and other poisons)

 iii. Contraindications

  (a) Intolerance to systemic heparinization

  (b) Labile cardiovascular status incompatible with rapid changes in extravascular fluid volume

 iv. Anticoagulation

  (a) Prior to procedure, heparinization is done to keep blood anticoagulated within hemodialysis machine ("regional heparinization")

  (b) For noncomplicated patients, 5000 U heparin are administered to start, and 2000 U per hour while on machine ("general heparinization"). Dosage may have to be adjusted to meet needs of individual patients

  (c) Patients should be monitored closely for signs of bleeding.

v. Shunt care
   (a) Auscultate bruit or palpate for thrill to assess shunt patency
   (b) Promptly report any suspicion of clotting, color change of blood, separation of serum from blood, or absence of pulsations in tubing
   (c) Provide adequate hydration to minimize clotting
   (d) Change sterile dressing over shunt at least daily. Reinforce dressing as necessary
   (e) *Do not*: perform venipuncture, give intravenous therapy, give injections, or take BP with cuff on shunt arm
   (f) Instruct patient in self-care of shunt site
vi. Arteriovenous fistula care
   (a) *Do not:* perform venipuncture, start intravenous therapy, give injections, or take BP with cuff on fistulized arm
   (b) Palpate thrill or auscultate bruit to confirm patency
   (c) Report bleeding, skin discoloration, drainage, or other signs of infection. Culture drainage
   (d) For profuse bleeding, follow technique outlined by your specific health agency

ELECTROLYTE IMBALANCES – POTASSIUM IMBALANCE: Hyperkalemia – serum potassium level above 5.5 mEq/L.

1. **Pathophysiology**
   a. Inability of kidney tubules to excrete potassium ions due to tubular damage, salt depletion, and increased potassium load from injured tissues
   b. Decreased renal perfusion diminishes potassium excretion owing to limited amount of sodium available for exchange with potassium (e.g., in cardiac failure)

2. **Etiology or precipitating factors**
   a. Acute and chronic renal disease
   b. Increased cellular destruction with K^+ release as occurs in burns, trauma, or crush injuries
   c. Excessive administration/ingestion of KCl
   d. Adrenal cortical insufficiency – hypoaldosteronism
   e. Low cardiac output or Na^+ depletion
   f. Acidosis

3. **Clinical presentation**
   a. Numbness of extremities
   b. Tall and peaked T waves → bradycardia → cardiac arrest
   c. Oliguria

d. Abdominal cramping and diarrhea
e. Apathy and mental confusion

4. **Diagnostic findings**
   a. History —
      i. General — difficult to obtain. Imbalances should be suspected in presence of renal and endocrine disease, in association with excessive loss of body fluid (vomiting, diarrhea, etc.), and in some special situations with drug intoxication (indiscriminate use of electrolyte replacement, hormonal therapy, and vitamins)
      ii. Specific — excessive intake of KCl supplement, or history of chronic renal failure and dietary abuse
   b. Physical examination — general: all electrolyte imbalances generally present with evidence of abnormal neuromuscular function such as irritability, hypo- or hyperreflexia, seizures, weakness, cardiac dysrhythmias, etc.
      i. Mental status — apathy and confusion
      ii. Cardiac — disturbances in cardiac conduction with development of dysrhythmias
      iii. Gastrointestinal — increased motility of GI tract with abdominal cramping and diarrhea
      iv. Genitourinary — oliguria
      v. Neuromuscular — irritability to flaccid paralysis and numbness of extremities
   c. Diagnostic studies — ECG reveals peaked and elevated T waves → widened QRS → prolonged P-R interval → flattened-to-absent P wave, and S-T segment depression

5. **Complications**
   a. Bradycardia
   b. Cardiac arrest

6. **Specific patient care**
   a. Observe for changes in heart rate and rhythm
   b. In emergency situations (e.g., serum potassium over 6.0 mEq/L or ECG change indicating hyperkalemia), administer
      i. IV glucose, insulin, and sodium bicarbonate to temporarily drive potassium into cells
         (a) Essential to follow up with some other measure for permanent removal of potassium (e.g., Kayexalate/sorbitol administration or dialysis).
         (b) If refractory hyperkalemia occurs, dialysis is indicated
      ii. IV calcium chloride or calcium gluconate to stimulate cardiac action — contraindicated in patient on digoxin
   c. Administer Kayexalate and sorbitol to reverse hyperkalemia

    i.   Action of Kayexalate (an exchange resin) — sodium is "exchanged" 1:1 for potassium in bowel cell wall; therefore, nurse must also assess gain in sodium as well as amount of potassium loss

    ii.   Sorbitol, a nonabsorbable sugar, induces an osmotic diarrhea that contributes to potassium loss from bowels

    iii.   Routes of administration — oral or by means of enema. In both cases, be certain all Kayexalate/sorbitol mixture is expelled, especially preoperatively, since retained Kayexalate can cause bowel obstruction and perforation

ELECTROLYTE IMBALANCES — POTASSIUM IMBALANCE:

Hypokalemia — serum potassium level below 3.5 mEq/L (frequently associated with other fluid and electrolyte disturbances).

1. **Pathophysiology**
   a. K^+ loss exceeding intake
   b. Alkalosis — stimulates secretion of K^+ in distal tubule

2. **Etiology or precipitating factors**
   a. Alkalosis
   b. Abnormal gastrointestinal losses
   c. Liver disease
   d. Diuretic therapy
   e. Renal tubular acidosis
   f. Increased adrenal corticosteroid secretion

3. **Clinical presentation**
   a. Muscle weakness to flaccid paralysis
   b. Hypotension
   c. Cardiac dysrhythmias
   d. Enhanced digitalis effect
   e. Paralytic ileus
   f. Anorexia
   g. Nausea and vomiting
   h. Drowsiness to coma

4. **Diagnostic findings**
   a. History
       i.   General — see section on Hyperkalemia above
       ii.   Specific — increasing muscle weakness and nausea. Occasionally may be muscular cramping due to unbalanced electrochemical effect on muscle cell membrane
   b. Physical examination — see section on Hyperkalemia above
   c. Diagnostic studies — ECG can reveal depressed S-T segment, presence of U wave, and ventricular dysrhythmias

5. **Complications**
   a. Paralytic ileus leading to bowel perforation
   b. Cardiac dysrhythmias
   c. Hypotension to cardiac arrest can result as direct effect of decreased potassium on heart muscle; occurs independently of dysrhythmias
   d. Respiratory arrest due to respiratory muscle weakness

6. **Specific patient care**
   a. Record amount of urine output and estimate degree of potassium lost in drainage (such as from gastric aspirate and diarrhea), to aid in calculating total body potassium balance
   b. Observe for ECG and other cardiac changes
   c. Check for serum potassium levels
   d. Be aware of signs and symptoms of alkalosis
   e. Administer oral potassium supplements, diluted to prevent GI irritation and facilitate absorption
   f. Never give IV potassium chloride rapidly – large concentrations can precipitate hyperkalemia and possibly induce ventricular fibrillation
   g. Determine if patient is receiving digitalis or diuretics. Replace potassium losses, since hypokalemia enhances effect of digitalis and can precipitate digitalis toxicity. Hypokalemia also decreases effectiveness of most diuretics
   h. Emergency treatment
      i. Slowly administer IV potassium chloride while patient is being monitored with ECG in order to observe dysrhythmias
      ii. Be aware of signs and symptoms of hyperkalemia
      iii. Maintain record of serum potassium levels to assess adequacy of replacement achieved

ELECTROLYTE IMBALANCES – SODIUM IMBALANCE:
Hypernatremia – serum sodium level above 145 mEq/L.

1. **Pathophysiology**
   a. Increased ECF volume; sodium and water retention
   b. Less total body water in relation to quantity of body sodium – with increased amounts of water loss in comparison to amount of sodium loss

2. **Etiology or precipitating factors**
   a. With normal kidneys – lack of ADH or neurohypophyseal insufficiency (e.g., diabetes insipidus, water loss in excess of salt)
      i. Potassium depletion – causes a concentrating defect in kidney leading to polyuria; thus, water loss can lead to hypernatremic dehydration

ii.   Hypercalcemia – polyuria and dehydration
iii. Drugs (e.g., osmotic diuretics or increased administration
      of sodium bicarbonate or sodium chloride solution)
iv.   Excessive adrenocortical secretion
v.   Loss of thirst mechanism (e.g., in comatose patient)
vi.   Uncontrolled diabetes mellitus with osmotic diuresis
      secondary to hyperglycemia

b. Abnormal renal function – inability of renal tubule to respond
    to ADH (nephrogenic diabetes insipidus), and decrease in GFR
    causing stimulation of aldosterone release

3. **Clinical presentation:** symptoms may be associated with edematous
    states (sodium and water retention) or dehydration (sodium
    retention and water loss)
    a. Edematous states – fluid retention may be associated with
        edema, weight gain, and hypertension; if severe imbalances occur,
        changes in mental status and dyspnea may be anticipated
    b. Dehydration states – mental irritability, tachycardia, low grade
        fever, flushed skin, dry mucous membranes, oliguria

4. **Diagnostic findings**
    a. History
        i.   General – see section on Hyperkalemia
        ii. Specific
             (a) Complaints associated with "edematous states" (salt
                  and water retention) and hypoproteinemia, such as in
                  presence of nephrosis or cirrhosis. Patients complain
                  of excessive weight gain, fluid retention, and possibly
                  shortness of breath
             (b) Complaints associated with "dehydration states" (Na^+
                  retention/H_2O loss), e.g., extreme thirst, febrile
                  conditions, decreased urine output, dry mucous
                  membranes
    b. Physical examination – see section on Hyperkalemia
        i.   If actual amount of total body Na^+ is increased in
             presence of increased ECF volume (increased H_2O), expect
             pitting edema, hypertension, and (in some instances)
             dyspnea
        ii. If increases in serum sodium occur in presence of decreased
             ECF volume (decreased H_2O), expect dry mucous
             membranes, flushed skin, oliguria, possibly tachycardia,
             and a febrile state
    c. Diagnostic studies – laboratory evaluation
        i.   Serum sodium above 145 mEq/L and elevated HCT
        ii. Urine specific gravity greater than 1.025, and low urine
             sodium

5. **Complications**
   a. If ECF volume (increased sodium and H_2O) is increased, edematous states leading to hypertension, high cardiac output, and pulmonary congestion will occur
   b. If sodium retention occurs in presence of H_2O loss, severe dehydration leading to hypotension and increased serum osmolality will result in shock and respiratory arrest

6. **Specific patient care**
   a. Determine precipitating factors and treat as ordered
   b. Administer water in excess of sodium if patient requires volume (e.g., D_5W or 1/2 normal saline or both)
   c. Monitor serum sodium

ELECTROLYTE IMBALANCES – SODIUM IMBALANCE:

Hyponatremia – serum sodium level below 130 mEq/L.

1. **Pathophysiology**
   a. Excess of water relative to amount of sodium in body produces a dilutional effect on sodium concentration
   b. Salt (NaCl) loss in excess of water loss

2. **Etiology or precipitating factors**
   a. Water excess – excessive water intake without salt, and syndrome of inappropriate ADH
   b. Sodium depletion
      i. Diuretics
      ii. Diarrhea
      iii. Nasogastric suction
      iv. Abnormal losses via diaphoresis
      v. Iatrogenic – losses such as in diuretic therapy
      vi. Salt-losing renal diseases – interstitial nephritis
      vii. Hyperglycemia (glucose-induced diuresis)
   c. CHF/cirrhosis of liver
      i. Decreased cardiac output increases water retention by kidneys
      ii. Kidneys may retain larger amounts of water in excess of sodium

3. **Clinical presentation**: symptoms may be associated with dehydration if salt and H_2O loss occurs, or symptoms may relate to water retention
   a. Dehydration (decreased salt, decreased ECF volume) – dry mucous membranes, orthostatic hypotension, tachycardia, azotemia to oliguria

b. Water excess (salt loss and water retention): headache, lassitude, apathy, nausea, vomiting, diarrhea, muscle cramps and spasms. Severe imbalance may cause convulsions

4. **Diagnostic findings**
    a. History
        i.   General – see section on Hyperkalemia
        ii. Specific
            (a) Can be associated with chloride imbalance, acid-base imbalance, and shifts in quantity of body water
            (b) Complaints associated with dehydration (sodium and water loss), e.g., a history of taking salt-losing diuretics or excessive vomiting and diarrhea without adequate fluid and salt replacement
            (c) Complaints associated with water excess (sodium loss with increased ECF volume), e.g., when sodium depletion exists and only water is replaced. Common history of body fluid losses and IV therapy consisting of replacement with D_5W
    b. Physical examination – see section on Hyperkalemia
        i.   If sodium and water losses coexist, expect lassitude, apathy, tachycardia, orthostatic hypotension possibly progressing to shock state, decreased gastric motility leading to constipation, azotemia to oliguria, muscle spasms
        ii. If sodium is lost in presence of water excess, patient will show signs of water intoxication, usually demonstrated by CNS involvement – confusion, headache, general weakness, coma to convulsions
    c. Diagnostic studies – laboratory evaluation
        i.   Serum sodium below 130 mEq/L and decreased HCT due to water excess
        ii. Urine volume and urine specific gravity can be normal

5. **Complications**
    a. Rare
    b. Severe imbalance may lead to shock, coma, convulsion, and death

6. **Specific patient care**
    a. Administer diet high in sodium with adequate fluid intake
    b. Anticipate replacement with normal saline or hypertonic saline IV – watch carefully for pulmonary edema when giving these solutions
    c. Observe for changes in signs and symptoms during treatment
    d. Obtain serum sodium concentrations
    e. Discontinue diuretics if implicated in etiology
    f. Measure and record urine output – report any decreases

    g. Do not give hypertonic saline in syndrome of inappropriate ADH secretion – this does not correct basic cause and may precipitate CHF in susceptible patients

    h. In syndrome of inappropriate ADH restrict all water intake, since decreased sodium is result of inability to excrete water normally

ELECTROLYTE IMBALANCES – CALCIUM IMBALANCE:
Hypercalcemia – serum calcium level above 10.5 mg/dl.

1. **Pathophysiology**
   a. Increased mobilization of calcium from bone occurs in primary hyperparathyroidism, immobilization, and thyrotoxicosis
   b. Increased intestinal reabsorption of calcium secondary to large dietary intake and excessive administration of vitamin D
   c. Altered renal tubular reabsorption of calcium

2. **Etiology or precipitating factors**
   a. Primary hyperparathyroidism seen in adenoma or carcinoma of parathyroids (rare), resulting in increased tubular reabsorption of calcium
   b. Metastatic carcinoma with "osteolytic lesions" and in multiple myeloma; hypercalcemia is result of lesions releasing calcium into plasma
   c. Hypophosphatemia
   d. Immobilization – prolonged bed rest causes calcium to be mobilized from bone, teeth, and intestines
   e. Alkalosis – increases calcium binding to protein, raising serum calcium levels
   f. Thyrotoxicosis
   g. Excessive doses of vitamin D, which increase reabsorption of calcium from intestine
   h. Drugs – chronic thiazide diuretic therapy inhibits calcium excretion
   i. Renal tubular acidosis

3. **Clinical presentation**
   a. Neuromuscular weakness to flaccidity
   b. Renal calculi (secondary to high excretion of Ca^{+2}
   c. Flank and thigh pain in presence of calcium calculi in urinary tracts
   d. Subtle personality changes occur before changes in consciousness
   e. Change in level of consciousness
   f. Polyuria and polydipsia (increased calcium inhibits action of ADH on distal tubules and collecting ducts)
   g. Gastrointestinal symptoms – nausea, vomiting, thirst, anorexia, constipation

4. **Diagnostic findings**
   a. History
      i.   General – see section on Hyperkalemia
      ii. Specific – note whether history of excessive intake of vitamin D, chronic thiazide diuretic therapy, hyperparathyroidism, bone disease, tumor, or prolonged immobilization
   b. Physical examination – see section on Hyperkalemia
      i.   Mental status – extreme hypercalcemia producing lethargy, confusion to coma
      ii. Cardiac – if patient is taking digitalis, excitability may occur secondary to enhanced digitalis effect from hypercalcemia
      iii. Gastrointestinal – nausea and vomiting may be secondary to hypercalcemia, acting as a stimulus for gastric acid secretion, and possible development of peptic ulcer disease. Inadequate peristalsis is related to hypotonicity of smooth muscle of the bowel, leading to constipation
      iv. Neuromuscular – hypotonicity/weakness of muscles
      v.   Skeletal – pathologic fractures, metastatic calcifications affecting extraosseous soft tissue seen in hyperparathyroidism
      vi. Genitourinary – polyuria
      vii. Ocular – observe for metastatic calcifications, usually calcium crystals deposited in cornea and visible by slit lamp examination.   If extensive they will be visible to naked eye as band keratopathy (semilunar whitish bands, beginning as parenthesis at lateral margins of cornea and extending in a band across cornea)
   c. Diagnostic studies
      i.   Laboratory
           (a) Serum calcium above 10.5 mg/dl
           (b) Sulkowitch urine test for calcium
      ii. Radiologic
           (a) Renal calculi
           (b) Calcium deposits on bone films
           (c) Nephrocalcinosis – calcium deposits in renal parenchyma
      iii. Special – ECG reveals shortening of S-T segment

5. **Complications**
   a. Renal calculi due to excessive urinary calcium
   b. Neuropathies or decreased level or consciousness due to depressant action of excess calcium on central and peripheral nervous systems
   c. Cardiac dysrhythmias due to stimulation of myocardium by excess calcium

6. **Specific patient care**
   a. Assessment
      i. Cardiac – monitor for ECG changes. If administering digitalis, do so cautiously – hypercalcemia enhances action of digitalis, and toxicity can result
      ii. Renal – ensure meticulous accuracy in recording intake and output
      iii. Neurologic – check signs frequently
   b. Anticipate use of therapies to reduce serum calcium level
      i. Normal saline infusion and diuretics increase GFR and calcium excretion
      ii. Corticosteroids decrease gastrointestinal absorption of calcium
      iii. Mithramycin therapy stimulates bone uptake of calcium
      iv. Phosphate binds calcium in gut and precipitates calcium when given IV

ELECTROLYTE IMBALANCES – CALCIUM IMBALANCE: Hypocalcemia – serum calcium level below 8.5 mg/dl.

1. **Pathophysiology**
   a. Excessive gastrointestinal losses of calcium secondary to diarrhea, effect of diuretics, and increased levels of lipoproteins
   b. Malabsorption syndromes such as vitamin D deficiency and hypoparathyroidism

2. **Etiology or precipitating factors**
   a. Hypoparathyroidism
      i. Surgical ablation of parathyroids
      ii. Parathyroid adenoma
      iii. Idiopathic
      iv. Depletion of magnesium – needed for effective action of PTH
   b. Chronic renal failure
      i. Hyperphosphatemia – potentiates peripheral deposition of calcium
      ii. Vitamin D resistance – inability to absorb calcium from intestine which is vitamin D-mediated
   c. Vitamin D deficiency secondary to chronic renal failure, hepatic failure, and rickets – "active" vitamin D is necessary for calcium absorption
   d. Chronic malabsorption syndrome resulting from
      i. Magnesium depletion
      ii. Gastrectomy
      iii. Fat diet – fat impairs calcium absorption
      iv. Small bowel disorders – inability to absorb vitamin D

    e. Increased thyrocalcitonin — stimulates osteoblasts to prevent calcium entry into serum

    f. Malignancy

        i. Osteoblastic metastases — calcium is consumed for abnormal bone synthesis

       ii. Medullary carcinoma of thyroid — abnormal secretion of thyrocalcitonin

    g. Acute pancreatitis — precipitation of calcium in inflamed pancreas and intra-abdominal lipids

    h. Hyperphosphatemia — calcium and phosphate bind together and precipitate in tissues

        i. Cytotoxic drugs (cytolysis of bone)

       ii. Increased oral intake of phosphates

      iii. Chronic renal failure (decreased excretion of PO_4^{-3})

3. **Clinical presentation**

    a. Neuromuscular irritability — muscle cramps to tetany

    b. Bronchospasm — tetany of laryngeal or respiratory muscles

    c. Biliary colic

    d. Tonic/clonic seizures

4. **Diagnostic findings**

    a. History

        i. General — see section on Hyperkalemia

       ii. Specific — hypoparathyroidism, acute pancreatitis, chronic nutritional derangements such as high protein diets, massive infection of subcutaneous tissue, chronic bone pain, chronic renal failure

    b. Physical examination

        i. Pulmonary — labored shallow breathing, wheezes and bronchospasm if respiratory musculature is involved. Neuromuscular irritability can cause airway obstruction and bronchial spasm

       ii. Neuromuscular — muscle tremors and cramps may accompany minor reductions in calcium level; tetany and generalized tonic/clonic seizures develop with severe reductions

           (a) Chvostek sign — tap finger over supramandibular portion of parotid gland, and observe twitches in upper lip on side of stimulation. This muscle spasm indicates a positive test. False responses can occur

           (b) Trousseau's sign — apply BP cuff to upper arm, and inflate cuff until carpopedal spasm develops. If spasm is present, test is positive; if no spasm appears in 3 minutes, test is negative. Remove cuff and tell patient to hyperventilate (30 times/minute). Respiratory alkalosis that develops can also produce carpopedal spasm (positive if occurs)

      iii. Gastrointestinal – paralytic ileus
      iv. Hematopoietic – bleeding secondary to changes in clotting
           mechanism, since calcium is necessary for normal clotting
  c. Diagnostic studies
      i. Laboratory – serum calcium below 8.5 mg/dl

5. Complications
  a. Bronchospasm may lead to respiratory arrest
  b. Decreased cardiac contractility may lead to cardiac arrest

6. Specific patient care
  a. Administer IV 10% calcium gluconate or calcium chloride
      i. Place patient on cardiac monitor
      ii. Rapid infusion may enhance digitalis
  b. If vitamin D deficiency is present, administer vitamin D
     supplements
  c. If phosphate deficiency is evident, replace phosphates before
     administering calcium
  d. Monitor serum calcium, phosphate, and potassium levels
  e. Assess and evaluate therapy by use of Chvostek and
     Trousseau signs, and ECG

ELECTROLYTE IMBALANCES – PHOSPHATE IMBALANCE:
Hyperphosphatemia – serum phosphate level above 5.5 mg/dl.

1. Pathophysiology
  a. Inability to excrete phosphate via kidney due to decreased GFR
     to one-tenth of normal, or to renal failure
  b. Excessive intake due to dietary or cathartic abuse and drugs
     (cytotoxic agents)

2. Etiology or precipitating factors
  a. Acute/chronic renal failure (inability to excrete phosphate)
  b. Hypoparathyroidism – PTH effect on kidney is to cause
     phosphatemia and lower body phosphate
  c. Cathartic abuse of phosphate-containing laxatives and enemas
  d. Cytotoxic agents for neoplasms – serum phosphate increases
     due to cytolysis; seen in leukemias or lymphomas
  e. Overadministration of IV or oral phosphates

3. Clinical presentation: same as for hypocalcemia

4. Diagnostic findings
  a. History
      i. General – see section on Hyperkalemia
      ii. Specific – presentation similar to that of hypocalcemia
         (see neuromuscular changes compatible with hypocalcemia,
         e.g., cramps, tetany, etc.). Since phosphate is necessary for

entry of calcium into bone, elevated phosphate level accelerates this process
  b. Physical examination — see specific history above
  c. Diagnostic studies
    i. Laboratory — serum phosphate greater than 5.5 mg/dl
    ii. Special — ECG changes comparable with those seen in hypocalcemia (e.g., prolongation of S-T segment)

5. **Complications**
  a. Signs and symptoms compatible with hypocalcemia
  b. Seizures — chronic phosphate elevation may depress calcium levels to point of precipitating seizures
  c. Metastatic calcification — precipitation of calcium phosphate in arteries, soft tissues, and joints

6. **Specific patient care**
  a. Administer aluminum hydroxide gels to bind phosphate in intestines, limiting its absorption, and thus reducing serum phosphate levels
  b. Teach patient purpose of gels (easy to confuse with antacid owing to similarity in drug preparation)

ELECTROLYTE IMBALANCES — PHOSPHATE IMBALANCE:
Hypophosphatemia — serum phosphate level below 3.5 mg/dl.

1. **Pathophysiology**
  a. Increased cell uptake to form sugar phosphates occurs during hyperventilation or increased glucose administration, e.g., parenteral hyperalimentation
  b. Decreased phosphate absorption from bowel
  c. Renal phosphate wasting (loss of proximal tubular function), seen in Fanconi's syndrome and vitamin D-resistant rickets

2. **Etiology or precipitating factors**
  a. Inadequate phosphate intake (seen in chronic alcoholism)
  b. Chronic phosphate depletion — occurs in osteomalacia and rickets
  c. Long-term hyperalimentation lacking in phosphates. Glucose phosphorylation utilizes phosphate, and can lead to phosphate depletion if no replacement is available
  d. Hyperparathyroidism — causes renal phosphaturia
  e. Malabsorption syndrome
  f. Abuse or overadministration of phosphate-binding gels, e.g., Amphojel
  g. Fanconi's syndrome — loss of phosphates in urine leading to osteomalacia (adults)

3. **Clinical presentation**
   a. Muscle weakness (lack of intracellular phosphates may prevent energy-producing metabolic processes)
   b. Hemolytic anemia
   c. Mental confusion

4. **Diagnostic findings**
   a. History
      i. General – see section on Hyperkalemia
      ii. Specific
         (a) Complaints of vague physical symptoms associated with muscle weakness. Symptoms result from acute depletion of intracellular ATP, which leads to a diffuse, muscle-wasting necrosis called "rhabdomyolysis"
         (b) Chronic depletion – complaints of anorexia, malaise, muscle wasting, weakness
         (c) Hypercalcemia and hypercalciuria, one of the indicators of acute phosphate depletion in hyperparathyroidism. PTH increases serum calcium by taking it from bone, and decreases serum phosphate by excreting it into urine
   b. Physical examination – see section on Hyperkalemia
      i. Muscle wasting and weakness
      ii. Hematopoietic – hemolysis and hypoxia resulting from deficit in RBC phosphate content necessary for 2, 3-diphosphoglycerate. A decreased intracellular level of 2,3-DPG is associated with a hemolytic reaction and a decrease in dissociation of oxygen from hemoglobin
   c. Diagnostic studies
      i. Laboratory – serum phosphate below 3.5 mg/dl, low serum alkaline pyrophosphate, high serum pyrophosphate.
      ii. Radiologic – skeletal abnormalities resembling osteomalacia (e.g., pseudofractures characterized by thickened periosteum and new bone formation over what appears to be an incomplete fracture)

5. **Complications**
   a. Osteomalacia – seen with long-standing hypophosphatemia. It is result of excessive losses of external phosphate
   b. Zieves syndrome – a severe intravascular hemolysis usually observed in alcoholics, and caused by phosphate depletion that results in decrease in RBC 2, 3-DPG

6. **Specific patient care**
   a. Replace phosphates IV, then orally
   b. Treat primary cause of hypophosphatemia
   c. Discontinue phosphate-binding gels

REFERENCES

Anderson, R.J., Berl, T., McDonald, K.M., and Schrier, R.W.: Clinical disorders of water metabolism. Kidney Int. *10:* 117, 1976.

Aronoff, G.: Antimicrobial therapy in patients with impaired renal function. Dialysis Transplant. 1 *8:*14, 1979.

Brundage, D.: Nursing Management of Renal Problems. C.V. Mosby Co., St. Louis, 1976.

Christopherson, L.K., and Gonde, T.A.: Patterns of grief: end-stage renal failure and kidney transplantation. J. Thanato. *3:*49–57, 1975.

Cleland, V., et al.: Prevention of bacteriuria in female patients with indwelling catheters. Nurs. Res. *20:*309, 1971.

Cobb, S.: Social support as a moderator of life stress. Psychosom. Med. *38:*300–314, 1976.

Dolan, P.O., and Greene, H.L.: Renal failure and peritoneal dialysis. Nursing *75:*40, 1975.

Drutz, D.: Altered cell-mediated immunity and its relationship to infection susceptibility in patients with uremia. Dialysis Transplant. 4 *8:*320, 1979.

Friedman, E.A.: Strategy in Renal Failure. John Wiley & Sons, New York, 1978.

Gambertoglio, J.: Pharmacokinetic principles and renal disease. Dialysis Transplant. 1 *8:*8, 1979.

Ganong, W.F.: Review of Medical Physiology. Lange Medical Publication, Los Altos, CA, 1971, p. 515.

Gebbie, K., and Lavin, M.: Classification of Nursing Diagnoses. C.V. Mosby Co., St. Louis, 1975.

Gibson, T.: Dialyzability of common therapeutic agents. Dialysis Transplant. 1 *8:*24, 1979.

Gulyassy, P.: Abnormal drug binding in uremia. Dialysis Transplant. 1 *8:*19, 1979.

Hall, R., et al.: Attitudes toward illness as a predictor of adjustment of chronic hemodialysis. Dialysis Transplant. 2 *8:*138, 1979.

Hariprasad, M., and Eisinger, R.: Experience with a one-bed acute hemodialysis unit. Dialysis Transplant. 6 *8:*596, 1979.

Hekelman, F.P., and Ostendarp, C.A.: Nephrology Nursing Perspectives of Care. McGraw-Hill Book Co., New York, 1979.

Judge, R.D., and Zuidema, G.D.: Physical Diagnosis — A Physiologic Approach to the Clinical Examination. Little, Brown, & Co., Boston, 1963.

King, P.: Legislation and stress in the renal patient. Dialysis Transplant. 10 *8:*952, 1979.

Kossoris, P.: Family therapy: an adjunct to hemodialysis and transplantation. Am. J. Nurs. *70:*1730, 1970.

Kroah, J.: An exploratory study of the strategies that renal nurses use in response to emotional reaction and behaviors of hemodialysis patients. Image *5:*16, 1972.

Leaf, A., and Cotran, R.: Renal Pathophysiology. Oxford University Press, New York, 1976.

Levinsky, N.G.: The interpretation of proteinuria and the urinary sediment. DM *3–40,* 1967.

Lipowski, A.J.: Physical illness: The individual and the coping process. Psychiatry in Med. *1:*91, 1970.

Merrill, R.H.: Review of vascular access. Dialysis Transplant. 6 *9:*22–28, 1977.

Normark, M., and Rohweder, A.: Scientific Foundations of Nursing. J.B. Lippincott Co., Philadelphia, 1975.

Papper, S.: Clinical Nephrology. Little, Brown & Co., Boston, 1971.

Rodriguez, D.: Moral issues in hemodialysis and renal transplantation. Nursing Forum *10:*201, 1971.

Rose, B.: Clinical Physiology of Acid-Base and Electrolyte Disorders. McGraw-Hill Book Co., New York, 1977.

Schlott, L.: Nursing and the Nephrology Patient. Medical Examination Publishing Co., Inc., New York, 1973.

Schrier, R.W.: Renal and Electrolyte Disorders. Little, Brown, & Co., Boston, 1976, pp. 304–305.

Schroeder, J., and Daily, E.: Techniques in Bedside Hemodynamic Monitoring. C.V. Mosby Co., St. Louis, 1976.

Stark, J.: Renal failure: imbalances inevitable. *In* Monitoring Fluid and Electrolytes Precisely. Nursing Skill Books, Philadelphia, 1978.

Stark, J.: BUN/creatinine — your keys to kidney function. Nursing 80 #5 *10:* 33, 1980.

Strout, V., Lee, C., and Schapen, C.A.: Fluid and Electrolytes. F.A. Davis Co., Philadelphia, 1977.

Teschan, P.: Neurologic aspects of renal disease. Dialysis Transplant. 6 *8*:646, 1979.

Thiele, N.F.: Clinical Nutrition. C.V. Mosby Co., St. Louis, 1976.

Ulrich, B.: Nephrology nurse: teaching the teachers to teach. Dialysis Transplant. 7 *8*:744, 1979.

Valtin, H.: Renal Dysfunction: Mechanisms Involved in Fluid and Solute Imbalance. Little, Brown, & Co., Boston, 1979.

Villazon, A., Portos, J., and Sierra, A.: Polyuric syndromes in the critically ill patient. Crit. Care Med. *4*:25, 1976.

Widmann, F.: Clinical Interpretation of Laboratory Tests. F.A. Davis Co., Philadelphia, 1973.

Zschoche, D.: Comprehensive Review of Critical Care. C.V. Mosby Co., St. Louis, 1976.

THE ENDOCRINE SYSTEM

prepared by

HELEN HOLLMANN, R.N., B.A., CCRN

BEHAVIORAL OBJECTIVES

Functional Anatomy

1. Describe the anatomic location and the parts of each endocrine gland.
2. List the hormones produced by each endocrine gland.
3. Explain the mechanisms that regulate the secretory functions of each gland.

Physiology

1. Describe the effects of each hormone on its respective target cells.
2. Describe the endocrine responses to stress

Assessment

1. Describe a systematic process for assessment of the endocrine system, using the history and physical examination.
2. Identify and justify the diagnostic studies used in assessment of the endocrine system.

General Patient Care Management

1. Discuss the influence of selected endocrine disorders on other body systems.
2. Develop a general nursing care plan that will enable the nurse to care for a patient with an endocrine disorder.

Pathologic Conditions and Management

For each of the following: diabetes insipidus, inappropriate secretion of ADH, thyrotoxic crisis, hypoparathyroidism, acute adrenal insufficiency, diabetic ketoacidosis, hyperosmolar coma, and hypoglycemic reaction:

1. Describe the physiologic derangements of the disorder.
2. Describe a systematic approach to diagnosis based on clinical presentation, the presence of etiologic or precipitating factors, and the results of diagnostic testing.
3. Identify and justify the treatment modalities used in the management of the disorder.
4. Outline the essential elements of a nursing care plan formulated to meet the needs of patients with the disorder.

THE ENDOCRINE SYSTEM

─────────── **FUNCTIONAL ANATOMY** ───────────

PITUITARY GLAND (HYPOPHYSIS)

1. **Location:** at base of brain, inferior to hypothalamus, in sella turcica of sphenoid bone

2. **Consists of two lobes**
   a. Anterior (adenohypophysis)
      i. Joins hypothalamus via a portal vascular system
      ii. Produces at least seven known hormones
         (a) Growth hormone (GH)
         (b) Adrenocorticotropic hormone (ACTH)
         (c) Thyroid-stimulating hormone (TSH)
         (d) Melanocyte-stimulating hormone (MSH)
         (e) Follicle-stimulating hormone (FSH)
         (f) Prolactin (PRL)
         (g) Luteinizing hormone (LH) – females
         (h) Interstitial cell-stimulating hormone (ICSH) – males
      iii. Secretory activities are controlled by tropic hormones produced by and transmitted from hypothalamus in response to negative feedback mechanisms
   b. Posterior (neurohypophysis)
      i. Is connected to hypothalamus by neural tissue
      ii. Produces two hormones
         (a) Antidiuretic hormone (ADH, vasopressin)
         (b) Oxytocic hormone (oxytocin)
      iii. Secretion is regulated by nerve impulses originating in hypothalamus in response to stimuli from other parts of body

THYROID GLAND

1. **Consists of two lobes:** connected by strip of tissue called the isthmus

2. **Location:** lies across second and third tracheal rings in anterior middle portion of neck

3. **Produces three hormones**
   a. Thyroxine (T_4)
   b. Triiodothyronine (T_3)
   c. Thyrocalcitonin (calcitonin)

4. **Secretion**: regulated by TSH from anterior pituitary, which in turn is regulated by thyrotropin-releasing hormone (TRH) from hypothalamus

PARATHYROID GLAND

1. **Consists of four flattened bodies**: located on posterior surface of thyroid, one at upper and lower poles of each thyroid lobe

2. **Produces parathyroid hormone (PTH, parathormone)**

3. **Secretion**: controlled by a negative feedback mechanism that operates between glands and blood calcium level

ADRENAL GLANDS

1. **Paired, triangular-shaped bodies**: lying retroperitoneally at apex of each kidney

2. **Composed of two divisions**
   a. Cortex (80% of gland)
      i.   Outer portion of gland consisting of three different histologic zones
      ii. Produces three categories of hormones – glucocorticoids, mineralocorticoids, and androgens
      iii. Regulatory mechanisms
         (a) ACTH stimulates secretion of large amounts of glucocorticoids, small amounts of mineralocorticoids (not prime regulator), and androgen production
         (b) Renin-angiotensin system is sensitive to changes in blood volume, and responds by stimulating secretion of large amounts of mineralocorticoids
   b. Medulla
      i.   Inner portion of gland that produces catecholamines – epinephrine and norepinephrine
      ii. Regulated by neural stimuli that result in increased catecholamine production

PANCREAS

1. **Location**: lies transversely across posterior abdominal wall between duodenum and spleen

2. **Composed of head, body, and tail**

3. **Has two main cell types**
   a. Acinar cells that have an exocrine function (see GI section)
   b. Islet cells that serve an endocrine function

    i.   Alpha cells secrete glucagon, which raises blood glucose by increasing hepatic glycogenolysis and glyconeogenesis. Secretion is stimulated by hypoglycemia, starvation, increased catecholamine secretion, excessive muscle exercise, and pheochromocytoma

    ii.   Beta cells secrete insulin, which enhances rate of glucose metabolism, decreases blood glucose levels, and increases glycogen stores in tissues. Secretion is stimulated by hyperglycemia, GH, ACTH, secretin, gastrin, glucagon, and amino acids

PHYSIOLOGY

HORMONES OF THE ANTERIOR PITUITARY GLAND (ADENOHYPO-PHYSIS): These control the activity of the thyroid, adrenal cortex, gonads, and mammary glands. They also affect general cellular metabolism and reproduction, as well as pigmentation of the skin.

1. **Growth hormone (GH):** also known as somatotropic hormone (STH)
   a. Release-stimulating factors
      i. Growth hormone releasing factor (GRF) from hypothalamus
      ii. Hypoglycemia
      iii. Decrease in amino acids
      iv. Exercise
   b. Release-inhibiting factors
      i. Growth hormone inhibiting factor (GIF, somatostatin) from hypothalamus
      ii. Hyperglycemia
      iii. Prolonged, excessive corticosteroid levels
   c. Target – body cells
   d. Normal effects
      i. Stimulation of protein anabolism
      ii. Mobilization of fat stores
      iii. Conservation of carbohydrates
      iv. Indirect stimulation of bone and cartilage growth
   e. Effects of increased levels – gigantism in childhood, acromegaly in adulthood
   f. Effects of decreased levels – dwarfism in childhood, decreased organ weight in adulthood

2. **Adrenocorticotropic hormone (ACTH)**
   a. Release-stimulating factors
      i. Corticotropin releasing factor (CRF) from hypothalamus
      ii. Stress
      iii. Hypoglycemia
      iv. Decreased cortisol levels

    b. Release-inhibiting factor — increased cortisol level

    c. Target — cells of adrenal cortex

    d. Normal effects

        i.   Regulation of growth and function of adrenal cortex

        ii. Control of production and release of glucocorticoid hormones

        iii. Stimulation of androgen production

        iv. Stimulation of mineralocorticoid production (not primary regulator)

    e. Effect of increased levels — Cushing's disease

    f. Effects of decreased levels — adrenal atrophy, decreased steroid production

3. **Thyroid-stimulating hormone (TSH)**

    a. Release-stimulating factors

        i.   Thyrotropin-releasing hormone (TRH) from hypothalamus

        ii. Cold

        iii. Decreased thyroid hormone levels

    b. Release-inhibiting factors

        i.   Sympathetic stimulation

        ii. Increased thyroid hormone levels

    c. Target — cells of thyroid gland

    d. Normal effect — stimulation of increased growth and function of thyroid cells

    e. Effects of increased or decreased levels — enhancement or inhibition of thyroid growth and function, respectively

4. **Melanocyte-stimulating hormone (MSH)**

    a. Release-stimulating factors

        i.   Hypothalamic releasing factor (possibly linked to CRF)

        ii. Decreased cortisol levels

    b. Release-inhibiting factors

        i.   Possible inhibitor factor from hypothalamus

        ii. Increased cortisol level

    c. Targets — skin cells

    d. Normal effect — regulation of amount of skin pigmentation deposited

    e. Effects of increased or decreased levels — increased or diminished pigmentation of skin, respectively

5. **Follicle-stimulating hormone (FSH)**

    a. Release-stimulating factor — follicle hormone releasing factor (FRF) from hypothalamus

    b. Targets — cells of ovaries or testes

    c. Normal effect — stimulation of growth of ovarian follicles or sperm

    d. Effects of increased or decreased levels — development of early or late puberty, respectively

6. **Prolactin (PRL):** formerly known as lactogenic hormone (LTH)
   a. Release-stimulating factor
      i. Suckling
      ii. Inhibition of hypothalamic prolactin-inhibiting factor (PIF)
   b. Target — cells of breast
   c. Normal effect — stimulation of lactation

7. **Luteinizing hormone (LH) in females; interstitial cell-stimulating hormone (ICSH) in males**
   a. Release-stimulating factor — luteinizing hormone releasing hormone (LHRH)
   b. Targets — cells of ovaries or testes
   c. Normal effects
      i. Stimulation of growth of corpus luteum, increased secretion of estrogen and progesterone
      ii. Stimulation of increased testosterone production and development of male sex characteristics

HORMONES OF THE POSTERIOR PITUITARY GLAND (NEUROHYPOPHYSIS)

1. **Antidiuretic hormone (ADH, vasopressin)**
   a. Release-stimulating factor — increased serum osmolality, causing stimulation of osmoreceptors in hypothalamus
   b. Release-inhibiting factors
      i. Decreased serum osmolality
      ii. Inflammatory conditions within hypothalamus or pituitary
      iii. Surgery of pituitary
   c. Targets
      i. Distal renal tubules and collecting ducts
      ii. Smooth muscle of arterioles and GI tract
   d. Normal effects
      i. Constriction of arterioles in shock
      ii. Increased water reabsorption by kidney tubules
      iii. Abdominal cramping
   e. Effects of increased levels — hyponatremia and/or water intoxication
   f. Effects of decreased levels — diuresis and dehydration

2. **Oxytocic hormone (oxytocin)**
   a. Release-stimulating factors — childbirth and/or suckling
   b. Targets — cells of uterus and breasts
   c. Normal effects — stimulation of uterine contraction and lactation

HORMONES OF THE THYROID GLAND

1. **Thyroxine (T_4):** a combination of iodine and tyrosine that binds with plasma protein upon entering circulation; comprises 90% of secreted thyroid hormones
   a. Release-stimulating factors — TSH, TRH, or cold temperature
   b. Release-inhibiting factors — increased glucocorticoids or TSH deficiency
   c. Target — all body cells
   d. Normal effects
      i. Increased protein synthesis, increased carbohydrate and fat metabolism
      ii. Increased cyclic AMP in muscle cells
      iii. Increased bone growth
   e. Effects of increased levels
      i. Increased gland size
      ii. Loss of weight with increased appetite
      iii. Diarrhea
      iv. Decreased tolerance to heat
      v. Tremors and muscle weakness
      vi. Menstrual irregularities
      vii. Tachycardia
      viii. Exophthalmos
      ix. Accelerated growth in children
   f. Effects of decreased levels
      i. Hypertrophy of gland
      ii. Decreased metabolic activity
      iii. Cardiomegaly and heart failure
      iv. Lethargy and fatigue
      v. Increase in weight
      vi. Intolerance to cold
      vii. Dry skin and hair; decreased perspiration
      viii. Constipation
      ix. Memory lapse and decreased concentration
      x. Periorbital edema

2. **Triiodothyronine (T_3):** a combination of iodine and tyrosine that binds with plasma protein for transport. Four times more potent than T_4; comprises 10% of secreted thyroid hormones. Release-stimulating and inhibiting factors, target, normal effects, and effects of increased or decreased levels are all same as for thyroxine

3. **Thyrocalcitonin (calcitonin)**
   a. Produced in C cells of thyroid gland
   b. Release-stimulating factors
      i. Increased serum calcium
      ii. Administration of magnesium or glucagon

    c. Targets — bone cells

    d. Normal effects

        i. Reduction of plasma calcium by inhibiting bone resorption (lysis and assimilation of bone)

        ii. Increased urinary phosphate, sodium, chloride, magnesium, and calcium excretion

HORMONE OF THE PARATHYROID GLANDS:

This needs adequate vitamin D levels to exert hormonal effects at gastrointestinal and bone sites.

1. **Parathyroid hormone (PTH, parathormone)**
   a. Release-stimulating factors
      i. Low serum calcium
      ii. Elevated magnesium or phosphate level (indirect effect)
   b. Release-inhibiting factors — increased calcium levels or increased vitamin D intake
   c. Targets — bone, GI tract, and kidney cells
   d. Normal effects
      i. Increased bone resorption of calcium
      ii. Increased gastrointestinal absorption of calcium
      iii. Increased absorption of ionized calcium, decreased reabsorption of phosphate, increased bicarbonate excretion in renal tubule
   e. Effects of increased levels
      i. Fatigue, lethargy, weakness
      ii. Headache
      iii. Hypercalcemia, renal calculi, polyuria
   f. Effects of decreased levels — hypocalcemia, tremors, tetany

HORMONES OF THE ADRENAL CORTEX

1. **Glucocorticoids:** cortisol most important
   a. Release-stimulating factors
      i. ACTH
      ii. Stress
      iii. Trauma
      iv. Infection
      v. CRF
   b. Release-inhibiting factor — negative feedback mechanism to hypothalamus (e.g., exogenous corticosteroids)
   c. Targets — all body cells, including liver cells
   d. Normal effects
      i. Stimulation of glyconeogenesis in liver; inhibition of glucose utilization in cells; inhibition of rate of protein synthesis; promotion of fatty acid mobilization from adipose tissue, resulting in increased blood glucose concentrations
      ii. Inhibition of inflammatory process

        e. Effects of increased levels
            i.   Deposition of fat in face and trunk
           ii.   Wasting of extremities, with thinning of skin
          iii. Weakness and fatigue
          iv. Irritability and depression
           v.   Increased blood sugar
          vi. Increased blood pressure
         vii. Interference with immune response
        f. Effects of decreased levels
            i.   Decreased blood pressure
           ii.   Weight loss and weakness
          iii. Hypoglycemia
          iv. Increased skin pigmentation

2. Mineralocorticoids: aldosterone
    a. Release-stimulating factors
        i.   Renin-angiotensin mechanism
        ii.   Decreased serum sodium, increased serum potassium
       iii. ACTH (supportive effect only – not essential for
             aldosterone release)
    b. Targets
        i.   Distal and collecting tubules of kidney
        ii.   Sweat glands
    c. Normal Effect
        i.   Increased sodium reabsorption and potassium excretion
        ii.   Increased ECF volume
    d. Effects of increased levels – hypertension, decreased potassium
       levels, weakness
    e. Effects of decreased levels – decreased serum sodium, increased
       water loss

3. Androgens
    a. In normal amounts, have minimal body effects
    b. Effects of increased levels – precocious sexual development in
       male, virilization in female

HORMONES OF THE ADRENAL MEDULLA (CATECHOLAMINES):

These are also synthesized by sympathetic nerve endings, peripheral tissue, and the brain. They are stored in "granules" in various tissues.

1. Epinephrine (Adrenalin): 80% of medullary secretion
    a. Release-stimulating factors
        i.   Sympathetic nerve stimulation
        ii.   Hormonal stimulation – insulin and histamine
    b. Targets – body cells, vascular beds, smooth muscle
    c. Normal Effects
        i.   Dilatation of pupils

    ii.   Positive chronotropic and inotropic effects on heart, with resultant increase in systolic pressure and cardiac output

    iii. Dilatation of blood vessels in heart and skeletal muscles; constriction in abdominal viscera and skin

    iv. Increase in perspiration

    v.   Dilatation of bronchioles, increased rate and depth of breathing

    vi. Decrease in peristalsis and secretion in GI tract

    vii. Contraction of urinary sphincter

    viii. Increased blood sugar

  d. Effects of increased levels – exaggeration or prolongation of normal effects

  e. Effects of decreased levels – slight or none

2. **Norepinephrine:** 20% of medullary secretion

  a. Release-stimulating factors – same as epinephrine

  b. Targets – body cells, vascular beds

  c. Normal effects – similar to epinephrine, but differs in following ways

    i.   Has lesser effect on cardiac and metabolic activities

    ii. Has greater vasoconstrictor activity in muscles – thus, increases peripheral vascular resistance

HORMONES OF PANCREAS

1. **Insulin**

  a. Release-stimulating and synthesis factors – increase in blood sugar and growth hormone levels

  b. Targets – body cells, especially liver cells

  c. Normal effects

    i.   Enhancement of glucose transport across cell membrane

    ii. Stimulation of protein synthesis

    iii. Inhibition of triglyceride breakdown in cell

    iv. Promotion of fatty acid storage

  d. Effect of increased levels – hypoglycemia

  e. Effects of decreased levels – hyperglycemia, ketosis, acidosis

2. **Glucagon**

  a. Release-stimulating factors

    i.   Decreased blood glucose

    ii. Elevated blood amino acids

  b. Targets – body cells, especially liver cells

  c. Normal effects

    i.   Stimulation of glycogenolysis, inhibition of glycolysis

    ii. Increased urea formation and fatty-acid oxidation

  d. Effect of increased levels – hyperglycemia

  e. Effect of decreased levels – idiopathic hypoglycemia

_____ **ASSESSMENT** _____

HISTORY

1. **Medical history:** current and significant past
    a. Cardiac and peripheral vascular disease
    b. Pulmonary disease
    c. Hypertension
    d. Renal disease
    e. CNS disease/condition
    f. Pre-existing endocrine disorders

2. **Symptoms:** important to establish onset, duration, intensity, frequency, and change in patterns. Signs and symptoms of endocrine disorders are extremely complex owing to many body systems that may be involved in any disorder
    a. Headache and vertigo
    b. Visual disturbances
        i. Blurring
        ii. Dimming of vision
        iii. Blind spots
    c. Change in taste, smell
    d. Changes in ability to phonate, difficulty in speech articulation
    e. Dysphagia
    f. Dyspnea and palpitations
    g. Polydipsia and polyphagia
    h. Polyuria, nocturia, oliguria
    i. Gastrointestinal disturbances, weight change
    j. Muscular weakness, cramping, tremors
    k. Changes in skin texture and color
    l. Changes in hair distribution and texture
    m. Changes in energy levels
    n. Intolerance to heat, cold
    o. Changes in personality
        i. Confusion
        ii. Irritability
        iii. Depression
        iv. Nervousness

3. **Medication history**
    a. Tranquilizers, narcotics
    b. Hypoglycemic agents, steroids
    c. Electrolyte supplements
    d. Cardiotonics, antiarrhythmic agents
    e. Oral contraceptives
    f. Synthetic hormones
    g. Chemotherapy

PHYSICAL EXAMINATION

1. **Inspection**
   a. General appearance
      i. Stature and distribution of subcutaneous fat relative to maturation level
      ii. Appearance relative to age, sex
      iii. Facial expression, body movement, stature
   b. Distribution of hair — scalp, facial, body
   c. Eyes
      i. Sunken
      ii. Exophthalmos
      iii. Periorbital edema
      iv. Visual acuity
   d. Facial features — bone structure
   e. Mouth
      i. Mucous membranes
      ii. Tongue — thickness, color, tremors
   f. Neck — as patient swallows, observe for motion of thyroid cartilage or lack of motion of any detectable masses
   g. Level of consciousness, general behavior
   h. Skin — turgor, pigmentation, lesions, vascularity, texture

2. **Palpation**: check for
   a. Enlarged thyroid — palpate neck first while standing in front of patient; also palpate with thumbs while standing behind patient
   b. Thrills over thyroid arteries
   c. Enlargement of masses above kidney or in abdomen

3. **Auscultation**: check thyroid gland for bruits

4. **Vital signs and temperature**

DIAGNOSTIC STUDIES

1. **Laboratory**
   a. Blood
      i. Electrolytes
      ii. T_3, T_4, cortisol, and other hormone assays
      iii. Glucose and glucose tolerance
      iv. BUN, cholesterol, calcium, phosphate, alkaline phosphatase, creatinine
      v. CBC, culture and sensitivity
   b. Urine
      i. Routine urinalysis
      ii. Sugar and acetone
      iii. Adrenal hormone assays (e.g., 17-ketosteroid)

      iv.   Culture and sensitivity
      v.   Catecholamines
      vi.   Osmolality, electrolytes

2. **Radiologic**
   a. Chest x-ray
   b. Thyroid scan
   c. Pancreatic scan
   d. Abdominal x-rays
   e. Long bone x-rays
   f. Skull x-rays
   g. Adrenal arteriography
   h. Computerized axial tomography (CT)

3. **Special:** 12-lead ECG

GENERAL PATIENT CARE MANAGEMENT*

1. **Maintenance of fluid and electrolyte balance:** see pp. 283–285
   a. Monitor intake and output; weigh daily
   b. Monitor vital signs; identify trends
   c. Monitor and interpret dysrhythmias
   d. Administer and maintain parenteral therapy
   e. Monitor and interpret laboratory data
   f. Test urine for specific gravity, sugar, acetone, and protein
   g. Assess physical parameters and interpret findings
      i.   Skin turgor, color, temperature
      ii. Muscle tone, coordination

2. **Maintenance of patent airway and ventilation:** see pp. 31–39

3. **Maintenance of acid-base balance:** see pp. 19–22

4. **Assessment of neurologic status:** see pp. 197–204

5. **Provision of emotional and psychologic support:** for patient and family

6. **Assessment of patient's health and illness status:** to prevent complications or recognize them early

---

*Patients with endocrine system disorders are not routinely admitted to the critical care unit, unless they are in crisis and have multiple system failure, or definitive therapy is planned.

7. **Provision of patient and family education**: regarding
   a. Patient's disorder, status, and limitations
   b. Medication regime
   c. Complications

PATHOLOGIC CONDITIONS AND MANAGEMENT

DIABETES INSIPIDUS

1. **Pathophysiology**: defect in release or synthesis of ADH or a defect in renal tubular response to ADH, causing impaired renal conservation of water

2. **Etiology or precipitating factors**
   a. Hereditary — rare
   b. Traumatic
      i. Skull fracture causing disruption of supraoptic axons within pituitary stalk or loss of osmoreceptor function
      ii. Surgery in area of neurohypophyseal system
   c. Inflammatory/degenerative
      i. Tubercular meningitis
      ii. Syphilis
      iii. Sarcoidosis
      iv. Hodgkin's disease
      v. Histiocytic granuloma (childhood)
      vi. Tumors of hypothalamo-neurohypophyseal system
      vii. Hypothalamic, metastatic lesions, primarily from breast or lung
   d. Idiopathic

3. **Clinical presentation**: often of sudden onset
   a. Polyuria (6–24 liters/day) with resultant dilute urine
   b. Polydipsia

4. **Diagnostic findings**
   a. History
      i. Head trauma, surgery, or other intracranial pathology
      ii. More common in young adult males
   b. Physical examination — marked dehydration may be seen
   c. Diagnostic studies
      i. Laboratory
         (a) Urine osmolality decreased, serum osmolality increased
         (b) Serum sodium and proteins elevated
         (c) Urine specific gravity 1.001–1.005 (diluted)
         (d) Serology positive (if syphilis is cause)
      ii. Radiologic

(a) Skull x-rays may show metastatic disease or skull fracture

(b) Chest x-rays may reveal metastatic disease

(c) CT scan may show intracranial pathology

iii. Special

(a) Spinal tap may reveal causative agent

(b) Visual fields – bitemporal field loss

(c) Sternal marrow aspiration may reveal neoplastic involvement

(d) Water deprivation/vasopressin infusion test – urine osmolality rises by 9% or more after vasopressin administration

5. **Complications**

a. Dehydration leading to hypovolemic shock

b. Dilatation/hypertrophy of bladder with megaloureter

c. Resistance to vasopressin therapy (sometimes caused by inadequate warming or agitation of vasopressin in oil)

6. **Specific patient care**: the critical care nurse usually encounters diabetes insipidus (DI) either in patients undergoing a physiologic crisis who incidentally have had a previous diagnosis of DI, or in those who potentially may develop DI as a result of the specific pathologic condition they are currently experiencing

a. Observe for signs and symptoms that may indicate

i. Developing DI

ii. Interruption of replacement therapy of previously diagnosed DI patients

b. Anticipate potential problems – recognize

i. Concomitant anterior pituitary insufficiency

ii. Rapidly developing hypovolemia

iii. Exhaustion of alert, unregulated patient – may occur through inability to rest owing to urinary frequency

c. Recognize that DI can be transitory or permanent

d. Recognize that diuresis of DI can be masked by

i. Previously administered cerebral dehydrating agents

ii. Steroid therapy

e. Assist with diagnostic procedures

i. Water deprivation test (most widely used)

(a) Maintain fluid restriction

(b) Monitor weight, vital signs

(c) Observe for dehydration, shock

(d) Collect timed samples (urine/blood)

ii. Saline infusion test

(a) Monitor vital signs and obtain timed samples (blood/urine)

(b) Observe for fluid overload and other untoward reactions

f. Administer therapy
   i. Replacement therapy – vasopressin
       (a) Vasopressin tannate in oil must be warmed and agitated vigorously – may cause swelling and pain at injection site
       (b) Lysine vasopressin (nasal spray) may be erratically absorbed in presence of respiratory infection or allergic rhinitis, and must be used with caution in patients with hypertension or heart disease
       (c) Deamino-D-arginine vasopressin (DDAVP), a nasal spray, has minimal side effects and prolonged antidiuretic activity
       (d) Observe for increased water retention
   ii. Chlorpropamide – stimulates ADH release and potentiates its effects
       (a) Observe for hypoglycemia
       (b) To prevent hypoglycemia, have patient adhere to a regular schedule for meals
g. Ensure meticulous recording of intake and output

INAPPROPRIATE SECRETION OF ADH (SIADH)

1. **Pathophysiology:** either increased delivery or increased secretion of ADH, which is unrelated to plasma osmolality and which results in increased total body water

2. **Etiology or precipitating factors**
   a. Tuberculous meningitis/tumors
   b. Extracranial malignant tumors, especially bronchogenic and pancreatic cancer
   c. Skull fracture, subdural hematoma, subarachnoid hemorrhage
   d. Drugs – chlorpropamide, vincristine, thiazides, clofibrate
   e. Vasopressin therapy
   f. Pneumonia, tuberculosis, other respiratory infections
   g. Addison's disease, hypopituitarism, hypothyroidism

3. **Clinical presentation**
   a. Headache, mental sluggishness, disorientation
   b. Weakness, decreased tendon reflexes
   c. Nausea, vomiting, diarrhea, anorexia
   d. Seizures

4. **Diagnostic findings**
   a. History
      i. Intracranial pathology
      ii. Recent respiratory infection
      iii. Extracranial malignancies
      iv. Vasopressin therapy

    b. Physical examination
       i.   Confusion
      ii.   Weakness
     iii.   Lassitude
     iv.   Diminished tendon reflexes
    c. Diagnostic studies
       i.   Laboratory
          (a) Serum sodium, potassium, chloride, proteins, and osmolality decreased
          (b) Urine sodium and osmolality increased
          (c) Urine specific gravity increased
      ii.   Radiologic
          (a) Skull x-rays may show tumor process or injury
          (b) Chest x-rays may show tumor or infectious process
          (c) Abdominal x-rays may show tumor process
     iii.   Special
          (a) Spinal tap — meningeal infection, intracranial process
          (b) Tumor assays
          (c) Waterloading test — patients fail to excrete less than half of water load, and fail to dilute urine
          (d) Adrenal and thyroid function tests

5. **Complications**
    a. Coma
    b. Seizures
    c. Death

6. **Specific patient care:** the critical care nurse is most likely to encounter this disorder in patients with imminent water intoxication
    a. Administer therapy aimed at prevention of water intoxication and correction of electrolyte disturbances
       i.   Fluid restriction
      ii.   Hypertonic saline and furosemide IV (acute episode)
          (a) Collect timed urine and blood samples for sodium and potassium
          (b) Administer potassium chloride supplements
     iii.   Demeclocycline interferes with action of vasopressin on kidney
    b. Closely observe and monitor patient's general and electrolyte status during therapy
    c. Anticipate nursing interventions needed to deal with manifestations of water intoxication if they occur. Remember that edema is not necessarily present during water intoxication
       i.   Weakness
      ii.   Confusion and disorientation
     iii.   Vomiting
     iv.   Seizures
      v.   Coma

    d. Assist with diagnostic, waterloading test
       i.   Collect timed urine samples
      ii.   Monitor vital signs
     iii.   Observe for water intoxication
    e. Maintain gastrointestinal function — avoid tap water enemas as these may be absorbed and increase water intoxication
       i.   Auscultate bowel sounds
      ii.   Prevent constipation/impaction
    f. Prevent complications of decreased mobility (e.g., atelectasis, decubiti)
    g. Monitor intake/output

THYROTOXIC CRISIS

1. **Pathophysiology**: biochemical and physiologic complex that results when cells are presented with excessive quantities of thyroid hormones that cause marked increase in systemic adrenergic activity

2. **Etiology or precipitating factors** •
    a. Decompensation of pre-existing hyperthyroid condition subsequent to trauma, infection, or stress
    b. Subtotal thyroidectomy
    c. Ketoacidosis
    d. Increased intake of thyroid hormone
    e. Vigorous palpation of thyroid gland in hyperthyroid patient
    f. Abrupt withdrawal of antithyroid drugs

3. **Clinical presentation**
    a. Hyperthermia, flushing, diaphoresis
    b. Hypertension, tachycardia, systolic murmurs
    c. Delirium, psychosis, emotional lability, stupor, coma
    d. Hyperkinesis, tremors, weakness
    e. Nausea, vomiting, diarrhea, weight loss
    f. Palmar erythema

4. **Diagnostic findings**
    a. History
       i.   Pre-existing hyperthyroidism of less than 2 years' duration
      ii.   Recent respiratory infection
     iii.   Cessation of thyroid therapy
    b. Physical examination
       i.   Hair and skin changes
      ii.   Hyperactive, flushed, diaphoretic appearance
     iii.   Emotional lability may be noted
     iv.   Thyroid enlargement and bruit may be present
      v.   Widened pulse pressure, third heart sound, systolic murmur, hyperdynamic heart

    c. Diagnostic studies
        i. Laboratory
            (a) Serum glucose and calcium normal or elevated
            (b) WBC, hemoglobin elevated
            (c) T_4 and protein-bound iodine (PBI) elevated
            (d) T_3 resin uptake elevated
        ii. Radiologic
            (a) Thyroid scan – over 90% of sodium iodide (^{131}I) from blood stream will be absorbed by thyroid gland
        iii. Special
            (a) ^{131}I uptake elevated
            (b) ^{131}I excretion decreased

5. **Complications**
    a. Dehydration leading to hypovolemic shock
    b. CHF
    c. Exhaustion, coma, death

6. **Specific patient care**
    a. Decrease hypermetabolic state
        i. Institute hypothermic measures, provide hydration
        ii. Administer antipyretics, sedation, and corticosteroids, as ordered
        iii. Modify environmental stimuli and limit visitors
        iv. Avoid aspirin, which increases free thyroxine levels
    b. Diminish increased sympathetic effects and support myocardial function
        i. Administer, and monitor response to, positive inotropic agents
        ii. Administer, and monitor response to, antihypertensive agents and beta-adrenergic blocking agents
        iii. Monitor cardiac rate, rhythm, and vital signs
    c. Decrease hormone synthesis and release through administration of iodine agents and antithyroid agents
    d. Maintain adequate nutrition – administer carbohydrates, protein, and B complex vitamins
    e. Support respiratory function – elevate head of bed and give oxygen therapy
    f. Avoid iodine preparations (skin prep, contrast media, etc.) prior to ^{131}I studies, as these invalidate results

HYPOPARATHYROIDISM

1. **Pathophysiology**: defect in release of PTH, with consequent hypocalcemia and altered neuromuscular activity

2. **Etiology or precipitating factors**
    a. Idiopathic

    b. Surgery of thyroid or parathyroid glands
    c. Radiation injury secondary to thyroid therapy with ^{131}I
    d. Acute pancreatitis

3. **Clinical presentation**
    a. Numbness and tingling in fingers and toes
    b. Muscle cramps of hands and feet, carpopedal spasm
    c. Nausea, vomiting, abdominal pain
    d. Laryngeal stridor, dyspnea, cyanosis
    e. Confusion, lethargy, emotional lability
    f. Generalized convulsions

4. **Diagnostic findings**
    a. History – recent thyroid or parathyroid surgery
    b. Physical examination – signs of tetany or hypocalcemia
       i. Positive Chvostek's sign – twitching of muscles along facial nerve when latter is tapped (may be absent)
       ii. Positive Trousseau's sign – carpopedal spasm when circulation is interrupted with BP cuff (may be absent in over one-third of patients)
    c. Diagnostic studies
       i. Laboratory
         (a) Serum calcium is decreased (below 8.5 mg/dl) and serum phosphate is increased
         (b) Urine calcium and phosphate are decreased
       ii. Radiologic – bone x-rays may reveal increased bone density
       iii. Special
         (a) 12-lead ECG – prolonged Q-T interval
         (b) EEG – normal, or nonspecific abnormalities

5. **Complications**: seizures and tetany

6. **Specific patient care**: the critical care nurse is most likely to see hypoparathyroid patient if tetany is suspected
    a. Re-establish normal serum calcium
       i. Administer oral calcium supplements
         (a) Give with caution to patient on digitalis since both have similar effects on myocardium
         (b) If patient has GI upset, give with meals, but not with dairy products, as phosphorus may lessen calcium absorption
         (c) Administer vitamin D to increase calcium absorption
       ii. Administer IV calcium
         (a) Use intracath line since calcium is irritating to blood vessels
         (b) Avoid infiltration to prevent tissue irritation, necrosis, and sloughing

(c)   Administer slowly to avoid high serum concentrations and associated cardiac conduction delays

(d)   Monitor patient closely for changes in cardiac rhythm, rate, and BP

(e)   Do not mix in saline for infusion, as this causes calcium excretion

(f)   Monitor serum calcium levels

iii. Prevent stressors that may precipitate tetany — hyperventilation that accompanies stress may cause an alkalotic state that precipitates tetany

(a)   Modify environmental stimuli

(b)   Limit visitors

iv. Anticipate nursing interventions if laryngeal spasm or seizures occur

ACUTE ADRENAL INSUFFICIENCY (ADRENAL CRISIS)

1. **Pathophysiology**: a rapid, overwhelming exacerbation of a chronic, primary adrenal insufficiency (Addison's disease) in which there is a lack of aldosterone and cortisol, causing
   a.   Fluid and electrolyte imbalances
   b.   Protein, fat, and carbohydrate metabolism disturbances
   c.   Circulatory collapse

2. **Etiology or precipitating factors**
   a.   Hemorrhage, infection, trauma, or infarction of adrenal cortex
   b.   Adrenalectomy
   c.   Meningococcal, pneumococcal, staphylococcal, or Hemophilus meningitis (Waterhouse-Friderichsen syndrome)
   d.   Stress — in persons with no adrenal reserve (e.g., after trauma, infection, anesthesia, or surgery)
   e.   Abrupt cessation of steroid therapy
   f.   Autoimmune response
   g.   Hypopituitarism, hypothalamic disease
   h.   Tumor chemotherapy

3. **Clinical presentation**
   a.   Hypotension; rapid, thready pulse; cool, clammy skin; oliguria
   b.   Abdominal pain, weight loss, flaccid extremities
   c.   Nausea and vomiting, anorexia, dehydration, weakness, lethargy
   d.   Increased pigmentation (Addison's)
   e.   Confusion, restlessness, decreased level of consciousness

4. **Diagnostic findings**
   a.   History
      i.   Decreased adrenal reserve
      ii. Recent surgery

        iii. Trauma
        iv. Infection
        v.   Abrupt cessation of steroid therapy
  b. Physical examination may reveal
        i.   Increased pigmentation
        ii. Weakness and fatigability
        iii. Flaccid extremities
        iv. Dehydration
        v.   Ill-defined abdominal pain
  c. Diagnostic studies
        i.   Laboratory
            (a) Serum potassium and BUN elevated
            (b) Serum sodium and plasma cortisol decreased
            (c) Serum creatinine elevated
            (d) Hemoglobin decreased
            (e) Serum glucose decreased
            (f) Blood 17-hydroxycorticoids low
            (g) Urine 17-ketosteroids and 17-hydroxycorticoids low
            (h) Plasma ACTH and MSH elevated (Addison's)
            (i)   Plasma ACTH low (ACTH lack)
        ii. Radiologic
            (a) Adrenal arteriogram may reveal thrombosis
            (b) Chest x-ray may show heart smaller than normal
        iii. Special
            (a) ECG may show hyperkalemic changes
            (b) ACTH test — no cortisol rise after administration
            (c) EEG — marked slowing

5. **Complications**
  a. Dysrhythmias
  b. Dehydration and hypovolemic shock
  c. Coma and death

6. **Specific patient care**
  a. Restore adequate blood volume
        i.   Hydrocortisone is administered as a bolus dose or added to
           dextrose in isotonic saline
        ii. Plasma administration may be indicated
        iii. Vasopressors in dosages titrated according to BP may be
           used
  b. Monitor vital functions
        i.   Check vital signs, CVP, intake/output
        ii. Check urinary specific gravity hourly to ascertain
           hydration status and renal function
        iii. If hyperkalemia exists, monitor cardiac function
  c. If hyperpyrexia persists in spite of cortisol therapy, initiate
     nursing interventions to reduce fever

     d. Reduce physical and psychologic stress
        i.   Strict bed rest
        ii. Quiet environment
        iii. Reassure patient about procedures by giving short explanations
     e. Provide nursing interventions related to underlying cause of crisis

DIABETIC KETOACIDOSIS (DKA)

1. **Pathophysiology:** characterized by relative or absolute lack of circulating insulin, causing hyperglycemia due to peripheral underutilization or hepatic overproduction and ketonemia
   a. Without insulin, breakdown of glycogen is activated and its synthesis inhibited, and "free form" glucose readily diffuses into blood. Also, new glucose is synthesized by liver when amino acids are released from protein stores and glycerol from fat stores
   b. Impaired glucose uptake by adipose tissue causes impaired triglyceride synthesis and liberation of free fatty acids into blood ·
   c. Excessive fatty acids enter liver, resulting in accelerated synthesis of acetyl-CoA
   d. The acetyl-CoA conversion to citrate for fatty acid resynthesis is inhibited, and there is increased oxidation of acetyl-CoA to keto, acetoacetic, and β-hydroxybutyric acids. These accumulate faster than they can be metabolized, and readily dissociate into ketoneanions and hydrogen ions
   e. Some β-hydroxybutyric and acetoacetic acid are oxidized to acetone and lost via exhalation

2. **Etiology or precipitating factors**
   a. Omission of insulin, resistance to insulin
   b. Conditions increasing insulin demand (e.g., surgery, trauma, infection)
   c. Heredity
   d. Pancreatitis
   e. Vascular accidents, atherosclerotic heart disease
   f. Pregnancy

3. **Clinical presentation**
   a. Altered level of consciousness
   b. Abdominal pain
   c. Polydipsia, polyuria
   d. Kussmaul breathing
   e. Nausea and vomiting, weakness, weight loss
   f. Flushed face; dry, warm skin; poor skin turgor
   g. Hypotension, tachycardia, hypothermia
   h. Acetone breath

4. **Diagnostic findings**
   a. History
      i. Pre-existing diabetes with recent illness or trauma
      ii. Infection
   b. Physical examination
      i. Decreased sensorium
      ii. Kussmaul breathing
      iii. Abdominal tenderness and distention
      iv. Acetone breath
      v. Decreased deep tendon reflexes
   c. Diagnostic studies
      i. Laboratory
         (a) Serum glucose elevated (300–1000 mg)
         (b) Urine glucose positive (greater than 2^+)
         (c) Urine acetone positive (greater than 4^+)
         (d) Urine protein – trace amounts
         (e) Urine sodium and chloride decreased
         (f) Urine specific gravity elevated
         (g) Serum ketones increased
         (h) Plasma free fatty acids increased
         (i) BUN normal or increased
         (j) Serum bicarbonate decreased (metabolic acidosis)
         (k) Arterial PCO_2 decreased
         (l) Arterial pH decreased (acidemia)
         (m) HCT normal or increased
         (n) White cells normal or increased
         (o) Serum potassium elevated (decreased in 5% of patients), but may fall precipitously if acidosis is rapidly corrected
         (p) Serum sodium and phosphate decreased
      ii. Special – 12-lead ECG may reflect hyperkalemic or hypokalemic changes

5. **Complications**
   a. Shock, cardiac dysrhythmias, acute renal failure
   b. Pulmonary edema, cerebral edema, seizures
   c. Hypoglycemia, hypokalemia, hypophosphatemia
   d. Hyperkalemia during acidosis
   e. CSF acidosis, coma, death

6. **Specific patient care**
   a. Restore fluid balance
      i. Prepare for initial infusion of isotonic or hypotonic saline, to foster glucose excretion
         (a) Rapid administration may be ordered (1000 ml/hour initially)
         (b) Vital signs must be monitored closely

      ii.   When plasma glucose falls to 250 mg/dl, IV fluids should be changed to 5% glucose half-normal saline by physician, to prevent hypoglycemia, hypokalemia, and cerebral edema

      iii. CVP should be monitored in any patient with cardiac or renal impairment, to determine volume status

b. Restore normal carbohydrate, fat, and protein metabolism

      i.   Prepare for administration of rapid-acting insulin

         (a) Methods of administration

            (1) Loading doses – IM or IV, approx. 20 units

            (2) Continuous infusion IV, 4–8 units/hr (preferred method)

            (3) IV bolus, 10–25 units/hr

            (4) IM, 5–10 units/hr or SQ, 10–100 units/hr

         (b) Monitor hourly blood and urine glucose and ketone values

      ii. Correction of acidosis

         (a) Give sodium bicarbonate preparations as ordered.

         (b) Treat underlying cause of acidosis, hyperglycemia

         (c) Assess level of consciousness continuously

c. Restore electrolyte balance

      i.   Monitor serum electrolyte levels

      ii. Administer electrolyte supplements (phosphate, potassium, chloride) as ordered

      iii. Pay particular attention to potassium levels. As ketosis and volume problems are corrected, be alert for fluctuations from hyper- to hypokalemia

      iv. Monitor ECG for hyper/hypokalemic changes

d. Maintain function of related systems

      i.   Support ventilation and oxygenation

      ii. Observe for and relieve gastric dilatation

      iii. Observe for seizures and institute measures to protect patient from injury

      iv. Monitor adequacy of urinary output

e. Identify factor(s) causing ketoacidosis – usually infection

      i.   Inspect all body surfaces for sources of infection

      ii. Auscultate the lungs

      iii. Examine abdomen for distention or painful areas

      iv. Be alert for hidden infections, e.g., cholecystitis, pyelonephritis, or appendicitis

      v.   Suspect impending influenza or other upper respiratory tract infections

f. Observe for indices of improvement – increased urinary output, growing alertness, restored skin turgor, brightness of eyes

HYPEROSMOLAR COMA — NONKETOTIC (HHNK)

1. **Pathophysiology**
   a. Relative insulin deficiency causes hyperglycemia, hyperosmolality of ECF, cellular dehydration, and diuresis while insulin is sufficient to prevent ketone body formation. As hyperglycemia becomes marked, an osmotic gradient develops between brain and plasma, causing a loss of brain water and leading to CNS dysfunction
   b. Decreased GFR causes azotemia

2. **Etiology or precipitating factors**
   a. Mild diabetes (often undiagnosed or of recent onset)
   b. Acute illness, trauma, stress
   c. Diuretics, steroids, hypertonic solutions
   d. Patient usually 50 years of age or older

3. **Clinical presentation**
   a. Dehydration, poor skin turgor, dry mucous membranes
   b. Lethargy, stupor, coma
   c. Polyuria, polydipsia
   d. Nausea and vomiting, weight loss
   e. Hypotension, tachycardia, hyperthermia, tachypnea
   f. Hyperreflexia, disorientation, seizures (focal type)

4. **Diagnostic findings**
   a. History
      i. Recent use of hypertonic solutions, steroids, or diuretics
      ii. Recent trauma, stress in older individual
      iii. Cardiovascular or renal disease
   b. Physical examination
      i. Dehydration may be seen — dry skin and mucous membranes, hypotension, soft eyeballs
      ii. CNS dysfunction — dull sensorium, areflexia, vestibular dysfunction, focal neurologic disturbances, hallucinatory behavior
      iii. Fever, tachycardia, rapid respirations
   c. Diagnostic studies
      i. Laboratory
         (a) Serum glucose elevated (often greater than 1000 mg)
         (b) Serum osmolality elevated
         (c) Serum sodium normal or elevated
         (d) Serum potassium normal or decreased
         (e) HCT elevated
         (f) Arterial pH normal or decreased (if lactic acidosis)
         (g) BUN elevated
         (h) Urine glucose positive (greater than 2^+)

          (i)   WBC count elevated

          (j)   Arterial PCO_2 and bicarbonate decreased

     ii.   Special — 12-lead ECG may reflect hypokalemic changes

5. **Complications**
   a. Hypovolemic shock and acute tubular necrosis
   b. Vascular thrombosis, coma, death
   c. Iatrogenic hypoglycemia

6. **Specific patient care**
   a. Restore normal blood volume and osmolality, and normal metabolism
      i. Administer IV fluids — 10–20 liters may be necessary within 24–48 hrs (a controversy exists as to value of hypotonic vs isotonic fluids)
      ii. Correct insulin levels using "loading" IV dose and subsequent IV infusions of 4–10 units/hr
      iii. Use insulin judiciously, as fluid repletion initially is paramount
      iv. Observe for indices of improvement (e.g., improving sensorium, decreasing diuresis)
   b. Restore electrolyte balance
      i. Monitor serum electrolytes
      ii. Administer supplements of potassium (200–400 mEq may be needed in first 48 hours) and phosphate
      iii. Monitor ECG for hypo/hyperkalemic changes

HYPOGLYCEMIC REACTION

1. **Pathophysiology**
   a. Reduction in blood glucose due to defect in process of
      i. Increasing blood glucose by
         (a) Forming "new glucose" from nonglucose sources (glyconeogenesis)
         (b) Mobilizing glucose from glycogen (glycogenolysis)
         (c) Absorbing ingested carbohydrates
      ii. Removing blood glucose through use by adipose tissue, liver, muscle, etc.

2. **Etiology or precipitating factors**
   a. Reactive hypoglycemia (exogenous causes)
      i. Functional idiopathic
      ii. Fructose, galactose, amino acid intolerance
      iii. Postgastrectomy
      iv. Drugs — insulin, sulfonylurea, etc.
      v. Alcohol
   b. Fasting hypoglycemia (endogenous processes)
      i. Enzyme deficiencies (glycogen storage disease)

     ii.   Pancreatic disease
    iii.   Anterior hypopituitarism
    iv.   Hepatic disease
     v.   Severe CHF
    vi.   Glucagon, cortisol deficiencies
   vii.   Erythroblastosis fetalis
  viii.   Exercise, pregnancy, fever

3. **Clinical presentation**
   a. Headache
   b. Weakness
   c. Nervousness, tremors, palpitations, anxiety
   d. Hunger, nausea
   e. Personality changes — confusion, depression
   f. Blurred vision
   g. Pallor, diaphoresis
   h. Tachycardia, increase in systolic pressure
   i. Dilated pupils
   j. Lethargy, coma, seizures

4. **Diagnostic findings**
   a. History
      i. Pre-existing endocrine disorder
      ii. Alcohol abuse
      iii. Medication use
   b. Physical examination may show
      i. Anxiety
      ii. Tremors
      iii. Diaphoresis
      iv. Pallor
   c. Diagnostic studies
      i. Laboratory — serum glucose decreased
      ii. Radiologic
         (a) Celiac/mesenteric angiography may show diffuse acellular thickening of vessels
         (b) Liver scan may show enlargement from fat infiltration and parenchymal damage
         (c) GI series may reveal neoplasm
         (d) IVP may show general glomerular sclerosis with basement membrane thickening
         (e) C–T scan may show early tumor process
      iii. Special
         (a) Glucose tolerance test may show excessive decline in glucose levels
         (b) Insulin assays may reveal elevated plasma insulin activity
         (c) Tests of insulin secretion may show insulin sensitivity diminished
         (d) Glucagon levels increased

5. **Complications**
    a. Brain damage
    b. Myocardial ischemia
    c. Extension of myocardial infarction
    d. Death

6. **Specific patient care**
    a. Restore serum glucose to normal levels
        i. Administer carbohydrates
            (a) For unconscious patient, give 50 ml of 50% glucose IV. Epinephrine or glucagon may be given to stimulate liver to break down some of its glycogen. Upon regaining consciousness, patient should eat
            (b) For conscious patient, give sweetened orange juice, candy, or warm tea or coffee with honey
            (c) If in doubt as to whether hyper- or hypoglycemia exists in a comatose patient, draw blood sugar and give 50 ml of 50% glucose IV. Patient will respond within 1 minute if hypoglycemia is cause
    b. Identify possible cause and prevent recurrence
    c. Provide diet modifications and education regarding
        i. Restriction of simple sugars
        ii. Small, frequent meals (for alimentary hypoglycemia)
        iii. Restriction of caffeine-containing beverages and cigarettes in emotionally labile patients

REFERENCES

Something to sniff at. Emergency Med. 8:92, 1976.

Beeson, P.B., McDermott, W., and Wyngaarden, J.B.: Textbook of Medicine. W.B. Saunders Co., Philadelphia, 1979.

Bolinger, R.E.: Hypoglycemia. Crit. Care Q. 3:99, 1980.

Bondy, P.K., and Rosenburg, L.E.: Duncan's Diseases of Metabolism: Endocrinology. W.B. Saunders Co., Philadelphia, 1974.

Brunner, L.S., and Suddarth, D.S.: Textbook of Medical-Surgical Nursing. J.B. Lippincott Co., Philadelphia, 1980.

Brunner, L.S., and Suddarth, D.S.: The Lippincott Manual of Nursing Practice. J.B. Lippincott Co., Philadelphia, 1978.

Cataland, S.: Hypoglycemia: a spectrum of problems. Heart Lung 7:455, 1978.

Cryer, P.E.: Diagnostic Endocrinology. Oxford University Press, New York, 1979.

Ezrin, C., et al.: Systematic Endocrinology. Harper and Row, New York, 1973.

Fairchild, R.S.: Diabetes insipidus: a review. Crit. Care Q. 3:111, 1980.

Forsham, P.H.: Abnormalities of the adrenal cortex. Clin. Symp. 15:35, 1976.

Guthrie, D., and Guthrie, R.: Nursing Management of Diabetes. C.V. Mosby Co., St. Louis, 1977.

Guyton, A.C.: Textbook of Medical Physiology. W.B. Saunders Co., Philadelphia, 1976.

Hamburger, S.C., and Rush, D.R.: Syndrome of inappropriate secretion of antidiuretic hormone. Crit. Care Q. 3:119, 1980.

Hellman, R.: The evaluation and management of hyperthyroid crises. Crit. Care Q. *3:*77, 1980.

Jones, D., Dunbar, C., and Jirovec, M.: Medical-Surgical Nursing: A Conceptual Approach. McGraw-Hill Book Co., New York, 1978.

Kubo, W.M., and Grant, M.M.: The syndrome of inappropriate secretion of antidiuretic hormone. Heart Lung 7:469, 1978.

Kyner, J.L.: Diabetic ketoacidosis. Crit. Care Q. *3:*65, 1980.

Luckmann, J., and Sorensen, K.C.: Medical-Surgical Nursing: A Psychophysiologic Approach. W.B. Saunders Co., Philadelphia, 1980.

Rodman, M., and Smith, D.: Clinical Pharmacology in Nursing. J.B. Lippincott Co., Philadelphia, 1979.

Ryan, W.G.: Endocrine Disorders. Year Book Medical Publishers, Inc., Chicago, 1975.

Schimke, N.R.: Adrenal insufficiency. Crit. Care Q. *3:*19, 1980.

Schwartz, R.B., Ryan, W.G., and Berker, F.O.: The Year Book of Endocrinology. Year Book Medical Publishers, Inc., Chicago, 1973.

Skillman, T.G.: Diabetic Ketoacidosis. Heart Lung 7:594, 1978.

Sneid, D.S.: Hyperosmolar hyperglycemic nonketotic coma. Crit. Care Q. *3:* 29, 1980.

Sussman, K.E., and Metz, J.S.: Diabetes Mellitus. American Diabetes Association, New York, 1975.

Thorn, G., Adams, R., Braunwald, E., et al.: Harrison's Principles of Internal Medicine. McGraw-Hill Book Co., New York, 1977.

Tzagournis, M.: Acute adrenal insufficiency. Heart Lung 7:603, 1978.

Urbanic, R.C., and Mazzaferri, E.L.: Thyrotoxic crisis and myxedema coma. Heart Lung 7:435, 1978.

Williams, R.H.: Textbook of Endocrinology. W.B. Saunders Co., Philadelphia, 1974.

THE
HEMATOLOGIC
SYSTEM

prepared by

BONNIE MOWINSKI JENNINGS, R.N., M.S.

BEHAVIORAL OBJECTIVES

Functional Anatomy

1. Explain the functions of the six major cell types formed in bone marrow.

2. Discuss the hematologic functions of the spleen, liver, lymph system, and thymus.

Physiology

1. Identify and discuss factors that regulate erythropoiesis and hemolysis of mature and immature red blood cells.

2. Describe the process of hemoglobin synthesis.

3. Differentiate between humoral and cellular immunity in terms of B-cell and T-cell functions and their relationships to the immunoglobulins, Rh process, and delayed hypersensitivity.

4. Describe the three methods of hemostasis.

5. Explain the mechanisms that normally prevent clotting in the human body.

Assessment

1. Discuss systematically the major areas of data collection for hematologic assessment.

2. Explain the significance of findings elicited through history-taking that may indicate hematologic dysfunction.

3. Explain the significance of findings on physical examination that may indicate hematologic dysfunction.

General Patient Care Management

1. Discuss the underlying pathophysiology related to reductions in erythrocytes, leukocytes, or platelets.

2. Identify nursing interventions and underlying rationales aimed at decreasing potential complications that result from specific blood element deficiencies.

3. Discuss transfusion therapy in terms of purposes, potential reactions, and differences among blood administration products.

Pathologic Conditions and Management

1. Identify and explain appropriate nursing interventions for the anemic patient, relating each to etiologic factors, underlying pathophysiology, clinical signs, diagnostic criteria, and potential complications.

2. Differentiate between the four major types of leukemia.

3. Explain the meaning of "acute" and "chronic" as used in describing leukemia.

4. Describe and explain the correct technique for resuscitating a patient in anaphylaxis.

5. Explain disseminated intravascular coagulation succinctly in terms of etiology, pathophysiology, diagnosis, and treatment.

6. Explain the pathophysiology of sickle cell anemia and its relationship to the potential complications of pain, acidosis, and fluid and electrolyte imbalances.

7. Discuss the renal and skeletal complications of multiple myeloma in terms of pathophysiology.

8. Differentiate the various stages of Hodgkin's disease, using the "concept of staging."

9. Describe the nursing interventions and related rationales for the care of a patient receiving radiation therapy.

THE HEMATOLOGIC SYSTEM

———————— FUNCTIONAL ANATOMY ————————

BONE MARROW: This is the production site of the erythroid, myeloid, and thrombocytic components of the blood, and also one source of lymphocytes and macrophages. Several different morphologically distinct cells evolve during the maturation of erythrocytes, platelets, and leukocytes. Only certain differentiated cells will be discussed below; the reader should consult a hematology text for more complete details.

1. **Erythrocytes:** erythroid series or red blood cells
   a. Reticulocytes – erythrocyte precursors useful in assessing erythrocyte production
   b. Erythrocytes – mature cells, released to circulation because storage capacity of bone marrow is limited
   c. Primary task of RBCs is to transport oxygen to tissues; they also participate in maintenance of acid-base balance through hemoglobin's function as a buffer
   d. Red cell membrane
      i. Composed of two structures
         (a) Stroma – innermost structure of erythrocyte, composed primarily of lipids and proteins; a thick and spongelike substance to which hemoglobin attaches. Stroma contains antigenic material that defines A, B, O blood groups
         (b) Outer membrane – external portion of erythrocyte, composed primarily of lipoproteins; a thin and pliable substance on which antigens for blood types are located
      ii. Freely permeable to hydrogen, chloride, water, and bicarbonate ions
      iii. Less permeable to sodium and potassium ions, and maintains stable intracellular concentrations by active transport (concentrations are reversed in plasma)

2. **Thrombocytes**
   a. Megakaryocytes are precursor cells.
   b. Platelets (thrombocytes) are ultimate mature form
   c. In vitro – assist in adhesivity, aggregation, clot retraction
   d. In vivo – maintain endothelial integrity and help control traumatic bleeding

3. **Leukocytes**
   a. Granulocytes (myeloid series) – known as polymorphonuclear leukocytes (PMNs or polys)
      i. Neutrophils

(a) Immature form — characterized by granules, lobes, and strands of chromatin. Increase in these immature forms, which are called "segs" and "bands," is characteristic response to infection

(b) Mature form — phagocytic; active in inflammation and tissue damage

   ii. Eosinophils — sometimes phagocytic: active in detoxification in allergies and for parasites

   iii. Basophils — released in allergic responses, states of stress, and chronic inflammation

b. Lymphocytes — also produced in lymph nodes (see also section on Immunity)

   i. B cells — produce antibodies known as immunoglobulins, and mediate humoral immunity

   ii. T cells — produced when foreign tissue is recognized, and therefore provide for tissue immunity rather than antibody production; mediate cellular immunity

c. Monocytes — also produced in lymph nodes

   i. May differentiate into histiocytes

   ii. Show phagocytic activity in response to inflammation and chemotactic stimuli ("chemotaxis" refers to ability to attract granulocytes; such activity is critical at times of infection to facilitate movement of phagocytic cells to site of infection)

d. Histiocytes (macrophages)

   i. Fixed histiocytes

(a) Located within body structures other than bone marrow, e.g., spleen, Kupffer cells of liver, pulmonary alveoli, lamina propria of GI tract, peritoneal and pleural fluids

(b) Phagocytize microorganisms, cells, and cellular and noncellular debris

   ii. Free histiocytes

(a) Migrate from blood through endothelial membrane of vascular system to trap and localize material for phagocytosis

(b) Found at sites of inflammation and in peritoneal, pleural, and synovial fluids

e. Plasma cells — similar to lymphocytes

   i. Fully differentiated B cells that produce one specific antibody

   ii. Synthesize, store, and release all classes of immunoglobulins

SPLEEN

1. **Two compartments**

a. White pulp (lymphoid elements) — immunoglobulin synthesizing cells that produce antibodies

b. Red pulp (mass of vascular spaces) – contains phagocytic cells, and removes unwanted particles and defective cells from blood stream

2. **Extramedullary hematopoiesis**
    a. During fetal development, spleen is important site of hematopoiesis
    b. Postnatally, spleen produces primarily lymphocytes and monocytes

3. **Compartmental structure:** plays major role in removal of effete red cells from circulation

4. **Acts as cell reservoir:** contains 1–2% of circulating red cell mass

5. **Produces antibodies**

6. **Culling and pitting effect**
    a. Removes misshapen erythrocyres from circulation
    b. Removes unwanted parts of erythrocytes, and returns altered, undamaged cells to circulation

7. **Iron metabolism:** reticuloendothelial cells catabolize hemoglobin released from those erythrocytes that have been destroyed in spleen. Iron is then returned to bone marrow for reuse

LIVER (hematologic functions)

1. **Erythropoiesis:** takes place in liver during fetal development if bone marrow production is insufficient

2. **Bile production:** increased by erythrocyte destruction and bilirubin production

3. **Kupffer cells:** have a reticuloendothelial function as histiocytes with phagocytic activity and as important sites of iron storage

4. **Major site of synthesis of all plasma clotting factors:** vitamin K-dependent factors, i.e., II (prothrombin), VII, IX, and X; exception is factor VIII

5. **Synthesis of antithrombins:** substances that neutralize action of thrombin, thus restricting blood coagulation

LYMPHATIC SYSTEM

1. **Lymph:** a tissue fluid that diffuses through walls of lymphatic capillaries. Compared to blood, lymph

   a. Coagulates slowly
   b. Contains lymphocytes, granular leukocytes, enzymes, and
       antibodies
   c. Is deficient in erythrocytes, platelets, and fibrinogen

2. **Lymphatic capillaries**: thin-walled, endothelium-lined vessels,
   somewhat larger than blood capillaries and irregular in diameter

3. **Lymphatic vessels (formed by lymphatic capillaries)**
   a. Carry all lymph ultimately either to right lymphatic duct or to
       thoracic duct
   b. Do not supply nonvascular structures (e.g. cartilage)

4. **Lymph ducts**
   a. Right lymphatic duct is short — formed by several tributaries
       that carry lymph from right side of head, neck, and thorax;
       right upper extremity; right lung; right heart; and right upper
       surface of diaphragm
   b. Thoracic duct — largest terminal duct. Carries lymph from all
       parts of body except those drained by right lymphatic duct

5. **Lymph nodes**: small, flat, round- to bean-shaped organs of varying
   sizes located along lymph vessels
   a. Sites of B- and T-cell distribution
   b. Produce blood lymphocytes, monocytes, plasma cells, and
       histiocytes
   c. Filter bacteria and foreign particles carried by lymph
   d. Distribution — found throughout body, both superficially and
       deep. Superficial nodes can be palpated; deep nodes must be
       visualized on x-ray examination
       i.   Head and neck
            (a) Superficial — preauricular, posterior auricular,
                 occipital, tonsillar, submental, superior cervical,
                 posterior cervical, supraclavicular
            (b) Deep — submaxillary, deep cervical, infraclavicular
       ii. Upper extremities — all superficial
            (a) Axillary — lateral, central, subscapular (posterior),
                 pectoral (anterior)
            (b) Epitrochlear
       iii. Mediastinal — all deep
       iv. Abdominal — both superficial and deep
       v.   Lower extremities — all superficial — inguinal, femoral,
            popliteal

THYMUS GLAND

1. **Size changes with age**: rapid growth to 2 years of age, then slow
   growth to puberty, and degeneration after puberty

2. **Controls cellular immunity**: T-cell function or delayed hypersensitivity (see also section on Immunity)

────────────── **PHYSIOLOGY** ──────────────

ERYTHROCYTE PRODUCTION AND DESTRUCTION: Erythropoiesis and hemolysis.

1. **Erythropoiesis**: production of red cells requires energy
    a. Regulation
        i. Largely determined by relationship of cellular oxygen requirements and general metabolic activity
        ii. Stimulated by hypoxemia
        iii. Humoral control by erythropoietin, a hormone believed to be synthesized in kidney; various forms of cellular hypoxemia
        iv. Various endocrine glands, e.g., hypothalamus and pituitary, work on feedback system to stimulate release of erythropoietin from kidneys
    b. Nutritional requirements
        i. Nutrients (iron, vitamin B_{12}, folic acid) are necessary for erythrocyte and hemoglobin synthesis.
        ii. Deficiencies in nutrients result in decreased erythropoiesis
    c. Hemoglobin synthesis
        i. Takes place in bone marrow
        ii. Iron and a specific porphyrin combine to form heme molecule
        iii. Heme molecule then combines with one molecule of globin, a protein. Hemoglobin is formed by four connected chains of these subunits, a tetramer
        iv. Five distinct types of globin are responsible for producing the different varieties of normal hemoglobin — most common are fetal hemoglobin, which can be fully saturated with oxygen at a lower partial pressure, and adult hemoglobin

2. **Hemolysis**: destruction of red cells
    a. Destruction of immature red cells occurs in either bone marrow itself or in other reticuloendothelial organs, i.e., blood, general connective tissue, spleen, liver, lungs, and lymph nodes
    b. Destruction of mature red cells occurs in spleen
    c. Mechanisms resulting in premature destruction of erythrocytes
        i. Red cell membrane abnormalities
        ii. Hemoglobin abnormalities
        iii. Abnormal physical factors extrinsic to erythrocyte — primarily, glycolytic and enzymatic defects such as glucose-6-phosphate dehydrogenase (G6PD) and hexokinase deficiency

    d. Gross damage (e.g., that induced by trauma) results in intravascular destruction of red cells

    e. Extravascular hemolysis is removal of normal-aged red cells. It occurs in organs with large numbers of reticuloendothelial cells, e.g., spleen, liver, and (to some extent) bone marrow

IMMUNITY: Based on the body's recognition of a foreign substance.

1. **Humoral immunity:** antigens are processed by T cells and concentrated by macrophages; antibodies are then produced by B cells. Maximal effect which is active against extracellular pathogens is seen in minutes to hours

    a. Immunoglobulins

        i. IgG — the most common antibody

            (a) Major influence is against bacterial disease; some effect on viral

            (b) Functions in anamnestic responses, i.e., those that have immunologic memory as exemplified by events in secondary immune responses

            (c) Is major immunoglobulin in commercial gamma globulin

            (d) Is able to cross placenta, providing early form of antibody protection for neonates

       ii. IgA

            (a) Seen in two forms, serum and secretory — latter is most important

            (b) Found predominantly in saliva and secretions from GI and respiratory tracts

            (c) Appears to be major antibody protecting against antigen entry via respiratory tract

      iii. IgM

            (a) Like IgG, is most influential against bacterial disease, with some effect on viral

            (b) Is first antibody formed following exposure to an antigen, but its concentration diminishes rapidly as that of IgG increases

            (c) Does not cross placenta. An elevation of IgM levels in neonates indicates a viral or bacterial intrauterine infection, or mother/child ABO incompatibility

      iv. IgD — believed to protect fetus against infection

       v. IgE

            (a) Includes reagins, which cause many allergic reactions, involved in so-called "wheal-flare reaction." Reagins are antibodies that attach to tissue cells of same species from which they are derived, and that interact with their antigens to induce histamine release

            (b) May represent defense mechanism in respiratory tract

b. Blood groups — systems to determine type of antigens on surface
of red cells
   i.   ABO system
       (a) Basis of four blood groups (phenotypes), depending on
            presence or absence of A and B antigens
       (b) Antibodies that react with A or B antigens are found
            when corresponding antigen is absent from red cell
            surface (B antibodies are found in group A blood
            because B antigens are absent)
       (c) The four ABO blood groups are
            (1) O — so-called universal donor: genotype OO; has
                 no red cell antigens; serum contains both anti-A
                 and anti-B antibodies
            (2) A — genotypes AA and AO; has A antigens on red
                 cells; serum contains anti-B antibodies
            (3) B — genotypes BB and BO; has B antigens on red
                 cells; serum contains anti-A antibodies
            (4) AB — so-called universal recipient; genotype AB;
                 has both A and B antigens on red cells; serum
                 contains neither anti-A nor anti-B antibodies
       (d) Agglutination — basis for crossmatching of blood.
            Depends on presence of a serum antibody that reacts
            with antigens on red cells
            (1) Occurs in group A blood when B antigens are
                 introduced, because anti-B antibodies react with
                 B antigen
            (2) Indicates incompatibility when red cells of donor
                 and recipient are exposed to one another
   ii. Rh–Hr system — includes several Rh antigens; most potent
        is Rh D
       (a) Historically, an individual was considered Rh-positive
            if his red cells agglutinated when mixed with rabbit
            serum that had been immunized by red cells of rhesus
            monkey. Those whose blood did not agglutinate were
            considered to be Rh-negative. Terms "Rh-positive"
            and "Rh-negative" imply presence or absence of
            D respectively, since this is most immunogenic of
            Rh antigens
       (b) Antibody acting against Rh-Hr antigen generally is not
            in serum; antibody associated with A and B antigens *is*
            in serum
       (c) Antibody against Rh-Hr antigen is formed when
            Rh-negative person is sensitized to Rh-positive blood,
            usually as a result of transfusion therapy or maternal-
            fetal sensitization
c. Cold agglutinins — antibodies that cause erythrocytes to
    coagulate when blood plasma temperature is below normal body
    temperature

      i.   Commonly seen in blacks and patients with cirrhosis, severe anemia, hemolytic anemia, or other chronic disease

      ii.   When receiving cold blood, patients with chronic illnesses should be observed carefully for symptoms of cell hemolysis resulting from incompatibility of recipient and donor-cold agglutinins

      iii. Bank blood must be warmed before administration to patient who has cold agglutinins. Do not overheat blood — would result in denaturing of proteins

  d. Coombs' test

      i.   Used to determine presence of hemolyzing antibodies (e.g., Rh factor antibodies in Rh-negative person)

      ii.   Coombs' serum is prepared from rabbit serum sensitized against human globulins

      iii. Types of Coombs' tests

         (a) Direct — detects antibodies (IgG) attached to red cells

         (b) Indirect — detects antibodies (IgG) in serum

2. **Cellular immunity**: also known as thymic-controlled lymphocyte function; T-cell function; delayed hypersensitivity

  a. Does not involve immunoglobulins

  b. Important in antimicrobial defense (especially viruses, fungi, and protozoa), autoimmune disease, foreign tissue (graft) rejection, delayed hypersensitivity reactions, some allergies, and defense against cancer

  c. In fetus, T-cell precursors (lymphocytes) differentiate into clones within thymus, each programmed to recognize tissue as a "friendly" substance of "self" (basis of rejection phenomenon). T cells then migrate via lymphatics to lymph nodes, where they are stored

  d. When a foreign antigen enters system it attracts circulating T cells, which surround it and release the following factors (these factors cause the erythema and induration seen with positive delayed hypersensitivity reactions)

      i.   Interferon wraps around antigen

      ii.   Lymphocytotoxin assists in destruction of antigen

      iii. Macrophage attracting factor, from the tissues and in a circulating form, is mobilized

      iv. Migration-inhibiting factor (MIF) is released

      v.   B cells arrive (especially IgM) and facilitate neutralization of antigen

  e. When more T cells are needed, total WBC count rises. Laboratory data reflect

      i.   Increased neutrophils

      ii.   Increased bands

      iii. Immature (blast) forms on peripheral smear

3. **Phagocytic process**: a neutrophilic function involved with immunity, in which the following occur
   a. Adhesivity — macrophages slow down and adhere to vessel wall and site of antigen
   b. Penetration (also called diapedesis) — neutrophils begin to ooze through vessel wall into surrounding tissue
   c. Chemotaxis — macrophage migrates to site where antigen is located
   d. Phagocytosis — macrophage actually attaches to and engulfs antigen
   e. Killing — macrophage produces hydrogen peroxide, which destroys foreign substance
   f. Pus formation — from macrophages that also die after destroying foreign substance

4. **Complement system**
   a. Consists of distinct group of serum proteins (not antibodies) labeled C1 to C9. When activated, they function as mediators to enhance various aspects of inflammatory response, and to kill microorganisms directly without previous phagocytosis
   b. When foreign antigens are neutralized, certain factors related to complement must be present so that antigen and antibody can be bound to form an immune complex
   c. Complement-induced cell lysis produces a series of events that represent essential elements of an inflammatory response
      i. Increased capillary permeability
      ii. Chemotaxis of neutrophils
      iii. Immune adherence of antigen-antibody complexes
      iv. Promotion of phagocytosis
      v. Damage to membranes of mammalian cells, bacteria, and viruses, and possibly to basement membranes

5. **Autoimmunity**
   a. May be defined as appearance of antibodies that react against body's own tissue, as they would to foreign antigens
   b. Autoimmune disease is said to exist when either a humoral or cellular immune response causes tissue injury
   c. Mere presence of autoantibodies does not necessarily reflect autoimmune disease

6. **Consequences of immune responses**
   a. Immediate hypersensitivity reaction
      i. Cytotoxic — results in damage to a target cell selected because a complement-fixing antibody is directed against a cell surface antigen (e.g., acute hemolytic transfusion reaction)

      ii.   Anaphylactic — antigen-antibody interaction results in chemical mediators that act at secondary sites (particularly smooth muscle and vascular tissue)

   b. Subacute hypersensitivity reaction

      i.   Depends on immune complex deposits, activation of complement, and infiltration of PMNs

      ii.   Arthus lesions — a local skin reaction; serum sickness results when reaction is systemic

   c. Delayed hypersensitivity reaction — mediates reactions such as those seen with tuberculin skin testing and allograft rejection

INFLAMMATION: Sequence of events of white cell activity.

1. **Immediate increase in vascular permeability:** helps neutrophils get to site of inflammation

2. **Neutrophilia:** increased production of neutrophils starts 30–45 minutes after injury; peak phagocytic activity is reached in 6–8 hours

3. **Mononuclear cell (macrophages) exudation:** initiated 4 hours after injury; peak activity (phagocytic, formation of antibodies) is reached after 16–24 hours

4. **Leukocytosis:** usually secondary to neutrophilia, and often accompanied by increased sedimentation rate

5. **Isolation of inflammatory process:** may lead to abscess formation, thereby limiting spread of microorganisms
   a. Abscess is filled with pus that contains living bacteria and proteolytic enzymes, which can digest dead and living tissue
   b. Abscess may open by spontaneous rupture or by planned surgical incision and drainage

HEMOSTATIC MECHANISMS

1. **Vascular**
   a. Reflex vasoconstriction — arterioles contract when cut, thereby reducing blood flow to area of injury
   b. Larger vessels require collagen support for proper hemostasis. Defective collagen results in increased capillary fragility
   c. Disorders of blood vessel hemostasis
      i.   Acquired — usually secondary to or associated with septicemia, allergic vasculitis, drug-induced purpura
      ii.   Congenital — Ehlers-Danlos syndrome, abnormal collagen
   d. Evaluation of vascular mechanism
      i.   Bleeding time is prolonged

  ii. Good patient history is important because tests are not specific for vascular function

2. **Cellular (blood platelets)**
 a. Platelet plug is formed in capillaries by
  i. Adhesion — platelets are attracted to collagen, and so adhere to damaged vessel wall
  ii. Aggregation — platelets adhere to one another
 b. Disorders can be either acquired or congenital, and either quantitative (increased or decreased in number) or qualitative (diminished function)
 c. Thrombocytopenia — decreased numbers of platelets.* Major causes are
  i. Diminished production of platelets from bone marrow lesions secondary to drugs or disease, from aplastic anemia, or aspirin-induced thrombocytopenia
  ii. Increased destruction of platelets from drug-induced (e.g., quinidine) autoimmunity; viral disease; disseminated intra-vascular coagulation (DIC); or idiopathic thrombocyto-penic purpura (ITP)
  iii. Hypersplenism — often secondary to portal hypertension; results in increased sequestration of platelets in spleen
 d. Thrombocytosis — increased numbers of platelets (usually defined as more than 1 million per cubic ml). May lead to clot formation, necrosis of vessels distal to clots, or bleeding due to leakage from damaged vessels
 e. Evaluation of platelet function involves
  i. Careful observation for petechiae (may be first sign of platelet dysfunction)
  ii. Interpretation of laboratory data†
   (a) *In vivo* — bleeding time is best test
   (b) *In vitro* — platelet count; clot retraction

3. **Coagulation:** process by which plasma proteins in inactive form convert fluid blood to a clot
 a. Systems that initiate clotting
  i. Intrinsic system — initiated by contact activation following endothelial injury (i.e., "intrinsic" to blood vessel itself)
   (a) Factor XII initiates processes of intrinsic system as contact occurs between damaged vessel wall and plasma protein

---

*Since values vary from one institution to another, check with laboratory to determine values defining technical thrombocytopenia and prolonged bleeding time in your hospital.
†Significant values may vary from one institution to another.

(b) Factors VIII, IX, and XI all work as part of intrinsic system until it converges with common pathway

  ii. Extrinsic system – initiated by lipoproteins, known as tissue thromboplastins, which are released from injured tissue (i.e., "extrinsic" to blood vessels). Factor VII is part of extrinsic system, which then converges with common pathway

b. Common pathway – that part of coagulation cascade that is activated by either the intrinsic or the extrinsic pathways

  i. Platelet factor 3 (PF_3) and calcium react with factors X and V to accelerate clotting

  ii. Prothrombin is converted to thrombin (most powerful enzyme in coagulation process) by thromboplastin

  iii. Thrombin acts on fibrinogen to form soluble fibrin

  iv. Fibrin is essential portion of a clot; it is soluble until polymerized by factor XIII, which converts it to a stable (insoluble) fibrin clot

c. Screening tests for hemostatic function – group of tests that give information about both phases of hemostasis, and detect abnormalities in most cases

  i. Platelet count – tests number of platelets

  ii. Bleeding time – tests platelet plug formation

  iii. Partial thromboplastin time (PTT) – tests intrinsic and common pathways

  iv. Prothrombin time (PT) – tests extrinsic and common pathways

4. **Anticoagulant mechanisms in normal system:** to maintain blood in fluid state

a. Fibrinolytic system – clot-lysing activities maintain blood in fluid state

  i. Plasminogen is inert precursor of plasmin

  ii. Plasmin works to lyse fibrin clots. Found in two forms

  (a) Bound plasmin (in fibrin) – unaffected by antiplasmins, and carries out fibrinolysis (physiologic proteolysis)

  (b) Free plasmin (in plasma) – rapidly destroyed by antiplasmins, but if there is an excess of plasmin in comparison to antiplasmin, other plasma proteins and most coagulation factors may be destroyed, resulting in pathologic proteolysis

  iii. Fibrin split products (also called fibrin degradation products)

  (a) Breakdown products from fibrin and fibrinogen (known as fragments X, Y, D, and E)

  (b) When increased, highly suggestive of pathologic process in which coagulation factors are consumed

b. Antithrombin system – defends against excessive clotting

     i.   Antithrombin III — neutralizes clotting activity of thrombin; synthesized by liver

    ii.   Antithrombin II — plasma cofactor of heparin that acts with heparin to interfere in action of thrombin on fibrinogen (may be same as antithrombin III)

   iii.   Heparin — serine protease that inhibits all serine proteases in cascade, including XIIa, XIa, and Xa, as well as thrombin. Interferes with the action of thrombin on fibrinogen

---

ASSESSMENT

HISTORY: Much of the evaluation of this system depends on obtaining a thorough history.

1. **Family history:** may be positive for
   a. Jaundice
   b. Anemia
   c. Bleeding disorders — predisposition to bleed (as in hemophilia) and to clot (as in polycythemia)
   d. Malignancies
   e. Congenital RBC dyscrasias

2. **Medical history:** current and significant past
   a. Surgery
      i. Splenectomy
      ii. Tumor removal
      iii. Prosthetic heart valves
      iv. Surgical excision of portion of GI tract in which iron absorption occurs
   b. Allergies
      i. Multiple transfusions with blood or blood products
      ii. Known allergies and allergic reactions (including anaphylaxis)
   c. Mononucleosis
   d. Occupational exposure to radiation, or multiple treatments with internal or external beam radiation
   e. Occupational exposure to chemicals
   f. Recurrent infections
   g. Malabsorption syndrome
   h. Anemia
   i. Problems with wound healing

3. **Symptoms**
   a. General — fatigue, weakness, chills, fever, weight loss, heat intolerance, night sweats, poor wound healing, apathy, lethargy, malaise
   b. Specific

      i.   Skin — prolonged bleeding, excessive bruising, jaundice, pruritus, pallor

     ii.   Eyes — visual disturbances, blindness

   iii.   Ears — vertigo, tinnitus

   iv.   Nasopharynx and mouth — epistaxis, gingival bleeding, ulceration of tongue or oral mucosa, sore tongue, dysphagia, persistent hoarseness

     v.   Neck — nuchal rigidity

   vi.   Lymphadenopathy

  vii.   Chest — pulmonary emboli, exertional dyspnea, palpitations, angina pectoris, orthopnea, presence of prosthetic heart valves, respiratory tract infections, cough, hemoptysis, sternal tenderness, superior vena cava syndrome

 viii.   Gastrointestinal — melenic or hematochezic stools, liver disease, ulcers, abdominal pain, change in bowel habits, masses, vitamin K deficiency, alcohol abuse

   ix.   Genitourinary — hematuria, menorrhagia, amenorrhea, bladder dysfunction, urinary tract infections

     x.   Nervous system — confusion, impaired consciousness, headache, paresthesias, syncope

   xi.   Back and extremities — pain in joints, back, shoulder, or bone

4. **Medication history:** current
    a. Iron — oral and parenteral
    b. Vitamin B_{12}
    c. Pyridoxine
    d. Folic acid
    e. Corticosteroids
    f. Anticoagulants
    g. Antibiotics
    h. "Allergy" medication
    i. Aspirin or analgesics that contain aspirin
    j. Some antidysrhythmic agents
    k. Cryoprecipitate
    l. Antineoplastic agents
    m. Immunosuppressive agents

PHYSICAL EXAMINATION

1. **Inspection**
    a. Pallor or flushing of mucous membranes, nail beds, palmar creases
    b. Cyanosis
    c. Jaundice (best evaluated in daylight) of skin, conjunctivae, mucous membranes
    d. Bleeding
        i. Petechiae and ecchymoses

     ii.   Mucosal bleeding, including epistaxis
     iii. Retinal hemorrhages and exudates
     iv. Hemorrhage from any orifice
     v.   Plethora
  e. Ulcerations or lesions
  f. Swelling or redness (with particular attention to lymph nodes)
  g. Neuromuscular alterations
     i.   Pain and touch sensation
     ii.   Position and vibratory sensation
     iii. Tendon reflexes

2. **Palpation**
  a. Superficial lymph nodes — evaluate for
     i.   Location
     ii.   Size in centimeters
     iii. Tenderness
     iv. Fixation — movable or fixed
     v.   Texture — hard, soft, or firm
  b. Sternal tenderness
  c. Rib tenderness
  d. Joint mobility and tenderness
  e. Bone tenderness

3. **Percussion**
  a. Diaphragmatic excursion
  b. Hepatomegaly
  c. Splenomegaly

4. **Auscultation**
  a. Murmurs
  b. Bruits — cerebral, cardiac, splenic
  c. Rubs — pericardial, pleural
  d. Tachycardia
  e. Bowel sounds

DIAGNOSTIC STUDIES

1. **Laboratory**
  a. Blood
     i.   Complete blood count with differential and peripheral
        smear
        (a) RBC count with indices (MCV, MCH, MCHC) and
             peripheral smear
        (b) Hemoglobin
        (c) Hematocrit
        (d) WBC count with differential
        (e) Platelet count
        (f) Reticulocyte count

      ii.   PT
      iii. PTT
      iv. Erythrocyte sedimentation rate (ESR)
      v.   Serum protein electrophoresis
      vi. Serum bilirubin – direct and indirect
      vii. Serum iron
      viii. Total iron-binding capacity
      ix. Leukocyte alkaline phosphatase
      x.   Other, less common, studies – plasma protein assays; direct and indirect Coombs' tests; determination of fibrin split products

  b. Urine
      i.   Routine urinalysis
      ii. Bence-Jones protein assay
      iii. Hemetest
  c. Stool for guaiac

2. **Radiologic**
  a. Routine chest x-ray
  b. X-rays of other areas as indicated by history and physical examination (e.g., spine, flat abdomen)
  c. Lymphangiography
  d. Radionuclide scans

3. **Special**: bone marrow aspiration and biopsy

GENERAL PATIENT CARE MANAGEMENT

HEMATOLOGIC DISORDERS: These patients are not routinely admitted to the critical care unit unless they are in crisis or multiple system failure, or unless definitive therapy is planned.

PATIENTS WITH REDUCED NUMBERS OF ERYTHROCYTES

1. **Related problems**
  a. Fatigue and weakness – to alleviate, alternate periods of rest and activity should be encouraged
  b. Orthostatic hypotension – move patient slowly when changing his position
  c. Close monitoring of cardiopulmonary status is important because hypoxemia, oxygen saturation, and acid-base status are all affected by decreased number of erythrocytes. Tachypnea, orthopnea, tachycardia, palpitations, murmurs, or angina may be noted

2. **Administration of red blood cells:** may be part of therapeutic regime

PATIENTS WITH REDUCED NUMBERS OF WHITE CELLS

1. **Concurrent infection:** a major problem facing patient with compromised white cell function
    a. Significance of elevated temperature — when white cells are decreased, classic signs of infection (pus, redness, heat, pulmonary infiltrates) are not manifested; therefore, only fever may be present — a classic, hallmark sign
        i. Temperature pattern may be observed and recorded without treatment
        ii. Aspirin may interfere with normal platelet aggregation, thereby increasing possibility of hemorrhage. Acetaminophen is used only after evaluation of fever. Do not mask this important indicator
        iii. Hypothermia may be ordered to control excessively high body temperatures. Important to prevent shivering during this treatment, since shivering increases metabolic activity, produces heat, and may cause increased intracranial pressure (ICP), which predisposes to intracranial bleeding
        iv. Appropriate culture specimens should be obtained, using acceptable technique, to determine specific organism that needs treatment — critical to patient's survival
        v. If broad-spectrum antibiotics are being used until culture results return, prompt IV administration is preferred to oral route
    b. Complications may be indicated by certain complaints — sore throat; chest pain (possible pneumonia); burning on urination (possible urinary tract infection); chills and complaints of feeling cold when environment is warm; rectal pain (possible abscess)
    c. Meticulous perianal care is important, since irritated bowel mucosa may lead to perirectal abscess
        i. Character and number of bowel movements should be noted
        ii. Rectal thermometers, medications, or enemas should be avoided
        iii. Perianal area must be cleansed carefully after BMs
    d. Oral infections, e.g., *Candida albicans,* should be watched for closely
    e. IV antibiotics are important in severely neutropenic patients — orders for oral administration should be questioned
    f. IV administation — since these patients are particularly prone to infection, care should be used whenever venipuncture is

necessary. Special consideration should be given to reducing number of venipunctures, using metal or specially treated plastic needles, and employing an inline filter when appropriate. Institutional policy should be adhered to rigidly in regard to skin preps prior to venipuncture and to protocols for dressing changes

g. Patient should be encouraged in good personal hygiene — brisk hand washing, bathing, hair washing, perineal care, mouth care, skin inspection

h. Staff also should be instructed to follow exceptionally stringent hand washing techniques — this may preclude need for total reverse isolation

i. Skin irritation should be prevented since reddened areas may develop into cellulitis and lead to septicemia. Standard precautions for immobilized patients should be observed

j. Prevent infected or ill individuals (visitors, staff, other patients) from contacting patient

k. Administer antibiotics properly — dilute medication sufficiently to reduce irritation to vein, check for precipitates when more than one agent is used (clear line well in between drugs), evaluate for side effects such as nephrotoxicity and ototoxicity

2. **Granulocyte transfusions:** may be part of therapeutic regime

PATIENTS WITH DECREASED PLATELET FUNCTION

1. **Hemorrhage:** the major problem. Common sites of bleeding are gums, nose, bladder (hematuria); GI tract (bloody stools, hematemesis); and brain

a. Mouth care — reduction of friction on gums can be achieved by using baby bristle toothbrushes, cotton swabs, mild mouthwash, WaterPiks

b. Epistaxis may be life-threatening — patient should be placed in high Fowler's position; nose clips, ice, or nasal packing may be used to control hemorrhage

c. Maintain skin integrity
i.   Electric rather than straight-edged razors reduce possibility of accidental cuts
ii. After venipuncture, prolonged manual pressure is needed to avoid external bleeding and internal hematoma formation
iii. To reduce incidence of hematoma formation, medications should be given IV, not IM or SQ. If IV route is not possible, injections should be administered with a small gauge needle and pressure should be applied to puncture site for as long as necessary

      iv. Patients who receive oxygen via nasal prongs and endo-
tracheal tubes, or who have nasogastric or nasotracheal
tubes, should be observed for irritation of mucosa

      v. Protection from physical injury and trauma — take BP
carefully, as pressure from cuff can break superficial
capillaries and cause petechiae and ecchymoses; observe for
purpura; use restraints judiciously; pad bedrails and sharp
protuberances

  d. Instruct patient not to strain with BMs and when coughing

  e. Do not administer aspirin — it interferes with platelet aggregation
and may induce unnecessary gastric irritation

  f. Maintain careful record of number of sanitary napkins used
during menses, as menses may lead to hemorrhage

  g. Evaluate mental status carefully — confusion may also be due to
metabolic problems such as hypercalcemia, but may be first
signal of intracranial hemorrhage

2. **Platelet transfusions**: use proper techniques as indicated (this should
be included as transfusion therapy for other blood elements as
presented)

COMPLICATIONS ASSOCIATED WITH USE OF BONE MARROW SUPPRESSANTS

1. **Side effects**: most problems arise in anatomic areas where cell
division is rapid, e.g., entire GI tract, bone marrow, and hair
follicles

  a. Nausea and vomiting

      i. Antiemetics or sedatives may be necessary for control

      ii. Soda crackers, warm lemon-lime soda, or Coke syrup may
also offer relief from symptoms

      iii. Evaluate nutritional and hydration status

         (a) Modify oral diet — small, frequent meals; bland foods
of moderate temperature; pleasant environment

         (b) Institute total parenteral nutrition when necessary
unless patient is neutropenic

  b. Alopecia is a result of therapy, and is usually reversible —
patient may need reassurance that hair will grow back. Provide
patient with a head covering, if desired, such as a wig, scarf, or
hat

  c. Mouth sores — it is important to differentiate between *Candida
albicans* and stomatitis

      i. Modify diet — avoidance of acidic, spicy, or mechanically
irritating foods

      ii. Viscous lidocaine, oxethazaine, or other soothing agents may
be used for mouthwash

    d. Hyperuricemia results from cell breakdown
       i. Administration of allopurinol is common — skin rash indicates an allergic reaction to this agent
      ii. Alkaline urine helps prevent formation of renal calculi — may be maintained by encouraging fluid intake to 3 liters/day if this does not compromise cardiopulmonary status

2. **Bone marrow toxicity**: laboratory results may reveal presence of anemia, neutropenia, or thrombocytopenia

ADMINISTRATION OF BLOOD AND COMPONENT THERAPY

1. **Purposes of transfusion therapy**
    a. Facilitation of oxygen transport (RBCs)
    b. Expansion of volume (whole blood, plasma, albumin)
    c. Provision of proteins (fresh frozen plasma, albumin, plasma protein fraction)
    d. Provision of coagulation factors (cryoprecipitate, FFP, fresh whole blood)
    e. Provision of platelets (platelet concentrate, perhaps fresh whole blood)

2. **Blood and blood products**
    a. Citrate-phosphate-dextrose (CPD) whole blood
       i. Volume — about 500 ml/unit
      ii. If fresh, provides all components including platelets and coagulation factors
     iii. Large volume is a drawback — it takes 12–24 hours before Hb and HCT rise. Other sources of coagulation factors may be preferred, for similar reason
     iv. Possible complications
         (a) Hepatitis
         (b) Volume overload
         (c) Reaction to plasma proteins
         (d) Infusion of excess potassium and sodium
         (e) Infusion of anticoagulant (citrate)
    b. Red blood cells
       i. Volume — about 200–250 ml/unit
      ii. Replaces twice the amount of Hb as same amount of whole blood
         (a) Hb and HCT therefore rise faster than with whole blood replacement — Hb rises about 1–3 gm%/unit
         (b) Oxygen-carrying capacity is improved significantly
     iii. Indicated in anemia, slow blood loss, and CHF
     iv. Less risk of complications
    c. Fresh frozen plasma (FFP)
       i. Volume — approximately 200–250 ml/unit

    ii.   Contains all clotting factors except platelets

    iii.   Takes 20 minutes to thaw; is frozen to preserve factors V and VIII; stored at -30°C; good for 1 year

d. Cryoprecipitate

    i.   Volume of 10–20 ml/bag (coagulopathies such as DIC may require approximately 30 such bags)

    ii.   Contains factors VIII, fibrinogen, and XIII

    iii.   Should be used as soon as possible after thawing

    iv.   Indicated in hemophilia A, von Willebrand's disease, and DIC

e. Platelet concentrate

    i.   Volume – approximately 35–50 ml/unit

    ii.   Can be stored at room temperature for up to 3 days; bag should be agitated periodically.
Do not refrigerate

    iii.   Expected increase in platelets about $10,000/unit/m^2$. Failure to rise as expected may be due to fever, sepsis, splenomegaly, or DIC. Alloimmunization will also prevent increases in platelet count. Donor compatibility may be necessary

    iv.   Indicated in conditions caused by low platelet counts (below 10,000), e.g., ITP, DIC, dilutional thrombocytopenia, qualitative platelet disorders

f. Volume expanders

    i.   Albumin and plasma protein fraction (plasmanate) – chemically processed pooled plasma; treated with heat to kill hepatitis virus

       (a) Usually given in 250–500-ml increments in cases of shock

       (b) Solution is hyperosmolar, and acts by moving water from extravascular space to intravascular space – should not be used in dehydrated patients

       (c) Indicated for plasma volume expansion in shock, hypoproteinemia, cerebral edema, burns (reduces liquid and sodium losses, and prevents hemoconcentration)

    ii.   Salt-poor albumin

       (a) Usually given in 50–100-ml increments

       (b) Indicated in various hypoproteinemic states

g. Granulocytes

    i.   Available only in institutions with access to leukopheresis capability – requires special donors (or compatible donors)

    ii.   Each granulocyte suspension contains 200–300 ml

    iii.   Does not cause increase in WBC count; increases marginal pool (at tissue level – responsible for phagocytosis) rather than circulating pool

    iv.   Occurrence of fever and shaking chills during infusion is common and may not require cessation of transfusion –

prophylactic premedication with steroids and antihistamines may reduce the febrile response; meperidine may
control chills

3. **Transfusion reactions**
    a. Major types
        i. Hemolytic
        ii. Bacterial (febrile) — most common
        iii. Allergic (if severe, anaphylactic)
        iv. Circulatory overload
    b. Symptoms vary with type of reaction — all should be reported to
       blood bank and physicians — and may include
        i. Hives
        ii. Chills
        iii. Fever
        iv. Palpitations
        v. Chest pain
        vi. Flank pain
        vii. Headache
        viii. Flushing
        ix. Loss of consciousness
        x. Shortness of breath
        xi. Nausea/vomiting
        xii. Hypotension
        xiii. Tachycardia
        xiv. Increased warmth along vein in which IV catheter is
             inserted
    c. Nursing responsibilities — if a transfusion reaction occurs,
       blood should be stopped immediately and physician and blood
       bank notified. While physician's orders are awaited, patency of
       IV line should be maintained with saline solution, and BP and
       urinary output monitored. Subsequent nursing actions depend
       on type of reaction, treatment ordered by physician, and
       hospital policy. Nurses must be aware that reactions may be
       seen during blood administration or several days after blood
       transfusion

PSYCHOLOGIC SUPPORT OF PATIENT AND FAMILY

1. **Psychosocial adjustment:** most hematologic illnesses are chronic
   and require considerable adjustment as related to loss, sick role,
   role changes, coping behaviors, connotations of illness, etc.

2. **Psychologic effects of underlying hematologic condition:** these
   should be borne in mind even though patient may be in ICU for an
   unrelated disorder

3. **Other members of health team**: social worker, chaplain, dietician, physical therapist, and occupational therapist may all be involved in care of these patients

---------- **PATHOLOGIC CONDITIONS AND MANAGEMENT** ----------

ANEMIAS: This is a simplistic classification and overview. It is important to remember that anemia is a sign or symptom, not a disease entity.

1. **Pathophysiology**: reduced hemoglobin concentration of varying etiologies affects blood's oxygen-carrying capacity. Pathophysiologic effects are related to tissue hypoxia and compensatory mechanisms that try to maintain adequate oxygen delivery to meet cellular needs
   a. Oxyhemoglobin dissociation curve shifts right, thereby facilitating removal of more oxygen by tissues at same partial pressure of oxygen
   b. Blood is redistributed — it moves from tissues that have abundant blood supply but low oxygen need (skin, kidneys) to tissues that have high oxygen requirements (myocardium, brain, muscles)
   c. As severity of anemia increases, cardiac output must increase to meet oxygen demands of tissues
   d. 4–5 days after tissue hypoxemia increases erythropoietin production, rate of erythrocyte production increases

2. **Etiology or precipitating factors**
   a. Blood loss — may be acute or chronic
      i. GI tract
      ii. Menorrhagia
   b. Decreased production of erythrocytes
      i. Decreased hemoglobin synthesis
         (a) Iron deficiency
         (b) Decreased globin synthesis (thalassemias)
         (c) Decreased porphyrin — lead poisoning, sideroblastic anemia
      ii. Nuclear-cytoplasmic defect
         (a) Vitamin B_{12} deficiency
         (b) Folate deficiency
      iii. Decreased RBC precursors
         (a) Aplastic anemia
         (b) Replacement by tumor or myelofibrosis
   c. Increased destruction
      i. Intrinsic to erythrocytes

(a) Abnormal hemoglobins — Hb S, Hb C, unstable Hb
(b) Defective glycolysis (enzymes)
   (1) Pyruvate kinase deficiency
   (2) G6PD deficiency
(c) Membrane abnormalities
   (1) Hereditary spherocytosis
   (2) Hereditary elliptocytosis
   (3) Alpha-beta lipoproteinemias
   (4) Paroxysmal nocturnal hemoglobinuria (PNH)

ii. Extrinsic to erythrocytes
  (a) Physical
   (1) Prosthetic heart valves
   (2) Extracorporeal circulation
   (3) Abnormally small blood vessels (thrombotic thrombocytopenic purpura — TTP)
  (b) Antibodies
   (1) Autoregulation
   (2) Drug-related
  (c) Infectious agents and toxins
   (1) Malaria
   (2) Clostridia
   (3) Snake venom

3. **Clinical presentation**
  a. Skin and mucous membranes
   i. Pallor
   ii. Purpura
   iii. Jaundice
   iv. Pruritus
   v. Spider angiomas
  b. Eyes — blurred or impaired vision
  c. Ears — tinnitus
  d. Chest
   i. Exertional dyspnea
   ii. Tachypnea
   iii. Tachycardia
   iv. Palpitations
   v. Murmurs
   vi. Angina pectoris
   vii. Orthopnea
  e. GI tract
   i. Anorexia
   ii. Nausea
   iii. Splenomegaly
   iv. Melenic or hematochezic stools
   v. Dilated abdominal veins

    f. Genitourinary
      i.   Hematuria
      ii. Menorrhagia
    g. Nervous system
      i.   Headache
      ii. Vertigo
      iii. Irritability
      iv. Confusion
    h. Back and extremities
      i.   Bone tenderness, especially sternum
      ii. Joint pain
    i. Other
      i.   Fatigue
      ii. Weakness
      iii. Apathy

4. Diagnostic findings
    a. History
      i.   Precipitating causes, as described above
      ii. Developing clinical manifestations, as described above
      iii. Previous treatment for anemia
      iv. Use of drugs or exposure to toxins that could precipitate
           anemia
      v. Dietary history of iron deficiency, folic acid deficiency, and
          B_{12} deficiency
      vi. Underlying disease that could precipitate anemia, e.g.,
          chronic liver disease or uremia
    b. Physical examination − see Clinical presentation
    c. Diagnostic studies
      i.   Laboratory
         (a) CBC − erythrocyte count decreased
         (b) Hb decreased
         (c) HCT and red cell indices (MCV, MCH, MCHC)
             decreased
         (d) Leukocyte count with differential − after hemorrhage,
             neutrophils may be increased
         (e) Platelet count may increase after hemorrhage
         (f) Peripheral blood smear − immature cells
         (g) Reticulocyte count usually decreased, may be
             increased
         (h) Other studies employed after anemia has been
             classified include assays for
             (1) Vitamin B_{12} − absorption decreased
             (2) Folate − decreased
             (3) Pyridoxine − decreased
             (4) BUN − may be elevated
             (5) Creatinine − elevated when anemia is
                 secondary to chronic renal failure

        (6)   Serum iron-binding capacity — elevated only in iron deficiency anemia; usually normal or low in other types of anemia

        (7)   Coombs' test

            (a)   Direct — positive in acquired hemolytic anemia

            (b)   Indirect — usually negative

        (8)   Indirect bilirubin — elevated

        (9)   Stool guaiac — may be positive, especially if anemia is due to bleeding

      (10)   Urinalysis — nonspecific, possibly microscopic anemia

    ii.   Radiologic

       (a)   Chest x-ray nonspecific

       (b)   Upper and lower GI series will be positive during current or recent active bleeding

    iii.   Special — if indicated by classification

       (a)   Bone marrow — in pernicious anemia is hypercellular, containing a large number of red cell precursors with a characteristic megaloblastic pattern

       (b)   Gastric analysis — neutral pH and no titratable acidity in patients with pernicious anemia

5. **Complications**

    a.   Improper identification of etiology of anemia, which can lead to inappropriate treatment

    b.   Cardiopulmonary abnormalities in patients who try to compensate for hypoxemic effects of anemia

    c.   Infection and hemorrhage, common in aplastic anemia

6. **Specific patient care**: many of these conditions are chronic. Nursing intervention should be appropriate to the specific etiology of the anemia. See also General Patient Care Management

LEUKEMIA: A malignant hematologic neoplasm, affecting the bone marrow, lymph system, and spleen, characterized by disorderly, unregulated proliferation of white blood cells. The disease usually follows a progressive course that is eventually fatal, although the patient may live for decades with the disease. It is important to have some understanding of the specific types of leukemia, because of their different presentations and outcomes. Therefore, in addition to a general overview, the four major types of leukemia — chronic lymphocytic, chronic granulocytic, acute lymphoblastic, and acute granuloblastic — will be discussed separately below.

1. **Pathophysiology**
   a. Although cause is not yet entirely understood, there is either impaired maturation of WBCs or increased production of immature blood cells
   b. Whereas normal cells lose their mitotic ability as they mature, leukemic cells retain their ability to divide, and fail to mature and differentiate

2. **Etiology or precipitating factors**: exact etiology is unknown, but certain contributing factors may include
   a. Exposure to ionizing radiation in large doses
   b. Various chemical agents, e.g., benzene
   c. Genetic factors
   d. Viral influences
   e. Immunologic deficiencies

3. **Clinical presentation**
   a. Bone marrow failure
      i. Fatigue and symptoms of anemia (described above)
      ii. Hemorrhage, as reflection of thrombocytopenia
      iii. Infection, as indication of neutropenia
   b. Formation of masses composed of leukemic infiltrates
      i. Splenomegaly
      ii. Lymphadenopathy
      iii. Bone pain
      iv. Meningeal infiltration
      v. Oral lesions and gingival infiltrates
   c. General complaints
      i. Fever
      ii. Weight loss

4. **Diagnostic findings**: depend on type of leukemia – see descriptions below

5. **Complications**
   a. Infiltration of organs with leukemic cells
      i. Splenomegaly
      ii. Hepatomegaly
      iii. Lymphadenopathy
      iv. CNS involvement
      v. Renal infiltrates
      vi. Bone lesions
      vii. Skin infiltration

    b. Reduction in normal hematopoietic cells resulting in
       i. Anemia
       ii. Hemorrhage
       iii. Fever and infection
    c. Metabolic alterations leading to
       i. Hypercalcemia — as granulocytic elements in bone marrow proliferate, marrow changes occur that can lead to diffuse skeletal demineralization
       ii. Hyperuricemia — results from both increased metabolism secondary to rapid cell proliferation and death, and accumulation of cellular waste products secondary to effective therapy. If moderate, causes goutlike joint pain; if severe, can lead to impaired renal function and kidney failure

6. **Specific patient care**
    a. Recognize differences between various types of leukemia
       i. Classifications are based on cell type involved — granulocytic, lymphocytic, or monocytic, the latter being rare
       ii. Classifications are based on cell maturity — "acute" indicates that marrow infiltrate consists of mostly young, undifferentiated immature cells, often referred to as "blasts," whereas "chronic" implies that marrow is composed primarily of differentiated or mature cells
    b. Become familiar with various drug therapies and their side effects, which are potentially life-threatening
    c. Understand how steroids, although often a part of therapy, may mask symptoms of infection
    d. Prevent complications of pancytopenia, which are life-threatening
    e. Develop an understanding of remission as goal of therapy
       i. Induction — initial aggressive chemotherapy, when patient is more predisposed to complications
       ii. Maintenance — continued therapy that is less potent, used to facilitate continued remission
       iii. Complete remission — no evidence of disease in either bone marrow or peripheral blood
       iv. Partial remission — peripheral blood shows no disease, but disease is present in bone marrow

CHRONIC LYMPHOCYTIC LEUKEMIA (CLL)

1. **Pathophysiology**
    a. Disorderly proliferation of lymphoid tissue
    b. Normal B cells are reduced, leading to increased incidence of infections

2. **Etiology or precipitating factors:** see section on Leukemia

3. **Clinical presentation**
   a. Male predominance — 2.5:1
   b. Rare below age 45; patients usually are 50–70 years old
   c. Often found during examination for an unrelated disease — usually asymptomatic; gradual onset
   d. Lymphadenopathy and splenomegaly in 70% of patients
   e. Hepatomegaly in 25% of patients
   f. Sternal tenderness is rare

4. **Diagnostic findings**
   a. History — related to clinical presentation (see above)
   b. Physical examination — dictated by clinical presentation (see above); this type of leukemia is frequently discovered when evaluating a completely unrelated disease process
   c. Diagnostic studies
      i. Laboratory
         (a) Increased lymphocytes
         (b) Mild anemia as disease progresses
         (c) Mild thrombocytopenia as disease progresses
         (d) Increased incidence of Coombs'-positive hemolytic anemia
         (e) Increased reticulocyte count if hemolyzing cells present
      ii. Bone marrow contains more lymphocytes than normal

5. **Complications:** rare early, but develop as disease progresses. Occasionally, hemolytic anemia develops — if treated, infection and hemorrhage may result from cytotoxic therapy. Patients live well with this type of leukemia, and therefore concomitant illnesses are treated

6. **Specific patient care:** see section on Leukemia

CHRONIC GRANULOCYTIC LEUKEMIA (CGL): also called chronic myelogenous leukemia (CML).

1. **Pathophysiology**
   a. A common stem cell precursor of red cells, white cells, and platelets undergoes mutation
   b. An excessive development of neoplastic granulocytes in bone marrow replaces normal white cells and red cells
   c. These granulocytes move into peripheral blood in significant numbers
   d. All stages of cells (immature to mature) are found in bone marrow and peripheral blood, but mature cells are dominant peripherally

2. **Etiology or precipitating factors**: see section on Leukemia

3. **Clinical presentation**
   a. Predominantly found in young and middle-aged adults, ages 25–60
   b. Patient may be asymptomatic at first, but symptoms develop as disease progresses
   c. Weakness
   d. Weight loss
   e. Bone pain
   f. Fever
   g. Fatigue
   h. Moderate-to-massive splenomegaly
   i. Sternal tenderness
   j. Lymphadenopathy uncommon

4. **Diagnostic findings**
   a. History – related to clinical presentation (see above)
   b. Physical examination – dictated by clinical presentation (see above)
   c. Diagnostic studies
      i. Laboratory
         (a) Leukocytes – increased PMNs, decreased or normal monocytes, normal lymphocytes
         (b) Anemia
         (c) Platelet count – early in disease, thrombocytosis; late in disease, thrombocytopenia
         (d) Decreased leukocyte alkaline phosphatase
         (e) Philadelphia chromosome seen in 90% of patients with this disease – only disease in which it is present
      ii. Bone marrow demonstrates an increased myeloid: erythroid ratio

5. **Complications**: blastic crisis
   a. Increased myeloblasts in both blood and bone marrow
   b. Blastic crisis changes chronic leukemia to acute disease (cells are immature)
   c. Therapy can only be palliative, and complications (primarily infection and hemorrhage) usually accompany treatment

6. **Specific patient care**: see section on Leukemia

ACUTE LYMPHOBLASTIC LEUKEMIA (ALL): These individuals usually have a good response to treatment. There is a 95% chance of remission, and 50–60% of patients under age 15 achieve a 5-year survival (at present, cure is defined as 10-year survival).

1. **Pathophysiology**: proliferation of immature lymphocytes in bone marrow

2. **Etiology or precipitating factors**: see section on Leukemia

3. **Clinical presentation**
   a. Abrupt onset, usually before age 14, and infrequent beyond age 20; the most common leukemia of childhood
   b. Male predominance — 1.5:1
   c. Bone and joint pain
   d. Neurologic complaints due to CNS metastases
   e. Minimal hepatosplenomegaly
   f. Generalized lymphadenopathy
   g. Bleeding
   h. Headache
   i. Symptoms of increased ICP, secondary to meningeal infiltration

4. **Diagnostic findings**
   a. History — related to clinical presentation (see above)
   b. Physical examination — dictated by clinical presentation (see above)
   c. Diagnostic studies
      i. Laboratory
         (a) WBCs range from extremely low counts to above 100,000/mm^3. Characterized by many immature cells and presence of blasts
         (b) RBC counts decreased—anemia
         (c) Platelets decreased—thrombocytopenia profound
      ii. Radiologic — transverse lines of rarefaction at ends of long bones
      iii. Special — bone marrow is hypercellular, over half of cells being blast cells

5. **Complications**
   a. Most often secondary to antineoplastic therapy
   b. Intracranial bleeding may lead to death if WBC counts are extremely high
   c. Recurrence — sanctuaries for leukemic cells are found in CNS and reproductive organs

6. **Specific patient care**: see section on Leukemia

ACUTE GRANULOBLASTIC LEUKEMIA (AGL): Also called acute myeloblastic leukemia (AML). Patients live only 2–3 months without treatment. About 70% of those treated experience a remission lasting 6 months to 2 years.

1. **Pathophysiology**: uncontrolled proliferation of myeloblasts, the granulocytic precursors with hyperplasia of bone marrow and spleen

2. **Etiology or precipitating factors:** see section on Leukemia

3. **Clinical presentation**
   a. Usually affects people 20–24 years of age
   b. Uncontrollable bleeding
   c. Purpura
   d. Uncontrollable infection
   e. Fever
   f. Fatigue and weakness
   g. End stage of a variety of myeloproliferative diseases
   h. Minimal hepatosplenomegaly and lymphadenopathy
   i. Pallor
   j. Sternal tenderness
   k. Patients may not appear seriously ill at first

4. **Diagnostic findings**
   a. History – related to clinical presentation (see above)
   b. Physical examination – dictated by clinical presentation (see above)
   c. Diagnostic studies
       i. Laboratory
           (a) Leukocytes usually low or normal; may be high – classic myeloblasts contain Auer rods
           (b) Anemia – often severe
           (c) Platelet count very low unless disease is discovered very early
           (d) Reticulocyte count low
       ii. Bone marrow is usually markedly hypercellular as normal elements are replaced by a diffuse proliferation of immature granulocytes (mostly myeloblasts) and some atypical differentiated cells

5. **Complications**: usually secondary to therapy, but may be due to disease itself – control is important to ensure remission and survival
   a. Infection
   b. Hemorrhage

6. **Specific patient care:** see section on Leukemia

ANAPHYLAXIS: An exaggerated form of hypersensitivity that occurs within 1–20 minutes after introduction of the antigenic agent.

1. **Pathophysiology**
   a. Following sensitizing exposure, subsequent contacts with antigen activate an antibody-mediated reaction

b. Bronchospasm follows release of histamine, which has potent effect on smooth muscles of bronchioles and small blood vessels

c. As a result of vasodilation and increased vascular permeability, plasma leaves vascular space, resulting in vessel collapse and interstitial edema. Hypovolemia, resulting from loss of large amounts of fluid from intravascular space, leads to hypotension, shock, and circulatory compromise

2. **Etiology or precipitating factors**
   a. Drugs, especially penicillin
   b. Sera
   c. Insect stings, especially from bees and wasps
   d. Injected diagnostic reagents – intradermal skin tests, dyes, local anesthetics

3. **Clinical presentation**
   a. Arthralgia
   b. Generalized feeling of fear that increases with progressive difficulty in breathing and stridor
   c. Collapse
   d. Urticaria or other rashes
   e. Fever
   f. Lymphadenopathy
   g. Facial edema
   h. Profound hypotension
   i. Wheezing
   j. Cyanosis
   k. Palpitations

4. **Diagnostic findings**
   a. History
      i. Any existing allergic conditions
      ii. Any of the signs listed above under Clinical presentation, experienced in conjunction with any of the possible precipitating therapies
   b. Physical examination – dictated by clinical presentation (see above)
   c. Diagnostic studies – anaphylaxis is diagnosed on basis of symptoms. Following incident however, it is important to evaluate exact etiology in order to prevent recurrences

5. **Complications**
   a. Convulsions
   b. Cardiopulmonary arrest

6. **Specific patient care**: resuscitation to control circulation and ventilation
   a. Assess cardiac, respiratory, and neurologic status

    b. Immediately administer epinephrine SQ or IM (0.5–1.0 ml of a
1:1000 solution) – give IV if circulation is already compromised

    c. Maintain airway; provide supplemental oxygen

    d. Treat shock by replacing fluids rapidly to expand vascular
volume; vasopressors may be warranted; albumin may increase
vascular volume and help reduce edema

    e. Give aminophylline and corticosteroids IV, to diminish
bronchospasm

    f. Institute CPR if necessary

DISSEMINATED INTRAVASCULAR COAGULATION (DIC): A serious
bleeding disorder resulting from accelerated normal clotting, with a
subsequent decrease in clotting factors and platelets.

1. **Pathophysiology**

    a. Abundant intravascular thrombin is produced, which both
converts fibrinogen to a fibrin clot and enhances platelet
aggregation

    b. Naturally-occurring antithrombins, which inhibit thrombin, are
inactivated by plasmin

    c. Ultimately, as clots are lysed and clotting factors are destroyed,
blood loses its ability to clot

    d. A stable clot therefore, cannot be formed at injury sites,
predisposing patient to hemorrhage

2. **Etiology or precipitating factors**

    a. An abnormal syndrome that is always secondary to another
process

    b. Disorders in which DIC may be triggered include

        i. Obstetric – most common

            (a) Abruptio placentae

            (b) Retained dead fetus

            (c) Amniotic fluid embolism

       ii. Hemolytic processes

            (a) Transfusion of mismatched blood

            (b) Acute hemolysis with infection or immunologic
disorders

      iii. Tissue damage

            (a) Extensive burns and trauma

            (b) Rejection of transplants

            (c) Postoperative damage, especially following
extracorporeal circulation

            (d) Heat stroke

      iv. Neoplastic

            (a) Cancer of prostate

            (b) Acute leukemias – secondary to cell destruction from
chemotherapy

            (c) Giant cavernous hemangioma

     v.   Fat embolism
    vi.   Snake bites
   vii.   Acidosis

3. **Clinical presentation**
   a. Bleeding in a patient with no previous bleeding history
   b. Severity may vary from mild oozing at venipuncture sites to significant hemorrhage from all orifices (latter is most common)
   c. Signs and symptoms
      i. Acrocyanosis or signs of peripheral thrombosis
      ii. Purpura

4. **Diagnostic findings**
   a. History
      i. Evaluation of underlying diseases that may predispose patient to DIC
      ii. Related to clinical presentation (see above)
   b. Physical examination — dictated by underlying disease and clinical presentation (see above)
   c. Diagnostic studies
      i. Laboratory
         (a) PT prolonged
         (b) PTT prolonged
         (c) Thrombin time prolonged
         (d) Fibrinogen decreased
         (e) Platelet count decreased
         (f) Fibrin split products elevated
         (g) Schistocytes in peripheral smear
         (h) Bilirubin elevated
         (i) HCT low
         (j) Protamine sulfate test—strongly positive

5. **Complications**: uncontrollable hemorrhage

6. **Specific patient care**: in addition to emergency measures, treatment of underlying cause of DIC is necessary for effective management
   a. Give blood product support to convert serum to plasma
      i. FFP — to replenish consumed factors, and provide antithrombin if heparin is used; may preclude need for heparin
      ii. Cryoprecipitate, possibly, as source of fibrinogen
      iii. Platelets
      iv. Specific factor replacement
   b. Heparin — only IV route is acceptable. Use is controversial as efficacy difficult to prove
      i. Its antithrombin activity neutralizes free circulating thrombin and prevents propagation of thrombi that have formed in capillaries

       ii.   Has an inhibitory effect on activation of blood clotting

       iii. Factor replacement is also needed

  c. Epsilon aminocaproic acid — EACA (Amicar)

       i.   Inhibits fibrinolysis

       ii. Use is controversial — never give in DIC without first treating with blood products and heparin

  d. Correction or prevention of acidosis serves to diminish development of DIC

  e. Evaluate evidence of active hemorrhage. Carefully measure blood loss — weight bandages, pads, and linen, and record drainage

  f. Review laboratory data to evaluate DIC and its therapy

SELECT HEREDITARY BLEEDING STATES

1. **Hemophilias:** sex-linked recessive traits — seen almost exclusively in males, but female carriers transmit the disease
   a. Classic hemophilia (A) is a factor VIII deficiency
   b. Christmas disease (hemophilia B) is a factor IX deficiency

2. **Von Willebrand's disease:** an autosomal dominant trait seen in both sexes, characterized by platelet dysfunction as well as low levels of factor VIII

3. **Clinical presentation**
   a. Begins in childhood
   b. Uncontrollable hemorrhage from minor injuries, e.g., dental extractions and hematomas of unknown origin
   c. Neurologic manifestations, usually from nerve compression secondary to hemorrhage
   d. Hemarthrosis (not seen in von Willebrand's)
   e. Hematuria
   f. Epistaxis

4. **Diagnostic findings**
   a. History
      i. Familial history of bleeding disorders
      ii. Related to clinical presentation (see above)
   b. Physical examination — dictated by clinical presentation (see above)
   c. Diagnostic studies
      i. Laboratory
         (a) PTT prolonged
         (b) Factor VIII assay shows decrease in hemophilia A; also decreased, but not consistently, in von Willebrand's
         (c) Factor IX assay shows decrease in hemophilia B.
         (d) Platelet adhesivity and bleeding time — normal with hemophilia; decreased with von Willebrand's

    ii.   Radiologic — major joint destruction following repeated bleeds

5. **Complications**
   a. Uncontrollable hemorrhage
   b. Painful hemarthrosis

6. **Specific patient care**
   a. Management of hemorrhage
      i. Evaluate extent of hemorrhage
      ii. Replace factor VIII, IX, and platelets as needed to achieve and maintain adequate hemostasis
      iii. Administer antihemophilic factors
      iv. Avoid IM and SQ injections
      v. Firm pressure or ice on cuts and abrasions usually controls bleeding; in hospital use Gelfoam or fibrin foam packing
      vi. Pressure from a nasal catheter usually controls epistaxis
   b. Management of painful hemarthrosis in hemophiliacs may require use of potent analgesics; joint must be totally immobilized to prevent crippling deformities
   c. Reinforce patient and family education
      i. Patient and family should be able to recognize problems that require hospital treatment and how to prevent injuries
      ii. Home administration of antihemophiliac factors may be appropriate
      iii. Teach good dental care techniques to reduce need for oral surgery
   d. Psychosocial support — if not already accomplished, following should be initiated
      i. Referral to National Hemophilia Society
      ii. Assessment of patient and family adaptation to disease
      iii. Genetic evaluation and counseling
      iv. Psychotherapy and association with other patients who are managing successfully

SICKLE CELL DISEASE: A chronic, hereditary, hemolytic disease, seen almost exclusively in blacks.

1. **Pathophysiology**
   a. An Hb S gene is inherited from each parent, and therefore red cells lack Hb A. When deprived of oxygen, Hb S red cells assume various crescent shapes, e.g., sickle shapes
   b. Erythrostasis occurs when sickled red cells become trapped in small vessels
   c. Further sickling and increased blood viscosity result from deoxygenation and reduced pH
   d. Cycle develops as deoxygenation and reduced pH are perpetuated, leading to more sickling

e. Sickled red cells form solid masses that occlude blood vessels, thereby leading to thrombosis and infarction

f. When stasis is resolved, a certain portion of red cells released into free circulation will be more sensitive to mechanical trauma, even the normal trauma experienced during circulation

2. **Clinical presentation**
    a. Increased weakness
    b. Aching joint pain, especially in hands and feet (dactylitis)
    c. Bony deformities
    d. Chest pain
    e. ECG changes—related to chest pain
    f. Cardiomegaly — cardiac signs resemble mitral stenosis or mitral regurgitation; peripheral signs resemble aortic insufficiency
    g. Sudden, severe abdominal pain
    h. Chronic leg ulcers
    i. Icteric sclera
    j. Funduscopic vessel changes
    k. Impaired growth and development
    l. Retardation of secondary sex characteristics

3. **Diagnostic findings**
    a. History
        i. Documentation of familial blood disorders
        ii. Related to clinical presentation (see above)
    b. Physical examination — dictated by clinical presentation (see above)
    c. Diagnostic studies
        i. Laboratory
            (a) Leukocytosis
            (b) Hemolytic anemia
            (c) Hb S in erythrocytes. (It is important to distinguish sickle cell trait from the disease. In both the trait and the disease, sickle cell prep and sickledex will be positive. Hb electrophoresis will be all Hb S with the disease, and 50% Hb S with the trait. Peripheral smear will be normal with the trait, but will show sickle cells with the disease.)
            (d) Increased reticulocyte count
            (e) Increased platelets
            (f) Impaired ability to concentrate urine
        ii. Radiologic
            (a) IVP shows increased renal medullary blood flow and dilated tortuous medullary blood vessels
            (b) Bone x-rays show increased density or aseptic necrosis secondary to infarction (skull — radial striation; vertebral bodies — osteoporosis)

4. **Complications**
   a. Painful crises that characterize this disease
   b. Impaired circulation resulting in leg ulcers
   c. Infarction of various body organs and areas
   d. Shrinkage of spleen
   e. Hepatomegaly
   f. Aseptic bone necrosis
   g. Hematuria
   h. Priapism
   i. Pulmonary infarction
   j. CNS problems
   k. Shock secondary to crisis
      i. Abdominal — capillary hypoxia may result in plasma loss, hemoconcentration, and further stagnation
      ii. Cardiogenic — resembles myocardial infarction or acute myocarditis

5. **Specific patient care**
   a. Because of inherited nature, no cure is available, so care must be directed toward symptomatic relief
   b. Adequate hydration and electrolyte balance are essential
   c. Correct acidosis if it occurs
   d. Pain is usually severe — both oxygen and analgesics may be necessary
   e. Institute prompt antibiotic therapy for infections
   f. Administer blood or blood products during shock or aplastic crises
   g. Anticipate and develop strategies for dealing with repeated exacerbations and psychologic reactions of patient and family
   h. Refer for genetic counseling

MULTIPLE MYELOMA: A neoplastic disorder of plasma cells, usually arising in the bone marrow.

1. **Pathophysiology**
   a. Neoplastic plasma cells produce abnormal immunoglobulins (myeloma or M proteins), thereby diminishing body defenses
   b. In more advanced stages, proliferation of myeloma cells causes diffuse osteoporosis as protein destroys bone
      i. Bony lesions often are best seen in skull, vertebrae, and ribs
      ii. Hypercalcemia also accompanies advanced disease
      iii. Vertebral destruction may lead to collapse of vertebrae, with ensuing compression of spinal cord, nerve roots, or spinal nerves
   c. Hypercalcemia and excessive amounts of circulating protein may lead to kidney obstruction and renal failure

2. **Etiology or precipitating factors:** many hypotheses, but no identified cause

3. **Clinical presentation**
   a. Weakness
   b. Unexplained infection
   c. Relatively asymptomatic until disease is advanced
      i. Skeletal pain — predominant manifestation when patients become symptomatic
      ii. Susceptibility to infections
      iii. Hemorrhage
   d. Renal failure
   e. Amyloidosis
   f. Neurologic manifestations
   g. Arthritis

4. **Diagnostic findings**
   a. History — related to clinical presentation (see above)
   b. Physical examination — dictated by clinical presentation (see above)
   c. Diagnostic studies
      i. Laboratory
         (a) Increased ESR
         (b) Pancytopenia
         (c) Hyperuricemia
         (d) Uremia
         (e) Hypercalcemia
         (f) Sudden, high elevation in serum and urine protein electrophoresis
         (g) Positive urine for Bence-Jones protein
         (h) Elevated creatinine
      ii. Radiologic — osteolytic skeletal lesions, especially seen in skull, vertebrae, and ribs
      iii. Bone marrow shows increased plasma cells and abnormal forms

5. **Complications**
   a. Frequent and recurrent infections
   b. Renal disease resulting from infection, calcium precipitates, uric acid complications of multiple myeloma, Bence-Jones proteinuria
   c. Damage to liver, spleen, lungs, and various structures in nervous system
   d. Hypercalcemia
   e. Pathologic fractures
   f. Uric acid complications

6. **Specific patient care**
   a. Hypercalcemia and renal complications – provide for
      i.   Control of dietary protein and calcium
      ii. Adequate hydration – maintain urine output of 1½–2 liters/day
      iii. Ambulation
      iv. Analgesia – aspirin is more effective to diminish bone pain than more potent analgesics
      v.   Medications – allopurinol for hyperuricemia; steroids
      vi. Ongoing evaluation of kidney function
   b. Treatment of localized lesions – provide for
      i.   Radiation therapy
      ii. Analgesics
      iii. Orthopedic supports
      iv. Good body alignment
   c. Chemotherapy is treatment of choice to improve and prolong survival by reducing number of plasma cells

LYMPHOMAS

1. **Pathophysiology**: hyperplasia of lymphoreticular tissues
   a. These neoplasms can be differentiated by histopathologic appearance and different patterns of development and metastasis
   b. Classification – helpful in predicting patterns of presentation and dissimination; also has predictive value in terms of sites of involvement, tendency to remain localized, response to therapy, and prognosis
      i. Hodgkin's lymphomas (characterized by Reed-Sternberg cell)
          (a) Lymphocytic predominant (16%)
          (b) Nodular sclerosis (35%)
          (c) Mixed cellularity (33%)
          (d) Lymphocyte depletion (16%)
      ii. Non-Hodgkin's, lymphomas
          (a) Burkitt's tumor
          (b) Reticulum cell sarcoma
          (c) Lymphosarcoma
   c. Staging – determines extent of disease. Based on symptoms and location and node involvement
      i. Classification by symptoms
          (a) A – asymptomatic
          (b) B – symptomatic for certain general symptoms
              (1) Unexplained weight loss of greater than 10% body weight over 6 months

(2)   Unexplained fever with temperature above 38°C
(3)   Night sweats
ii.   Staging by extent of disease involvement
(a)   Stage I — one node group involved
(b)   Stage II — two nodal areas of involvement on same side of diaphragm
(c)   Stage III — nodes involved on both sides of diaphragm
(d)   Stage IV — disease has spread to organs outside lymphatic system
iii.   Important in terms of prognostic and treatment implications
(a)   In Hodgkin's disease, Stages I and II are usually treated with radiation therapy — and many patients are "cured"
(b)   In Hodgkin's disease, chemotherapy can provide 10-year survival for patients with stage III or IV disease
iv.   Exploratory laparotomy is often a part of staging procedure
(a)   Deep lymph nodes can be examined (i.e., retroperitoneal nodes)
(b)   Splenectomy is often done to facilitate examination for evidence of disease involvement
(c)   Radiopaque clips are often placed in abdomen to serve as landmarks for planning future radiation therapy
v.   Staging as a predictive guide is important because statistical chances for cure are greater in patients with more restricted disease. When other problems develop, they may be treated quite aggressively

2.   **Etiology or precipitating factors:** unknown

3.   **Clinical presentation**
a.   Lymphadenopathy — discrete and movable nodes that are also painless (unless nerves are involved) and nontender
b.   Mediastinal involvement results in cough, dyspnea, stridor, dysphagia
c.   Weight loss
d.   Fever
e.   Night sweats
f.   Pain with alcohol ingestion
g.   Splenomegaly —especially in Hodgkin's lymphoma
h.   Palpable liver
i.   Cachexia
j.   Jaundice
k.   Urticaria and other rashes

4.   **Diagnostic findings**
a.   History — related to clinical presentation (see above)

    b. Physical examination — dictated by clinical presentation (see above)

    c. Diagnostic studies

       i. Laboratory

          (a) Slight leukocytosis or leukopenia

          (b) Anemia

          (c) Increased platelets in Hodgkin's lymphoma

          (d) Presence of Reed-Sternberg cells in Hodgkin's lymphoma

       ii. Radiologic

          (a) Chest x-ray may reveal mediastinal or hilar node involvement

          (b) Bone x-ray may show involvement of skeletal system

          (c) Lymphangiography will show extent of involvement of lymphatic system

      iii. .Bone marrow — not characteristic, and rarely helpful

      iv. Excisional lymph node biopsy — offers definitive means to diagnose Hodgkin's disease

5. **Complications**: usually secondary to treatment; often life-threatening

    a. Fatigue, malaise, lassitude

    b. Anorexia, nausea, vomiting

    c. Diarrhea or constipation

    d. Obstruction

    e. Hematopoietic effects, pancytopenia

    f. Skin erythema or desquamation from radiotherapy

6. **Specific patient care**

    a. Radiotherapy — proper techniques for skin care

       i. Use tepid water for bathing area being radiated

       ii. Gently dry wet areas within radiation field

      iii. Wash around markings, leaving them intact

      iv. Instruct patient to avoid sun exposure

       v. Consult with radiotherapist before using mechanical irritants (ice bags, heating devices) or topical agents (especially those containing heavy metals, e.g., zinc or bismuth, and alcohol) — these substances may further irritate skin

    b. Be familiar with radiotherapy and its effects

       i. Setting for treatment and personnel involved

       ii. Fractionation

      iii. Fields and skin markings

      iv. Reaction of neighboring organs and use of lead blocks

       v. Side effects and intervention

      vi. Differences between various types of radiotherapy

c. Chemotherapy
   i. Combination therapy – multiple drugs used to augment antitumor effect without increasing side effects
   ii. Given in cycles

REFERENCES

Alavi, J. B., et al.: A randomized clinical trial of granulocyte transfusions for infection in acute leukemia. N. Engl. J. Med. *296:*706–711, 1977.

–––. *AMA drug evaluation.* AMA, Illinois, 1980.

Barlock, A. L., Howser, D. M., and Hubbard, S. M.: Nursing management of adriamycin extravasation. Am. J. Nurs. *79:*94–96, 1979.

Beard, J., and Fairley, G.: Acute leukemia in adults. Semin. Hematol. *9:*5–24, 1974.

Bellanti, J. A.: Immunology II. W. B. Saunders Co., Philadelphia, 1978.

Bellingham, A. J.: The red cell in adaptation to anemic hypoxia. Clin. Haematol. *3:*577–593, 1974.

Bingham, C. A.: The cell cycle and cancer chemotherapy. Am. J. Nurs. *78:*1201–1205, 1978.

Bodey, G., and Rodman, : Protected environment–prophylactic antibiotic programmes; microbiological studies. Clin. Haematol. *5:*395–408, 1976.

Boggs, D.: Physiology of neutrophil proliferation, maturation and circulation. Clin. Haematol. *4:*535–551, 1975.

Brulé, G., Eckhardt, S., Hall, T., and Winkler, A.: Drug Therapy of Cancer. World Health Association, Geneva, 1973.

Buickus, B. A.: Administering blood components. Am. J. Nurs. *79:*937–941, 1979.

Burkhalter, P. K., and Donley, D. L. (eds.): Dynamics of Oncology Nursing. McGraw Hill Book Co., New York, 1978.

Buschke, F., and Parker, R. G.: Radiation Therapy in Cancer Management. Grune & Stratton, New York, 1972.

Butler, J. H.: Nutrition and cancer: a review of the literature. Cancer Nurs. *3:*131–136, 1980.

Childs, J., Collins, D., and Collins, J.: Blood transfusion. Am. J. Nurs. *72:*1602–1605, 1972.

Clark, R. L., and Howe, C. D. (eds.): Cancer Patient Care at MD Anderson Hospital and Tumor Institute. Yearbook Medical Publishers, Chicago, 1976.

Cline, M. J., and Haskell, C. M.: Cancer Chemotherapy, 3rd ed. W. B. Saunders Co., Philadelphia, 1980.

Colman, R. W., Minna, J. D., and Robboy, S. J.: Disseminated intravascular coagulation: a problem in critical care medicine. Heart Lung *3:*789–796, 1974.

Cullins, L. C.: Blood therapy: preventing and treating transfusion reactions. *79:*935–936, 1979.

Desotell, S.: A brighter future for leukemia patients. Nursing *7(1):*19–24, 1977.

DeVita, V. T., et al.: Peritonoscopy in the staging of Hodgkin's disease. Cancer Res. *31:*1746–1750, 1971.

Dilworth, J. A., and Mandell, G. L.: Infections in patients with cancer. Semin. Oncol. *2:*349–359, 1975.

Doswell, W. M.: Sickle cell anemia: you can do something to help. Nursing *8(4):*65–70, 1978.

Dougherty, W. M.: Introduction to Hematology. C. V. Mosby Co., St. Louis, 1976.

Elliott, C.: Radiation therapy: how you can help. Nursing *6(9):*34–41, 1976.

Fagerhaugh, S. Y., and Strauss, A.: How to manage your patient's pain. . .and how not to. Nursing *10(2):*44–47, 1980.

Graham, V., and Rubal, B. J.: Recipient and donor response to granulocyte transfusions and leukapheresis. Cancer Nurs. *3:*97–100, 1980.

Graw, R., and Yankee, R.: Principles of hematologic supportive care. Med. Clin. North Am. *57:*441–461, 1973.

Greenberger, J. S., Come, S. E., and Weichselbaum, R. R.: Issues of controversy in radiation therapy and combined modality approaches to Hodgkin's disease. Clin. Haematol. *8:*611–624, 1979.

Gurewich, V., and Lipinski, B.: Low-dose intravenous heparin in the treatment of disseminated intravascular coagulation. Am. J. Med. Sci. *274:*83–86, 1977.

Guy, R. B., and Rothenberg, S. P.: Sickle cell crisis. Med. Clin. North Am. *57:*1591–1598, 1973.

Guyton, A. C.: Textbook of Medical Physiology. W. B. Saunders Co., Philadelphia, 1981.

Hardisty, R. M., and Weatherall, D. J.: Blood and its Disorders. Blackwell Scientific Publication, Oxford, 1974.

Henderson, E. S.: Treatment of acute leukemia. *In* Holland, J. F., Mischer, P. A., and Jaffe, E. R. (eds.): Leukemia and Lymphoma. Grune & Stratton, New York, 1969.

Henry, J. B. (ed.): Todd, Sanford, Davidsohn: Clinical Diagnosis and Management by Laboratory Methods. Vols. I and II. W. B. Saunders Co., Philadelphia, 1979.

Herzig, R. H., et al.: Successful granulocyte transfusion therapy for gram-negative septicemia. N. Engl. J. Med. *296:* 701–705, 1977.

Huggins, C.: Frozen blood components: the parts are something better than the whole. Am. J. Intrav. Ther. *7:*29–31, 1975.

Jennings, B. M.: Improving your management of DIC. Nursing *9(5):*60–67, 1979.

Jones, D., Dunbar, C., and Jirovec, M. (eds.): Medical Surgical Nursing: A Conceptual Approach. McGraw Hill Book Co., New York, 1978.

Jones, S. E.: Clinical features and course of the non-Hodgkin's lymphomas. Clin. Haematol. *3:*131–160, 1974.

Keaveny, M. E.: Hodgkin's disease: the curable cancer. Nursing *5(3):*48–54, 1975.

Klastersky, J.: The use of synergistic combinations of antibiotics in patients with haematological diseases. Clin. Haematol. *5(2):*361–377, 1976.

Kwaan, H. C.: Disseminated intravascular coagulation. Med. Clin. North Am. *56:*177–191, 1972.

LeBlanc, D. H.: People with Hodgkin's disease: the nursing challenge. Nurs. Clin. North Am. *13:*281–300, 1978.

Lerner, R. G.: The defibrination syndrome. Med. Clin. North Am. *60:*871–880, 1976.

Levine, A. S.: Protected environment—prophylactic antibiotic programmes; clinical studies. Clin. Haematol. *5:* 409–424, 1976.

Levine, A. S., Schimpff, S. C., Graw, R. G., and Young, R. C.: Hematologic malignancies and other marrow failure states: progress in the management of complicating infections. Semin. Hematol. *11:*141–202, 1974.

Linman, J. W.: Hematology. Physiologic, Pathophysiologic, and Clinical Principles. Macmillan, New York, 1975.

Lister, T. A., and Yankee, R. A.: Blood component therapy. Clin. Haematol. *7(2):*407–423, 1978.

Lovejoy, N. C.: Preventing hair loss during Adriamycin therapy. Cancer Nurs. *2:*117–122, 1979.

Luckmann, J., and Sorensen, K. C.: Medical-Surgical Nursing. A Psychophysiologic Approach. W. B. Saunders Co., Philadelphia, 1980.

Marino, E. B., and LeBlanc, D. H.: Cancer chemotherapy. Nursing *5(11):*22–33, 1975.

Mayer, G. G.: Disseminated intravascular coagulation. Am. J. Nurs. *73:*2067–2069, 1973.

Maxwell, M. B.: Scalp tourniquets for chemotherapy-induced alopecia. Am. J. Nurs. *80:*900–902, 1980.

McCaffery, M.: Nursing Management of the Patient with Pain. J. B. Lippincott Co., Philadelphia, 1972.

McCaffery, M., and Hart, L. L.: Undertreatment of acute pain with narcotics. Am. J. Nurs. 76:1586–1591, 1976.

Megliola, B.: Multiple myeloma. Cancer Nurs. 3:209–218, 1980.

Middleman, E., Watanabe, E., and Kaizer, H.: Antibiotic combinations for infections in neutropenic patients. Cancer 30:573–579, 1972.

Moschella, S. L., Pillsbury, D. M., and Hurley, H. J.: Dermatology. Vol. I. W. B. Saunders Co., Philadelphia, 1975.

Myhre, B. A. (ed.): Blood Component Therapy: A Physician's Handbook. American Association of Blood Banks, Washington, D. C., 1975.

O'Brian, B. S., and Woods, S.: The paradox of DIC. Am. J. Nurs. 78:1878–1880, 1978.

O'Loughlin, J. M.: Infections in the immunosuppressed patient. Med. Clin. North Am. 59:495–501, 1975.

Patterson, P.: Granulocyte transfusion: nursing considerations. Cancer Nurs. 3:101–104, 1980.

Patterson, P. C.: Hemophilia: the new look. Nurs. Clin. North Am. 7:777–785, 1972.

Priesler, H. D., and Bjornson, S.: Protected environment units in the treatment of acute leukemia. Semin. Oncol. 2:369–377, 1975.

Rapaport, S. I.: Introduction to Hematology. Harper & Row, New York, 1971.

Rodgers, J. M.: Hodgkin's disease: hope is the key to nursing care. Nursing 5(3):55–58, 1975.

Rodriguez, V., and Bodey, G. P.: Antibacterial therapy—special considerations in neutropenic patients. Clin. Haematol. 5(2):347–360, 1976.

Rodriguez, V., Burgess, M., and Bodey, G. P.: Management of fever of unknown origin in patients with neoplasms and neutropenia. Cancer 32:1007–1012, 1973.

Rorth, M.: Hypoxia, red cell oxygen affinity and erythropoietin production. Clin. Haematol. 3:595–607, 1974.

Ryden, S. E., and Oberman, H. A.: Compatibility of common intravenous solutions with CPD blood. Transfusion 15:250–255, 1975.

Satterwhite, B. E.: What to do when Adriamycin infiltrates. Nursing 8(2):37, 1980.

Schumann, D., and Patterson, P.: Multiple myeloma. Am. J. Nurs. 75:78–81, 1975.

Schumann, D., and Patterson, P. C.: The adult with acute leukemia. Nurs. Clin. North Am. 7:743–761, 1972.

Schwartz, L. M., and Miles, W.: Blood Bank Technology. Williams and Wilkins Co., Baltimore, 1977.

Sherman, L. A., Wessler, S., and Avioli, L. V.: Therapeutic problems of disseminated intravascular coagulation. Arch. Intern. Med. 132:446–453, 1973.

Smith, D. S., and Chamorro, T. P.: Nursing care of patients undergoing combination chemotherapy and radiotherapy. Cancer Nurs. 1:129–134, 1978.

Sutcliffe, S. B., Timoth, A. R., and Lister, T. A.: Staging in Hodgkin's disease. Clin. Haematol. 8:593–609, 1979.

Thomas, S. F.: Transfusing granulocytes. Am. J. Nurs. 79:942–944, 1979.

Vaz, D. D.: The common anemias: nursing approaches. Nurs. Clin. North Am. 7:711–725, 1972.

Wagner, D.: Body image and patients experiencing alopecia as a result of cancer chemotherapy. Cancer Nurs. 2:365–369, 1979.

Welch, D., and Lewis, K.: Alopecia and chemotherapy. Am. J. Nurs. 80:903–905, 1980.

Wiernik, P. H.: Treatment of acute leukemia in adults. Clin. Haematol. 7:259–273, 1978.

Williams, W. J., Beutler, E., Erslev, A. J., and Rundles, R. W. (eds.): Hematology. McGraw Hill Book Co., New York, 1977.

Wintrobe, M. M., Lee, G. R., Boggs, D. R., et al.: Clinical Hematology. Lea & Febiger, Philadelphia, 1974.

Young, R. C., and DeVita, V. T.: Chemotherapy of Hodgkin's disease. Clin. Haematol. 8:625–644, 1979.

THE GASTROINTESTINAL SYSTEM

prepared by

SUSAN VAN DeVELDE-COKE, R.N., M.A. and
ROSEANN N. LUTONSKY, R.N., B.S.N., CCRN

BEHAVIORAL OBJECTIVES

Functional Anatomy

1. Identify the major functions of each of the named divisions of the gastrointestinal system.

Physiology

1. Describe the major physiologic functions of each of the named divisions of the gastrointestinal system.

2. Discuss the mechanisms that promote swallowing in the esophagus.

3. Explain the mechanisms by which carbohydrates, amino acids, water, electrolytes, and fats are absorbed by the small intestine.

4. Describe the physiologic functions of the accessory organs of digestion.

Assessment

1. Describe a systematic process for assessment of the gastrointestinal system utilizing history-taking and physical examination skills.

2. Explain the rationales for diagnostic studies generally used in the assessment of the gastrointestinal system.

3. When given several common gastrointestinal disease processes, select the characteristic changes in inspection, palpation, percussion, and auscultation that occur with each.

General Patient Care Management

1. Develop a plan for nursing intervention to assist in the maintenance of optimal gastrointestinal functioning.

2. Describe factors that impair the nutritional status of the patient with a gastrointestinal disorder.

3. Describe the fluid and electrolyte problems frequently encountered in the patient with a gastrointestinal disorder.

4. Incorporate the care of other body systems into the management of the critically ill patient.

Pathologic Conditions and Management

For each of the following: gastric ulcer, duodenal ulcer, esophageal varices, cirrhosis of the liver, hepatic failure, and acute pancreatitis

1. Describe the specific physiologic derangements that characterize each dysfunction.

2. Select a systematic approach to the assessment of each, based on its clinical presentation, the presence of etiologic or precipitating factors, and the results of diagnostic testing.

3. Develop an effective plan of care for the client with a gastrointestinal dysfunction demonstrating an understanding of pathophysiology and related psychosocial concepts such as body image and family relationships.

THE GASTROINTESTINAL SYSTEM

FUNCTIONAL ANATOMY AND PHYSIOLOGY

UPPER GASTROINTESTINAL SYSTEM

1. **Oral cavity**
   a. Composed of lips, cheeks, gums, palate, teeth, tongue, and salivary glands
   b. Functions – ingestion, mastication, salivation, and first stage of deglutition (swallowing)
   c. Three stages of deglutition – primarily an involuntary reflex act requiring 25 muscles; lasts 1–2 seconds
      i. Voluntary – initiation of swallowing
      ii. Pharyngeal – involuntary passage into esophagus through hypopharyngeal sphincter
      iii. Esophageal – involuntary passage from esophagus into stomach through gastroesophageal sphincter
   d. Saliva – secreted by three salivary glands (parotid, submandibular, sublingual); approximately 1-2 L/day composed of 99% H_2O, 1% proteins (mucins, amylase). Secretion of saliva is controlled by nerves (no hormones involved)

2. **Pharynx**: composed of three divisions that participate in deglutition
   a. Nasopharynx – has immovable walls that extend from nasal cavity to soft palate; soft palate elevates during swallowing to prevent aspiration of food
   b. Oropharynx – has movable walls that extend from soft palate to hyoid bone
   c. Laryngeal pharynx – extends from hyoid bone to esophagus. Entire larynx is pulled upward and forward by muscles attached to hyoid bone. Epiglottis swings backward over superior opening of larynx to prevent passage of food into trachea

3. **Esophagus**
   a. Collapsible tube approximately 10 inches long that serves as pathway for food from pharynx to stomach
   b. Lies posterior to trachea and heart; shares common fibroelastic membrane with posterior trachea
   c. Attaches to stomach below level of diaphragm
   d. Contains two sphincters
      i. Hypopharyngeal – when skeletal muscles of sphincters are relaxed, sphincter is closed by passive elastic tension; when contracted, sphincter opens to allow bolus of food to enter esophagus (also contracts during act of vomiting)

       ii.   Gastroesophageal – remains tonically closed, but peristaltic wave from bolus of food relaxes sphincter and allows opening (similar to hypopharyngeal). This sphincter is important in keeping food in stomach. Most of esophagus is in thoracic region and is subject to subatmospheric pressure of -5 to -10 mm Hg. Stomach lying below diaphragm has internal pressure slightly above atmospheric (+5 to +10 mm Hg), due to its compression by contents of abdominal cavity. Thus, gastroesophageal sphincter prevents reflex of contents into esophagus. Without closure, condition referred to as achalasia occurs

   e.   Achalasia appears to be result of damage to or absence of myenteric nerve plexus in gastroesophageal sphincter

   f.   Cell layers of esophagus

       i.   Upper third of esophagus – skeletal (striated); lower two thirds of esophagus – smooth muscle

       ii.   Outer muscle layer of entire esophagus runs longitudinally; inner muscle layer is positioned transversely around lumen

       iii.   Mucosa layer – squamous epithelium cells lie over muscle layers

4. Stomach

   a.   Elongated pouch approximately 10–12 inches in length and 4–5 inches at maximal transverse diameter

       i.   Proximal receptacle relaxes and allows food to enter, secretes HCl, pepsin, intrinsic factor, mucus

       ii.   Distal pump mechanically mixes food via churning action, and delivers to duodenum

   b.   Occupies epigastric, umbilical, and left hypochondriac regions of abdomen

   c.   Anatomy (see Fig. 7–1)

   d.   Two sphincters – function is to control rate of food passage

       i.   Cardiac – located at opening from esophagus

       ii.   Pyloric – located at opening into duodenum

   e.   Layers of stomach wall

       i.   Mucosal – contain gastric, cardiac, pyloric glands (see above)

       ii.   Muscularis mucosa – muscle layer that folds mucosa into rugae

       iii.   Submucosal – loose, connective tissue and elastic fibers, blood vessels, and lymphatics in this layer

       iv.   Muscular coat – contains three layers that are thin at fundus, thicker at antrum

          (a)   External longitudinal layer – smooth muscle

          (b)   Middle circular layer – smooth muscle

          (c)   Inner oblique layer – smooth muscle

   f.   Gastric glands

       i.   Cardiac – secrete mucus

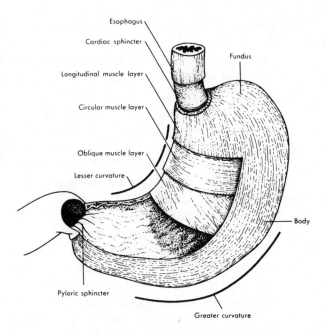

Figure 7–1. (From Given, B.A., and Simmons, S.J.: Nursing Care of the Patient with Gastrointestinal Disorders. C.V. Mosby Co., St. Louis, 1979.)

    ii.   Fundic
        (a)   Chief cells secrete pepsinogen and mucus
        (b)   Parietal cells secrete HCl and water
        (c)   Mucous neck cells secrete mucus
    iii. Pyloric – secrete mucus and pepsinogen
  g. Rugae – foldlike structures of stomach wall, composed of mucosal layer and muscularis mucosa, which provide increased surface area and allow for distention
  h. Gastric motility
    i.   Storage and mixing
        (a)   Receptive relaxation phenomenon – stomach stretches; volume of food does *not* result in increase in stomach pressure
        (b)   Mixing results from tonic and peristaltic contractions of fundus and body of stomach
        (c)   Control of motor function is primarily vagal (vagotomy results in decreased peristalsis and gastric tonus)
        (d)   Longitudinal muscle cells are under control of "pacemaker cells" located in region near entry of esophagus into stomach. Contractions initiated are about 3 per minute
    ii. Gastric emptying
        (a)   Dependent primarily on contractile activity of smooth muscle layers of antral portion of stomach

  (b) Pyloric sphincter is ring of smooth muscle and connective tissue
    (1) Normally, there is no pressure gradient to cause material to move from stomach into duodenum
    (2) Strong peristaltic waves of antrum cause small amounts of chyme to move through pyloric valve; antral contraction also causes valve to close, resulting in antral contents moving back into body of stomach. Contractions in antrum thus mix food as well as move it to duodenum

 iii. Control of gastric emptying
  (a) Stomach empties at rate proportional to volume of material in it at any one time
  (b) Most important factor is chemical composition of chyme, in duodenum, which contains chemoreceptors, osmoreceptors, and pressure receptors.
  (c) Factors that inhibit gastric emptying include
    (1) Fat – most potent inhibition stimulus
    (2) Contents high in osmolarity (protein and starch), owing to need for increased amounts of water to neutralize
    (3) Sadness, depression, fear, and intense pain, which decrease motility controlled by higher CNS centers
    (4) Hormones – secretin and cholecystokinin released from duodenum decrease motility
  (d) Factors that accelerate gastric emptying include
    (1) Liquids, increased volume
    (2) Aggression, anger

 iv. Vomiting – expulsion of contents of stomach and upper GI tract through mouth
  (a) Coordinated by vomiting center in medulla
  (b) Autonomic nervous system discharge – sweating, increased salivation, increased heart rate, and feelings of nausea precede act of vomiting
  (c) Stimuli that induce vomiting include tactile stimulation to back of throat, large distention of stomach or duodenum, increased pressure within skull, rotating movements of head leading to dizziness, intense pain

 i. Gastric secretion
  i. Parietal cells secrete hydrochloric acid; approximately 2 L/day of pH 1–3. Function of HCl is to
   (a) Denature protein and break intermolecular bonds
   (b) Activate some enzymes secreted by stomach
   (c) Kill bacteria
  ii. Precise mechanism of HCl secretion is unknown; hydrogen ions must be moved against high concentration gradient.

   iii Intrinsic factor is mucoprotein secreted by parietal cells and necessary for intestinal absorption of vitamin B_{12}.

     Intrinsic factor adheres to surface of epithelial cells of distal small bowel — resection of this part of bowel necessitates that patient receives vitamin B_{12} exogenously

   iv. Chief cells produce inactive proteolytic enzyme, pepsinogen, which is activated by HCl to form pepsin. Pepsin catalyzes splitting of bonds between particular types of amino acids in protein chains

   v. Mucous cells secrete mucus and water to lubricate stomach lining and contents

  j. Control of gastric secretion

   i. Basal secretion — 0.5 ml/min

    After meal — 3.0 ml/min

   ii. Three phases

    (a) Cephalic — mediated by parasympathetic system (vagus nerve); sight, taste, smell of food initiates release of HCl and hormone gastrin from antral cells

    (b) Gastric — distention elicits release of acid and enzyme secretion; presence of protein in stomach causes marked increase in secretion. Gastrin is stimulated primarily by protein digestion products, which in turn stimulate release of acid. Important to remember feedback mechanism — as hydrogen ion concentration increases, gastrin release is inhibited. If protein is still present and hydrogen ion concentration decreases owing to breaking down of protein, gastrin is again stimulated, and this in turn stimulates parietal cells to secrete more HCl.

    (c) Intestinal — distention, hypertonic solutions, acid, and fat within duodenum stimulate gastric secretion to a lesser degree. Since duodenum becomes filled quickly, stomach must slow down emptying, and this initiates enterogastric reflex. This reflex causes inhibition of gastrin release and acid secretion. The duodenal hormones secretin, cholecystokinin, and other yet unidentified hormones, the external nerves, and the internal nerve plexus are involved in this complex inhibition

LOWER GASTROINTESTINAL SYSTEM

1. **Small intestine**

  a. Coiled, convoluted, 20-foot-long tube that extends from pylorus to cecum, filling most of abdominal cavity

  b. Consists of three divisions

   i. Duodenum — 10 inches long

        ii.   Jejunum — 8 feet long

        iii. Ileum — 12 feet long

  c. Contains ileocecal valve located at terminal end of ileum at junction of cecum and colon; controls flow of contents into large intestine, and prevents reflux into ileum

  d. Layers of small intestinal wall

        i.   Mucosal — composed of epithelial and columnar cells, smaller blood vessels, nerve fibers, plasma and blood cells; separated from submocosa by muscularis mucosa

        ii.   Submucosal — contains larger blood vessels, connective tissue, nerves, ganglia, lymphoid elements

        iii. Muscular

            (a) Inner circular layer — smooth muscle

            (b) Outer longitudinal layer — smooth muscle

            (c) Myenteric plexus interspersed between two layers

  e. Structural features of small intestine

        i.   Villi — finger-like projections of mucosa and submucosa (discernible with hand lens) prominent in duodenum and jejunum. Purpose is to increase surface area for absorption (X 600)

            (a) Individual cells of villi contain small projections known as microvilli that greatly increase surface area of each cell

            (b) Villi contain at least 5 different types of cells whose function is to absorb fat, carbohydrate, or protein and/or secrete enzymes, mucus

            (c) Each villus contains single lymph vessel called a "lacteal" and a dense capillary bed to aid in absorption

        ii.   Crypts of Lieberkühn — located between villi; most absorptive and secretive cells in crypts are undifferentiated, have a high mitotic activity, and replace cells of villus

        iii. Peyer's patches — cells that lie in mucosa and submucosa. They consist of lymphoid follicles, carry out antibody synthesis, and are very important in contributing to immune response of body

        iv. Brunner's glands — cells that secrete mucus; located primarily in duodenum

  f. Small intestinal motility

        i.   Muscle layers of stomach have oscillating basic electrical rhythm originating in pacemaker cells located in proximal duodenum. Frequency is 11 cycles/min; speed approximately 20 cm/sec

            (a) Oscillations ("slow waves") do *not* cause contractions, but set interval when contractions can occur — 10–12 cycles/min in duodenum, 8 cycles/min in ileum

Figure A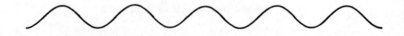

    ii.   Spike potentials or action potentials arise on crest of basic oscillation, and contraction of longitudinal and circular muscles follows immediately

Figure B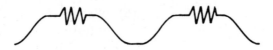

    iii. Two types of movement result from these contractions
      (a) Segmenting — localized ring contractions that divide lumen and its content into segments, resulting in mixing of chyme
      (b) Peristaltic — weak contractions that move chyme toward anus at a rate of a few centimeters distally per minute.
  g. Small intestinal functions
    i. Basic absorption mechanisms
      (a) Active transport — requires energy source (ATP) to move in and out of cell. Example — proteins, glucose, Na^+, K^+
      (b) Passive diffusion — molecules move passively from area of high concentration to area of low concentration. Example — free fatty acids, water
      (c) Facilitated diffusion — requires carrier to move into cell, but process does not require energy. Substance cannot move against electrochemical gradient. Example — fructose
      (d) Non-ionic transport — does not require energy source; substances move freely in and out of cell. Example — unconjugated bile salts, drugs
      (e) Absorption of other important substances
        (1) Water-soluble vitamins (folic acid, vitamin B_{12}, ascorbic acid, vitamin C) — absorption occurs in all parts of small intestine by passive diffusion. Vitamin B_{12} requires intrinsic factor from parietal cells and is absorbed in ileum
        (2) Fat-soluble vitamins (A, D, E, K) require bile salts for purpose of micelle formation (see Fat absorption)
        (3) Calcium — absorbed mainly in duodenum; requires vitamin D and 1,25-dehydroxycholecalciferol (activated in kidney) to be absorbed
        (4) Iron — uptake occurs in all areas of small intestine by active transport. Stored as protein-bound iron; 10–20 mg may be ingested daily, but only 0.5–1.0 mg is absorbed daily — absorption can increase as needed

(5) Electrolytes — sodium, potassium, chloride, bicarbonate, magnesium phosphate are absorbed by active transport mechanism — all areas of intestine

(6) Water — passive diffusion throughout small intestine

(a) 9 liters of water and electrolytes (isotonic fluid) are presented to proximal small bowel daily

(b) Overall absorption of water and electrolyte by small and large bowel is 98–99% efficient (only 100–200 ml normally should exist as stool)

(c) Absorption in each region of small and large intestine

(i) Proximal small bowel — high permeability to water and NaCl macromolecules. Efficiency of absorption — 50% (4–5 L)

(ii) Ileum — most nutrients have been absorbed; fluid is osmotically near that of plasma fluid. Efficiency of absorption — 75% (3–4 L)

(iii) Colon — efficiency of absorption 90%. Aldosterone also increases sodium absorption in colon

ii. Carbohydrate absorption

(a) Approximately 350 gm absorbed daily (60% starch, 30% sucrose, 10% lactose)

(b) Three basic sugars are fructose, glucose, galactose. Calories — 4 kcal/gm

(c) Starch — multiple glucose molecules broken down by maltase and amylase. Sucrose — glucose and fructose broken down by sucrase. Lactose — glucose and galactose broken down by lactase

(d) Glucose and galactose are transported actively across bowel wall into blood; fructose is transported via facilitated diffusion

iii. Protein absorption

(a) 70–90 gm absorbed daily; 4 kcal/gm broken down to 22 basic amino acids. Eight are essential — isoleucine, methionine, leucine, phenylalanine, lysine, threonine, valine, tryptophan

(b) Protein is degraded by multiple enzymes; most prominent are pepsin from chief cells of stomach, and trypsin and chymotrypsin from pancreas

(c) Amino acids absorbed by active transport

      iv. Fat
- (a) 60–100 gm absorbed daily; 9 kcal/gm, mostly in form of fat or triglycerides
- (b) Four phases of fat digestion and absorption
  - (1) Lipolysis of dietary triglycerides by pancreatic enzymes to glycerol and fatty acids
  - (2) Micellar solubilization of fatty acid with bile acid (micelle – fatty acids and bile salt)
  - (3) Absorption of micelle into jejunal cell
  - (4) Delivery of triglycerides to general circulation via lymphatic system

  h. Secretion in small intestine
     i. Intestinal secretion reaches about 3000 ml/day with a pH of approximately 7.0
     ii. Secretions are emitted from epithelial cells of mucosa lining; primarily made up of digestive enzymes – peptidases, sucrase, lactase, maltase, lipase, amylase
     iii. Control of secretion
- (a) Local stimuli produced by presence of chyme in small intestine increases secretion
- (b) Hormonal stimuli – vasoactive intestinal peptide stimulates release of secretion. Other hormone-like substances are being investigated for their effect on intestinal juices

2. **Large intestine (colon)**
  a. Tube 5–6 feet long and 2-1/2 inches in diameter that extends from ileum to anus; instrumental in absorption of nutrients/water and in elimination of waste products.
  b. Consists of
     i. Cecum, a cul-de-sac from which vermiform appendix is attached
     ii. Colon, which has four sections – ascending, transverse, descending, and sigmoid
     iii. Rectum, approximately 7 inches long, extending from sigmoid to anus. Distal 1–2 inches is the anal canal
  c. Has two flexures
     i. Hepatic – bend in colon, right upper quadrant of abdomen forming junction of ascending with transverse colon
     ii. Splenic – bend at junction of transverse with descending colon in left upper quadrant (ileocecal sphincter closes opening from small intestines)
  d. Houses two sphincters – internal and external anal sphincters that control anus, and open only to eliminate feces
  e. Walls of large intestine
     i. Mucosal – epithelial cells largely involved with absorption of water and electrolytes

       ii.   Submucosal — similar to small intestine

      iii. Muscular layer

          (a)   Circular layer deviates slightly from being strictly circular

          (b)   Longitudinal layer is gathered into three strips called "teniae coli" that are evenly spaced around circumference of bowel. These cause sacculations, or pouches, called haustra, which form because longitudinal strips are shorter than circular layer

f. Colonic motility

    i.   Pacemaker regions are present as in small intestine, but slow waves seem to occur in both directions rather than always aboral

    ii. Spike potentials may be prolonged and may cause powerful contractions, resulting in mass movement of contents of large intestine, occurring a few times daily

    iii. Defecation — normally initiated when mass movements force feces into rectum; approximately 150 gm of feces eliminated daily

        (a)   Distention of wall of rectum initiates defecation reflex; mediated primarily by internal nerve plexuses

        (b)   Reflex response consists of a contraction of rectum, relaxation of internal and external sphincters, and increased peristaltic activity in sigmoid colon

        (c)   Deep inspiration, followed by closure of glottis and contraction of chest and abdominal muscles, results in increased intra-abdominal pressure transmitted to large intestine

    iv. Factors that enhance colonic motility

        (a)   Drugs — morphine, magnesium sulfate

        (b)   Irritation of colon — osmotic overload, bacterial enterotoxins such as *Vibrio cholerae,* destruction of mucosa such as in ulcerative colitis, presence of increased bile salts

    v.   Factors that inhibit colonic motility

        (a)   Low bulk diet

        (b)   Anticholinergic drugs — atropine, propantheline bromide

g. Colonic functions

    i.   Absorption

        (a)   Mainly water and electrolytes. Ascending and transverse colon absorb approximately 1 L of water per day. Sodium is actively absorbed (also under influence of aldosterone). Potassium is secreted into lumen as sodium is absorbed. Chloride passively follows sodium. Bicarbonate is actively secreted into lumen.

        (b)   When presented with excessive volumes of fluid as result of proximal small bowel dysfunction, colon can increase its absorption threefold

ii. Bacteria
    (a) Main anaerobic bacteria — *Bacteroides fragilis.* Main aerobic — *Escherichia coli*
    (b) Function is to partially break down cellulose and to synthesize vitamins (folic acid, riboflavin, vitamin K, nicotinic acid)
iii. Urea breakdown — conservation of nitrogen
    (a) Blood urea, a metabolic waste product, is broken down to ammonia by mucosal cells of colon
iv. Elimination of fecal material
    (a) Composition of feces — 75% water and 25% solid matter composed of 30% dead bacteria, 10–20% fat, 10–20% inorganic material, 2–3% protein, 30% undigested roughage of food, and sloughed epithelial cells
    (b) Brown color of feces is caused by urobilin, derivative of bilirubin

GASTROINTESTINAL HORMONES

1. **Gastrin**: secreted from antral cells of stomach. Main effects are to
   a. Stimulate parietal cells, increasing HCl
   b. Stimulate chief cells, increasing pepsin
   c. Promote antral motility

2. **Secretin**: secreted from duodenal cells. Main effects are to
   a. Stimulate pancreatic and hepatic HCO_3^- and water secretion
   b. Augment action of cholecystokinin

3. **Cholecystokinin (CCK)**: secreted from duodenal cells. Main effects are to
   a. Increase gallbladder contraction
   b. Stimulate lipase, amylase, trypsin, and other enzyme secretion from pancreas
   c. Decrease stomach tone

4. **Vasoactive hormone**: main effects are to stimulate intestinal juice

5. **Intestinal peptide (VIP)**: secreted from small intestine
   a. Main effects are similar to those of secretin
   b. Is extracted from GI mucosa

6. **Gastric inhibitory hormone**: secreted from small intestine. Main effect is to release insulin

7. **Polypeptide (GIP)**: secreted from small intestine. Main effect is to inhibit gastric secretion

BLOOD SUPPLY to Gastrointestinal Tract

1. **Arterial**
   a. Aorta → aortic arch → thoracic arch → abdominal aorta → celiac artery
   b. Celiac branches
      i. Left gastric (supplies stomach, esophagus)
      ii. Hepatic → right gastric (supplies stomach)
      iii. Gastroduodenal (supplies stomach, duodenum)
      iv. Cystic (supplies gallbladder)
      v. Splenic (supplies stomach, pancreas, and spleen)
   c. Superior mesenteric artery (branches off abdominal aorta) supplies jejunum, ileum, cecum, ascending colon, and part of transverse colon
   d. Inferior mesenteric artery (branches off abdominal aorta) supplies transverse, descending, and sigmoid colon, and rectum

2. **Venous**
   a. Portal vein system — portal vein collects blood from entire venous drainage of GI tract and delivers blood to liver. Main branches that bring blood to portal vein are
      i. Gastric — returns blood from stomach, esophagus
      ii. Splenic — returns blood from stomach, esophagus, duodenum, pancreas, gallbladder
      iii. Superior mesenteric — returns blood from small intestine, ascending and transverse colon
      iv. Inferior mesenteric — returns blood from descending and sigmoid colon, rectum. Inferior mesenteric vein joins splenic vein, which in turn returns to portal vein
   b. Portal vein subdivides into liver sinusoids, which then unite with branches from hepatic artery to form hepatic vein, which empties into inferior vena cava

$$\begin{array}{c} \text{portal vein} \searrow \\ \text{hepatic artery} \nearrow \end{array} \text{hepatic vein} \to \text{inferior vena cava}$$

NERVOUS INNERVATION

1. **Extrinsic nerves of autonomic nervous system:** located outside wall of gut
   a. Parasympathetic — cranial X (vagus) and sacral nerves. Acetylcholine is neurostimulus from postganglionic fiber
   b. Sympathetic — vertebral ganglia situated on either side of vertebral trunk, which terminate in all organs of gut. Neurostimuli from postganglionic fibers include epinephrine, norepinephine, dopamine

2. **Intrinsic nerves of autonomic nervous system:** located inside wall of gut
   a. Consist of extensions from extrinsic nerves, and form two major and three minor networks of plexuses
      i. Major
         (a) Auerbach's plexus — lies between circular and longitudinal muscle layers
         (b) Meissner's plexus — located in submucosa
      ii. Minor
         (a) Subserosal — located beneath serosa (outer covering of wall)
         (b) Deep myenteric — situated within circular muscle layer
         (c) Mucous — widely innervates villi and glandular cells

ACCESSORY ORGANS OF DIGESTION

1. **Pancreas**
   a. Soft, lobulated, fish-shaped gland that lies behind duodenum and spleen
   b. Divisions include
      i. Head, which lies in C-shape curve of duodenum
      ii. Body
      iii. Tail — thin, narrow portion in contact with spleen
   c. Main pancreatic duct (duct of Wirsung) transverses length of organ from left to right. Joins common bile duct at right end of organ; short segment before entrance into duodenum is called the ampulla of Vater
   d. Pancreatic secretion — colorless fluid that approximates 1500–2000 ml/day; pH = 8.3
      i. Exocrine — acinar cells secrete a high concentration of sodium bicarbonate, H_2O, Na^+, K^+, and digestive enzymes, most prominent being
         (a) Lipase — breaks down triglycerides to fatty acids and glycerol
         (b) Amylase — breaks down polysaccharides to glucose and maltase
         (c) Trypsin — breaks amino acid bonds in interior of proteins
         (d) Ribonuclease, deoxyribonuclease — splits nucleic acids into free mononucleotides
      ii. Endocrine
         (a) Beta cells (from islets of Langerhans) secrete hormone insulin, which acts directly or indirectly on most tissues of body (except brain) by stimulating entry of glucose into cell. Glucose entry leads to glucose oxidation, fat synthesis, and glycogen synthesis

          (b) Alpha cells (from islets of Langerhans) secrete glucagon, which stimulates
              (1) Breakdown of hepatic glycogen to glucose, and adipose tissue to triglyceride
              (2) Glyconeogenesis from amino acids

e. Control of pancreatic secretion
    i.   Vagal — during cephalic and gastric phases, parasympathetic impulses result in moderate secretion of pancreatic enzymes
    ii.   Hormonal — entrance of food into small intestine greatly stimulates pancreatic secretion via hormonal influences of secretin and cholecystokinin (see section on GI hormones)

2. **Gallbladder**
    a. Pear-shaped organ (7–10 cm long, 2.5–3.5 cm wide) attached to undersurface of liver by areolar tissue, peritoneum, and blood vessels; capable of holding 50 ml of bile
    b. Has four divisions
        i.   Fundus (blind lower end of body)
        ii.   Body
        iii. Infundibulum
        iv. Neck, which joins body with cystic duct
    c. Supplied with oxygenated blood via hepatic and cystic arteries; venous drainage occurs via cystic vein
    d. Innervated by splanchnic nerve, right branch of vagus verve, and seventh thoracic segment of sympathetic nerve supply
    e. Serves as passageway for bile from liver to intestine — regulates bile flow, and collects, concentrates, and stores bile
    f. Sphincter of Oddi is terminal end of common bile duct, located at entrance into duodenum. Sphincter opens upon vagal and hormonal stimulation
    g. Bile composition — released by parenchymal cells of liver. Bile moves into liver canaliculi → hepatic duct → cystic duct → gallbladder for storage. Drainage of bile from gallbladder → cystic duct → common bile duct → duodenum
        i.   Bile pigments and bile salts, high concentration of cholesterol, some neutral fat, phospholipid, and inorganic salts
        ii.   Bile salts are primarily responsible for emulsification of fats, form micelle
        iii. 80% of bile salts are reabsorbed in intestinal tract and returned to liver; 20% are lost in feces
        iv. Major bile pigment is bilirubin, a breakdown product of hemoglobin. Presence of bile pigment gives feces brown color; absence produces gray-white feces. Blockage of bile duct results in accumulation of bile pigments in blood and body tissues, producing jaundice

h. Bile metabolism

   i. Heme portion of hemoglobin molecule is converted to bilirubin by reticuloendothelial cells and released into blood stream, where it binds to albumin (fat-soluble, indirect, or unconjugated bilirubin)

   ii. In liver, indirect bilirubin is bound with glucuronic acid to form water-soluble (direct, conjugated) bilirubin, which is then excreted into bile

   iii. In intestinal mucosa, water-soluble (conjugated) bilirubin is converted to a series of urobilinogen compounds mediated by intestinal bacteria and excreted primarily in stool; lesser portion is recycled to liver and returned to bile or excreted in urine

   iv. In jaundice state, both conjugated and unconjugated bilirubin blood levels are measured to help determine pathophysiology (e.g., high conjugated indicates biliary tract obstruction; high unconjugated indicates hepatocellular dysfunction)

3. **Liver**

a. Largest organ in body (3–4 lb), located in right upper abdominal quadrant, fitting snugly against right inferior diaphragm

b. Divided into four main lobes — right, left, caudate, and quadrate

c. Each lobe is divided into numerous lobules — functional units of liver

d. Each lobule or sinusoid is composed of branching plates of liver cells radiating from center to periphery. Sinusoid receives oxygenated blood from hepatic arterioles, and also blood rich in metabolic precursor (amino acids, fats, sugars, vitamins) from portal vein. Approximately 1500 ml of blood is delivered to liver each minute

e. Cellular functions

   i. Kupffer cells — phagocytes of reticuloendothelial system. Function is to destroy old blood corpuscles and detoxify toxic substances

   ii. Hepatocytes — secrete bile (600–1000 ml/day) and metabolize carbohydrates, fats, proteins

   iii. Synthesizes amino acids, albumin, alpha and beta globulins, prothrombin, fibrinogen, and other blood factors

   iv. Deaminates amino acids for glucose availability

   v. Forms urea in order to remove ammonia from blood

   vi. Vitamin storage (fat-soluble vitamins, vitamin B_{12}, copper, iron)

   vii. Converts glucose to glycogen, stores it, and breaks it down as needed

      viii. Synthesizes and catabolizes fatty acid and neutral fats to form ketone bodies and acetate. Also forms lipoproteins, cholesterol, phospholipids

      ix. Detoxifies drugs, hormones, toxic substances

ASSESSMENT

HISTORY: The examiner may make pertinent observations during the course of history-taking, e.g., abdominal protuberance, jaundice, and so forth.

1. **General symptoms**: state of nourishment, general weakness, easy fatigability, nervousness, change in sleep patterns, change in appetite, indigestion, use of laxatives or enemas, change in bowel habits

2. **Specific symptoms**
   a. Pain — nature, duration, site, intensity, character, positional, paroxysmal, length of symptoms, aggravating or relieving factors
   b. Nausea and vomiting — frequency, timing, positional, aggravating or relieving factors, description of vomitus
   c. Diarrhea — duration, frequency, amount, nature, color, aggravating or relieving factors
   d. Constipation — duration, nature, color, aggravating or relieving factors
   e. Heartburn — reflux of food contents before, during, or following meals; not related to eating
   f. Easier bruising or bleeding — onset, duration, extent
   g. Darker or orange urine — onset, duration, amount
   h. Difficulty in swallowing — onset, with liquids or solids
   i. Shortness of breath — positional, duration
   j. Increased itching — onset, time of day, body area
   k. Weight loss

3. **Medical history**: current and significant past
   a. Gastrointestinal diseases, hemorrhage
   b. Hepatic disease
   c. Pancreatic disease
   d. Anemia
   e. Debilitating disease, chronic disease
   f. Allergic states
   g. Previous surgery, injuries, hospitalizations
   h. Medication history
   i. Alcohol habits
   j. Exposure to contagion, e.g., salmonella
   k. Occupational history
   l. Change in food patterns or eating habits

PHYSICAL EXAMINATION

1. **Anatomic landmarks:** used in describing location of pain, tenderness, and other abnormal findings
   a. Subcostal margins
   b. Epigastric hollow
   c. Midline
   d. Umbilicus
   e. Lateral borders of rectus abdominis
   f. Poupart's ligaments (inguinal)
   g. Anterior superior spine
   h. Costovertebral angle
   i. Flanks

2. **Abdominal regions:** quadrants
   a. Right upper
   b. Left upper
   c. Right lower
   d. Left lower

3. **Vital signs**

4. **Inspection**
   a. Skin – scars, striae, dilated veins, rashes and lesions, unusual pigmentation, spider angiomata
   b. Umbilicus – contour, location, signs of inflammation or hernia, caput medusae, eversion
   c. Contour of abdomen – flat, rounded, protuberant, or concave
   d. Symmetry
   e. Masses – movable or stationary
   f. Peristalsis – may be visible in thin people, children
   g. Pulsations – aortic pulsation frequently visible in epigastrium
   h. Pubic hair distribution – diamond-shaped in males, triangular in females
   i. Presence of cutaneous angiomata – associated with liver disease
   j. Presence of draining wounds, fistula, or ostomy

5. **Auscultation**
   a. Basic points
      i. Should be done prior to percussion and palpation since these may alter frequency of bowel sounds
      ii. Diaphragm should be placed lightly against abdominal wall to avoid artifacts resulting from friction and compression of vessels
      iii. Listen in all four quadrants – note frequency, character, and location of bowel sounds
      iv. May be necessary to listen full 2–5 min to detect

  b. Normal bowel sounds

   i. More rapid than respiratory cycle

   ii. Continuous succession of clicks and gurgles

  c. Abnormal bowel sounds

   i. Loud gurgles (borborygmi) indicate hyperperistalsis, usually heard when meal overdue or when person is tense or nervous

   ii. Absence or extreme weakness and infrequency of sounds indicates immobile bowel of peritonitis or paralytic ileus

   iii. Loud, rushing, high-pitched tinkling sounds occur proximal to an intestinal obstruction — may be accompanied by pain, severe cramping, and visible peristalsis

   iv. Succession splash — caused by increased air and fluid in stomach, as in pyloric obstruction

  d. Other auscultatory findings

   i. Bruit — resembles systolic murmur; created by turbulence in flow of blood through a partially occluded artery

   ii. Venous hum — heard over upper portion of abdomen or liver; associated with liver disease or with portal or splenic vein thrombosis

   iii. Friction rubs — quite soft and associated with respiration. May be heard over spleen, indicating inflammation or infarction, and liver, indicating primary or metastatic tumor

 6. **Percussion:** used to establish presence of distention, tumors, fluid, and enlargement of solid viscera

  a. Normal liver — dullness; both lower and upper borders should be ascertained to detect enlargement

  b. Normal spleen — dullness

  c. Normal stomach — tympany when empty

  d. Abnormal abdominal sounds

   i. Liver dullness may be decreased or absent when free air is present below diaphragm, as from a perforated hollow viscus

   ii. Increased tympany of stomach with upper abdominal distention indicates gastric dilatation

   iii. Change in percussion from tympany to dullness on inspiration suggests splenic enlargement

 7. **Palpation:** most important part of examination

  a. Information obtained

   i. Pain or discomfort elicited

   ii. Change of tone in abdominal wall

   iii. Firmness and mobility of masses or organomegaly detected

  b. Location of painful area

   i. Visceral — arises from organic lesions or functional disturbance within abdomen, e.g., obstructive lesion of intestine with accompanied distention. It is a dull, poorly localized pain

     ii. Somatic – involves structure such as peritoneum. Pain is
        described as sharp and well localized, e.g., appendicitis
  c. Rebound tenderness indicates peritoneal inflammation
  d. Involuntary rigidity or spasm indicates peritoneal inflammation
  e. Enlarged, smooth, nontender liver may indicate cirrhosis
  f. Enlarged, smooth, tender liver may indicate hepatitis
  g. Enlarged, irregular liver suggests malignancy
  h. Spleen must be enlarged about three times its original size to be
      palpable

DIAGNOSTIC STUDIES

1. **Laboratory**
   a. Gastric analysis
      i. Basal analysis
      ii. Nocturnal analysis
      iii. Stimulation analysis
      iv. Hypoglycemic analysis
      v. Cytology
   b. Fecal fat analysis
   c. Laboratory procedures that provide direct or indirect support
       for diagnosis
      i. Hematology
      ii. Serology
      iii. Blood chemistries
      iv. Microbiologic studies
      v. Serum enzymes
      vi. Blood gas analysis
      vii. Urinalysis
   d. ECG

2. **Radiologic**
   a. Routine – posteroanterior, lateral chest
   b. Special – depends on nature of problem
      i. Flat plate abdomen
      ii. Upper GI tract
      iii. Lower GI tract
      iv. Barium enema
      v. Cholangiogram

3. **Special**
   a. Endoscopy
      i. Esophagoscopy
      ii. Gastroscopy
      iii. Sigmoidoscopy
   b. Biopsy/cytology
   c. Radionuclide uptake scan

GENERAL PATIENT CARE MANAGEMENT

GASTROINTESTINAL FACTORS THAT IMPAIR GENERAL NUTRITION

1. **Intake**
   a. Nausea, vomiting
   b. Anorexia, depression
   c. Pain
   d. Alcoholic intake
   e. Disease entities, e.g., cancer, obstruction

2. **Increased tissue destruction**
   a. Trauma, burns
   b. Ulcerative conditions
   c. Cancer
   d. Sepsis

3. **Malabsorption**
   a. Decrease or absence of digestive secretions or bile salts
   b. Hypermotility
   c. Drug therapy
   d. Metabolic disorders

4. **Decreased utilization and storage**
   a. Impaired liver function
   b. Neoplasms

5. **Increased excretion or loss**
   a. Hemorrhage
   b. Ascites
   c. NG drainage, nausea, vomiting, diarrhea
   d. Surgical procedures
   e. Neoplasms
   f. Excessive protein loss

6. **Increased nutritional requirements**
   a. Increased metabolism — hyperthyroidism, fever, cancer
   b. Trauma, sepsis, burns

MAINTAIN ADEQUATE NUTRITION

1. **Signs of inadequate nutritional state**
   a. Anorexia
   b. Nervousness, irritability
   c. Fatigue, apathy
   d. Headache

    e. Integumentary changes, e.g., dry, scaly skin; poor skin turgor; absence of subcutaneous fat; pallor of oral mucosa

    f. Weight loss, cachexia, diminished skinfold and arm circumference measurements

2. **Nitrogen balance**: nitrogen intake and excretion are equal

    a. Negative – nitrogen is being lost more rapidly than can be supplied

    b. Positive – nitrogen intake is greater than output

    c. Factors promoting negative nitrogen balance

        i.   Major catabolic response – increased protein breakdown and utilization

        ii. Protein depletion, e.g., liver disease

        iii. Decreased nutritional intake

        iv. Failure in absorption of nutrients

        v.   Immobilization

        vi. Corticosteroid therapy

        vii. Inability to metabolize one or more amino acids

    d. Major clinical manifestations associated with negative nitrogen balance

        i.   Weakness, muscle wasting

        ii. Weight loss

        iii. Mental stupor, apathy

        iv. Hypoalbuminemia – edema

        v.   Poor wound healing

        vi. Anemia

        vii. Fatty liver

        viii. Respiratory failure – sepsis

3. **Nutritional intake**

    a. Provide environment and foods conducive to eating

    b. Ensure proper oral hygiene; dentures if necessary

    c. Be aware of cultural, socioeconomic, and religious patterns

    d. Instruct patient in appropriate dietary regime

4. **Elemental diets** (Vivonex, Isocal, Complete-B, Ensure)

    a. Maintain caloric and nitrogen balance over extended periods

    b. More readily and rapidly absorbed than general diets

    c. Should be low in residue

    d. Should be available in suspension or stable solutions

    e. Monitor serum chemistries on a weekly basis

    f. Weigh daily

    g. Monitor intake and output

5. **Total parenteral nutrition (TPN)**: intravenous solution of protein as amino acids (nitrogen), hypertonic glucose, and additives (vitamins,

electrolytes, minerals, and trace elements). May be given peripherally or centrally. However, owing to hypertonicity of fluids required for adequate nutrients in a tolerable volume, peripheral nutrition is acceptable but limited in use

a. Peripheral parenteral nutrition
   i. Patients with high fluid requirements, e.g., high output fistula
     (a) $D_{10}W$–$D_{20}W$ combined with nitrogen obtained from 7% amino acid and electrolytes as required. Administered concomitantly with Intralipid
     (b) Fluid volumes of approximately 5 liters/day may be required to supply necessary nutrients. Trace element formula of 0.03 ml/kg/day is also included
   ii. Patients who may benefit from hypocaloric therapy for short periods – e.g., postoperative patients with adequate fat stores for 1 week
     (a) 3.5% amino acid solution and necessary electrolytes, with or without addition of dextrose or lipid, has had positive effect on nitrogen balance
     (b) Trace element formula of 0.03 ml/kg/day – dosage adjusted through biweekly serum testing

b. Central venous parenteral nutrition – therapy of choice when enteral and peripheral venous hyperalimentation are not possible
   i. Catheter insertion – a surgical procedure accomplished with special attention to asepsis, anatomy, patient position, and insertion technique
     (a) Complications during insertion
       (1) Arterial puncture
       (2) Pneumothorax
       (3) Lymphatic leak
       (4) Arm pain or paresthesias
       (5) Air embolism
       (6) Catheter embolism
     (b) TPN catheter is inviolate; only purpose should be administration of hyperalimentation fluid
   ii. Catheter care – proper care is critical, since sepsis is most dangerous and most frequent complication of TPN

c. Formulation and preparation of fluids
   i. Protein provided in form of crystalline amino acid mixtures, e.g., Aminosyn, Freamine, Travasol
   ii. Calories provided in form of hypertonic glucose $D_{50}W$ – optimal calorie-to-nitrogen ratio is 150 kcal:1 gm nitrogen. Additional calories are provided by Intralipid
   iii. Specific electrolyte requirement varies. Need for intracellular electrolytes is greatly increased – anabolism will not proceed if not present in sufficient quantities

    iv.   Vitamins – exact minimal daily requirements (MDRs) under conditions of stress are unknown. Vitamin K, vitamin B_{12}, and folic acid, owing to their instability or interaction with TPN solution, should be administered by alternative routes

    v.   Trace elements – Zn^{++}, Ca^{++}, Mn^{++}, I^- are provided when TPN is administered for longer than 2–3 weeks

    vi.   Each TPN order is evaluated for incompatibilities prior to preparation

    vii.   Extra aseptic precautions are required during preparation since solution is excellent growth media for bacteria

d. Complications of TPN therapy

    i.   Metabolic

       (a)   Hyperglycemia – may indicate onset of sepsis or hyperosmolar nonketotic coma. Prompt cessation of infusion and administration of insulin and K^+ is appropriate therapy to drive glucose into body cells

       (b)   Hypoglycemia – cause not fully understood, but decreasing the rate appears to be appropriate therapy

       (c)   Hypomagnesemia – indicated by tingling in extremities and agitation

       (d)   Hypophosphatemia – not a complication per se, but rather a deficiency secondary to inadequate IV phosphate administration. Manifested by lethargy, slurred speech, and rapid progression to coma

       (e)   Use of TPN in liver disease, renal failure, and cardiac failure requires specially prepared solutions

    ii.   Technical (*Note:* Insertion complications have already been addressed)

       (a)   Sepsis – most dreaded complication of TPN*

          (1)   Replace infusion with $D_{10}W$

          (2)   All IV tubing and extensions should be changed

          (3)   Fluid and blood withdrawn from catheter should be sent for culture

          (4)   If fever and other symptoms continue for more than 12–24 hours, discontinue catheter and send tip to lab for culture

       (b)   Subclavian thrombosis – may be source of pulmonary emboli

          (1)   Remove catheter immediately

          (2)   Institute anticoagulation therapy with heparin

          (3)   Cannulation site on affected side usually cannot be used again

---

*Protocol may vary from one institution to another.

MAINTAIN FLUID AND ELECTROLYTE BALANCE: See Renal System for normal physiology of fluid and electrolytes.

1. **Fluid and electrolyte assessment**
   a. Current intake and output
   b. Medications that may affect fluid and electrolyte balance
   c. Losses – vomiting, NG suction, fistulas, hemorrhage
   d. Gains – Na^+ retention, ascites, decreased urinary output
   e. Serum and urine electrolyte values recorded serially

2. **Common gastrointestinal electrolyte imbalances**
   a. Hyponatremia
      i. Potent diuretics
      ii. Vomiting, GI suction
      iii. Wounds and fistula drainage
      iv. H_2O enemas/irrigations
      v. Specific disease entities – peritonitis, pancreatitis
   b. Hypernatremia
      i. Excessive loss of H_2O, e.g., watery diarrhea
      ii. Inadvertent infusion of hypertonic saline
   c. Hypokalemia
      i. Prolonged gastric fluid loss
      ii. Hemorrhage
      iii. K^+ wasting diuretics
      iv. Prolonged hyperalimentation
      v. Specific disease entities – peritonitis
   d. Metabolic alkalosis
      i. Soluble antacid administration
      ii. Vomiting, NG suction (loss of gastric acid)
      iii. K^+ depletion
      iv. Drugs – diuretics, adrenocortical steroids
      v. Specific disease entities – peritonitis, pancreatitis
   e. Metabolic acidosis
      i. Sepsis
      ii. Diarrhea
      iii. Extreme catabolic states, inadequate nutritional intake
      iv. Specific disease entities – diabetes mellitus
   f. Hypocalcemia
      i. Fistula drainage
      ii. Increased infusion of citrated blood
      iii. Specific disease entities – peritonitis, pancreatitis

ESTABLISH AND MAINTAIN ADEQUATE BLOOD VOLUME: See Cardiovascular System for pathophysiology and management of hypovolemic shock.

1. **Assess severity of acute vs chronic blood loss:** tilt test for vasomotor instability

2. **Type and crossmatch immediately**

3. **Check vital signs frequently:** including CVP, PA, and wedge pressures if Swan-Ganz catheter is in place

4. **Administer O_2 if patient is in shock**

5. **Gastric intubation**
    a. Suctioning may be alternated with iced saline lavage (if cardiac pathology is present, tap H_2O may be indicated)
    b. In unconscious patient, advance tube between respirations to prevent entry into larynx
    c. Patient should be in low or semi-Fowler's position; avoid Trendelenburg position
    d. Auscultate breath sounds
    e. Maintain accurate record of irrigation fluid to ascertain exact amount of drainage

6. **Ensure prompt consultation:** for possible surgical intervention

PREVENT COMPLICATIONS: Those arising from patient's medical condition or from hospital care.

1. **Infection**
    a. Prime sources
        i.   Extensive surgical wounds
        ii. Indwelling tubes and catheters
        iii. Cross-contamination between patients
        iv. Debilitated patients
    b. Preventive measures
        i.   Strict hand washing or use of gloves
        ii. Use of aseptic technique in dressing changes
        iii. Special care in disposal of soiled dressings
        iv. Isolation technique as required
        v.   Antibiotics as indicated

PROVIDE PHYSICAL AND PSYCHOLOGIC SUPPORT

1. **Exercise:** to preserve muscle tone and prevent vascular complications of immobility

2. **Prevent sensory overload and sleep deprivation:** use narcotics with caution — they may cause further nausea and vomiting with possible aspiration

3. **Lessen anxiety:** give brief and clear explanations of procedures and environment

4. **Allow visits:** family members

5. **Make adequate preparations for transfer from ICU**

_____ PATHOLOGIC CONDITIONS AND MANAGEMENT _____

GASTROINTESTINAL HEMORRHAGE — PEPTIC ULCERS: Gastric or duodenal.

1. **Pathophysiology**
   a. Ulceration occurs when there is excess secretion of gastric juice (HCl and pepsin) in relation to degree of protection afforded by mucous secretion and neutralization of gastric acid by duodenal juices
   b. Decreased blood flow to mucosa may alter defensive barrier, allowing ulceration and necrosis to occur
   c. Aggressiveness of peptic activity is also dependent on parietal cell mass and mucosal trauma
   d. Endocrine hormones, e.g., ACTH and cortisone, may alter amount and type of mucous production and diminish protection by mucous barrier
   e. Bleeding may arise from single or multiple acute erosions in stomach or duodenum, or from artery at base of an acute duodenal ulcer
   f. Gastric ulcers can become cancerous; duodenal ulcers do not
   g. Gastric ulcers are commonly seen in later years; duodenal ulcers usually occur in third or fourth decade
   h. Gastric ulcers are more likely to bleed, and to bleed more frequently
   i. Approximately 80% of ulcers are duodenal, and 20% gastric

2. **Etiology or precipitating factors**
   a. Stress
      i. Physiologic
         (a) Burns
         (b) Surgery
         (c) Trauma
         (d) Excessive temperature changes
         (e) Sepsis
      ii. Psychic influence
         (a) Emotional stress
         (b) Type A personality
   b. Hormonal influence
      i. Sympathetic stimuli increase constriction of duodenal vasculature, making it more susceptible to HCl and pepsin activity
      ii. Increased activity of adrenal cortex may impair mucus production and stimulate gastric secretion
   c. Hereditary factors
      i. Increased frequency among parents and siblings
      ii. Activity of ABH antigens in saliva and gastric juice
   d. Drugs
      i. Alteration of mucosal barrier
         (a) Alcohol
         (b) Aspirin
         (c) Bile salts
         (d) Para-aminosalicylic acid (PAS)
      ii. Decreased gastric mucosal cell renewal
         (a) Corticosteroids
         (b) Phenylbutazone
      iiii. Acid stimulation
         (a) Caffeine, nicotine
         (b) Reserpine
      iv. Decreased mucosal blood flow
         (a) Vasopressors
         (b) Catecholamines

3. **Clinical presentation**
   a. Hematemesis – bright red or coffee-ground appearance
   b. Melena – more common with duodenal ulcers
   c. If bleeding is rapid in onset
      i. Faintness, pallor
      ii. Tachycardia, thready pulse, decreased blood pressure
      iii. Diaphoresis, thirst
      iv. Apprehension

    d. If bleeding is severe
       i. Hypotension (positive tilt test)
      ii. Rapid, shallow respirations
     iii. Cold, clammy skin
    e. If bleeding is gradual, faintness, fatigue and pallor may be the only complaints

4. **Diagnostic findings**
    a. History
       i. Presence of precipitating causes, as listed previously
      ii. Determine source of bleeding — patient with chronic alcoholism is more likely to bleed from esophogeal varices; patient with previous ulcer history frequently bleeds from peptic ulcer
     iii. Recent medication history and dietary habits
     iv. Previous bleeding; gastric distress or pain
    b. Physical examination: see Clinical presentation
       i. Inspect for vascular nevi to rule out liver disease
      ii. Palpate for masses to rule out cancer
     iii. Palpate for epigastric tenderness and muscle guarding
    c. Diagnostic studies
       i. Laboratory
         (a) Stool positive for guaiac
         (b) Decreased HCT, Hb, RBCs (not always reliable early in course)
         (c) Increased BUN
         (d) Prolonged prothrombin time (PT) if patient undergoing anticoagulant therapy, or in presence of liver disease
         (e) Arterial blood gases — with shock, expect
            (1) Decreased PO_2
            (2) Increased PCO_2
            (3) Decreased pH
         (f) ECG may detect myocardial ischemia, especially in presence of coronary artery disease
      ii. Radiologic
         (a) Upper GI series — positive for ulcer disease
         (b) Chest radiograph — nonspecific
     iii. Special — endoscopy — positive for ulcer disease

5. **Complications**
    a. Perforation with peritonitis and sepsis
    b. Myocardial infarction
    c. Transfusion reaction
    d. Pyloric obstruction
    e. Hypovolemic shock

6. **Specific patient care**
   a. All the objectives listed under General Patient Care Management apply, especially those that
      i. Establish and maintain adequate blood volume
      ii. Maintain fluid and electrolyte balance
      iii. Maintain adequate nutrition
   b. Intra-arterial infusion of vasopressin
      i. Administer after bleeding is demonstrated by angiography (mesenteric vessels)
      ii. Vasoconstriction of distal branches of perfused vessel with flow into capillary beds must be demonstrated by angiography prior to transfer from X-ray unit back to ICU
      iii. Observe carefully for bradycardia, water intoxication, post-vasopressin diuresis, hypotension, and tachydysrhythmias
   c. If bleeding is not stopped and complications occur (e.g., perforation, obstruction), surgery may be indicated

BLEEDING ESOPHAGEAL VARICES

1. **Pathophysiology**
   a. A hardened and distorted liver offers resistance to normal venous drainage into portal vein
   b. With portal hypertension, small plexus of veins at esophagogastric junction is forced to receive large amounts of shunted blood, producing distention and hypertrophy
   c. Fragility of vessels, acid pepsin erosion, or mechanical trauma will result in bleeding; sudden increase in abdominal venous pressure may also do so

2. **Etiology or precipitating factors**
   a. Portal hypertension resulting from cirrhosis
   b. Circulation abnormalities in splenic vein or superior vena cava

3. **Clinical presentation:** see also Clinical presentation of gastrointestinal hemorrage — peptic ulcers
   a. Sudden and painless hemorrhage
   b. Large quantities of blood lost in form of hematemesis
   c. Signs of shock

4. **Diagnostic findings**
   a. History
      i. Possible previous bleeding episodes
      ii. Alcohol intake and abuse
      iii. Weight loss
      iv. Poor dietary habits
      v. Family or personal crises
      vi. Some form of physical exertion (e.g., coughing or vomiting may have occurred immediately prior to bleeding)

    b. Physical examination: if patient has liver disease, the following findings may be present in addition to those listed previously under Clinical presentation
- i. Increased abdominal girth
- ii. Generalized muscle wasting
- iii. Vascular nevi
- iv. Jaundice
- v. Ascites
- vi. Splenomegaly
- vii. Anemia

    c. Diagnostic studies
- i. Laboratory
  - (a) Stool positive for guaiac
  - (b) Decreased HCT, Hb, RBC's, WBC's
  - (c) Increased BUN
  - (d) Increased LDH, SGOT, SGPT
  - (e) Prolonged PT
  - (f) Increased alkaline phosphatase
  - (g) Thrombocytopenia
  - (h) Increased Bromsulphalein (BSP) retention
  - (i) Arterial blood gases — with shock, expect
    - (1) Decreased Po_2
    - (2) Decreased pH
  - (j) ECG may detect myocardial ischemia, especially in presence of coronary disease

5. Complications
- a. Myocardial infarction secondary to ischemia
- b. Renal failure
- c. Congestive heart failure
- d. Hepatic coma
- e. Hepatorenal syndrome

6. Specific patient care
- a. All the objectives listed under General Patient Care Management apply, especially those that
  - i. Establish and maintain adequate blood volume
  - ii. Maintain fluid and electrolyte balance
  - iii. Maintain adequate nutrition
- b. Initiate esophageal and gastroesophageal tamponade
  - i. Sengstaken-Blakemore tube
  - ii. Linton tube
- c. Use cathartics through tube, to prevent ammonia intoxication, e.g., sorbitol, citrate of magnesia
- d. Use nonabsorbable antibiotics that prevent breakdown of protein by normal intestinal bacteria, e.g., neomycin
- e. Administer vitamin K to reverse prolonged PT

f. Institute intra-arterial infusion of vasopressin to lower portal venous pressure and control bleeding
   i. Administer via femoral artery or peripheral vein
   ii. Usually effective for 4–6 hours
   iii. Caution in patients with coronary artery disease: potent vasoconstrictor (keep amyl nitrite at bedside)
   iv. Titrate doses
g. If bleeding is not controlled, surgical ligation may be indicated; however, mortality is extremely high

CIRRHOSIS OF THE LIVER

1. **Pathophysiology**: general
   a. Liver parenchymal cells are progressively destroyed and replaced with fibrotic tissue
   b. Regeneration with overgrowth occurs, with resultant lobules very irregular in shape
   c. Because of distortion, twisting, and constriction of central sections of lobules, vascular flow is impeded
   d. After long periods of damage and regeneration, necrosis and atrophy occur
   e. Approximately three-fourths of liver can be destroyed without symptoms of impairment

1a. **Pathophysiology**: specific
   a. Laennec's, alcoholic, nutritional, fatty
      i. Fibrosis and nodule formation
      ii. Fatty changes, increased number of inflammatory cells, hepatomegaly
      iii. Mallory body or alcoholic hyaline and liver cell necrosis
      iv. Initially central lobular rather than portal in distribution
   b. Postnecrotic, posthepatic
      i. Broad bands of scar tissue with lobular collapse
      ii. Liver size may remain normal
   c. Biliary, cholangitic, obstructive
      i. Scarring around ducts and lobules
      ii. May be a disturbance of immune mechanisms
      iii. Proliferation of bile ducts

2. **Etiology or precipitating factors**
   a. Laennec's, alcoholic, nutritional, fatty
      i. Chronic alcohol abuse
      ii. Nutritional deficiencies
      iii. Male population more often affected
   b. Postnecrotic, posthepatic
      i. Hepatitis – usually not acute
      ii. Halothane (anesthetic agent)

    c. Biliary, cholangitic, obstructive
      i. Chronic biliary infection
      ii. Extrahepatic obstruction, e.g., biliary atresia

3. **Clinical presentation**: remainder of this discussion will be general, and only major differences specific to a type of cirrhosis will be listed
    a. Jaundice
    b. Dependent edema
    c. Vascular nevi
    d. Altered hair distribution, pectoral alopecia
    e. Palmar erythema
    f. Testicular atrophy — gynecomastia
    g. Fetor hepaticus (musty-sweet breath)
    h. Ascites

4. **Diagnostic findings**
    a. History
      i. Lassitude, anorexia
      ii. Indigestion, flatulence, irregular bowel habits
      iii. Nausea, vomiting
      iv. Weight loss
      v. Epigastric or right upper quadrant pain — usually described as dull, heavy, aching
      vi. Exposure to jaundiced persons, recent injections or transfusions, ingestion of drugs such as chlorpromazine, thiouracil, tolbutamide, chlorothiazide, halothane (causes of jaundice)
      vii. Heavy alcohol intake
      viii. Patient bruises or bleeds easily
    b. Physical examination
      i. Jaundice
      ii. Yellow sclera
      iii. Vascular nevi, palmar erythema
      iv. Skin lesions, bruises, gingival bleeding
      v. Gynecomastia, testicular atrophy
      vi. Edema of ankle, thigh, scrotum; ascites
      vii. Pectoral alopecia, muscular atrophy
      viii. Asterixis
      ix. Splenomegaly, hepatomegaly
      x. Possible presence of esophageal varices
    c. Diagnostic studies
      i. Laboratory
        (a) Decreased HCT or Hb
        (b) Hypoalbuminemia
        (c) Prolonged PT
        (d) Elevated serum, bilirubin; bilirubinuria

       (e)   Increased alkaline phosphatase
       (f)   Hypocholesterolemia
       (g)   Increased LDH, SGOT, SGPT
       (h)   Increased globulin
       (i)   Positive bile in stool
       (j)   BSP retention

   ii. Radiologic
       (a)   Upper GI may reveal esophogeal varices
       (b)   Splenoportal venography may detect portal hypertension
       (c)   Transhepatic cholangiography will reveal site, cause, and extent of obstruction

   iii. Special
       (a)   Liver scan reveals hepatomegaly and splenomegaly
       (b)   Liver biopsy reveals microscopic lobular changes, and assists in diagnosing specific type of cirrhosis

5. **Complications**
   a. Portal hypertension
   b. Esophageal varices
   c. Ascites
   d. Hydrothorax
   e. Hepatic coma

6. **Specific patient care**
   a. Ensure high caloric, minimal-to-moderate protein intake
   b. Restrict salt intake
   c. Prohibit alcohol intake
   d. Administer bile salts to increase absorption of vitamin A and synthesis of vitamin K in jaundiced patients
   e. Provide fat-soluble vitamins to compensate for liver's inability to store them
   f. Assess mentation and neurologic status frequently
   g. Instruct patient and family about diet, drugs, alcohol, and prevention of complications

HEPATIC FAILURE

1. **Pathophysiology**: see Pathophysiology of cirrhosis
   a. Exact mechanism of hepatic coma is poorly understood. It is related to inability of liver to conjugate ammonia, which leads to marked elevation of ammonia levels in circulatory system and CSF
   b. Essentially all clotting factors are produced in liver; hepatic failure results in inadequate levels for hemostasis
   c. Increased amount of NH_4^+ dissociation to $NH_3 + H^+$, due to diarrhea, hypokalemia, and alkalosis, results in acidosis and elevated ammonia (NH_3) levels

2. **Etiology or precipitating factors**
    a. Chronic liver disease with superimposed stress
        i.   Acute ingestion of alcohol
        ii. Toxicity from GI bleeding
        iii. Shock states
        iv. Rapid diuresis
        v.   Sedatives
    b. Hepatitis — acute viral or toxic
    c. Biliary obstruction
    d. Neoplasm
    e. Drugs — anesthetics, antibiotics, chemotherapeutic agents to which patient may have idiosyncratic susceptibility
    f. Portacaval shunt surgery
    g. Acute infectious process
    h. Severe dehydration
    i. Paracentesis due to loss of sodium and K^+ as well as a decrease in effective volume

3. **Clinical presentation**: see Clinical presentation of cirrhosis for contributing signs and symptoms
    a. Early manifestations — may be difficult to recognize unless patient is well known to staff
        i.   Slowness of mentation and affect
        ii. Slurred speech
        iii. Slight tremor
    b. Progressive manifestations
        i.   Inappropriate behavior
        ii. Inability to maintain sphincter control
        iii. Patient sleeps most of time, but is rousable
        iv. Speech incoherent, marked confusion
        v.   Tremor usually present if patient can cooperate
    c. Late manifestations
        i.   Patient may be unresponsive even to noxious stimuli
        ii. Tremor usually absent

4. **Diagnostic findings**
    a. History
        i.   Cirrhosis of liver with recent
             (a) Dietary indiscretion
             (b) Alcohol abuse
             (c) Surgery
             (d) Infection
             (e) Paracentesis
             (f) GI bleed, with or without transfusion
        ii. Acute hepatitis
        iii. Drug abuse
    b. Physical examination
        i.   Jaundice

  ii.   Vascular nevi
  iii. Palmar erythema
  iv.   Testicular atrophy
  v.   Gynecomastia
  vi.   Edema — ascites, ankle, scrotum
  vii. Bruises, bleeding gums
  viii. Asterixis and apraxia
  ix.   Positive Babinski; hyperactive reflexes
  x.   Deep, rapid respirations
  xi.   Elevated temperature
  xii. Alterations in pulse
  xiii. Coma
  xiv. Hepatomegaly, splenomegaly
  xv.   Corneal reflex may be absent
c. Diagnostic studies
  i.   Laboratory — these will help to differentiate the cause, and therefore guide treatment
    (a) Obstructive jaundice (potentially correctable surgically)
      (1) Marked elevation of alkaline phosphate
      (2) Mild elevation of SGOT, LDH
      (3) Significant bile in urine
      (4) Minimal to no urobilinogen in urine and feces
    (b) Hemolytic jaundice
      (1) Marked decreased HCT, Hb
      (2) Reticulocytosis
      (3) Marked increase in urobilinogen in urine
      (4) Normal-to-minimal elevations in enzymes
    (c) Hepatocellular jaundice
      (1) LDH, SGOT frequently in excess of 1,000 μ
      (2) Slight elevation of alkaline phosphatase
      (3) Urine may contain both bile and urobilinogen
      (4) Decreased fibrinogen
      (5) Prolonged PT even with vitamin K therapy
  ii. Special
    (a) EEG — abnormal, generalized slowing
    (b) Spinal tap — elevated glutamine

5. **Complications**
a. Hepatorenal syndrome
b. Disseminated intravascular coagulation (DIC)
c. Thrombocytopenia
d. Systemic infection
e. Intracranial hemorrhage

6. **Specific patient care**
a. Hemodynamic monitoring to assess fluid and electrolyte balance
b. Neurologic assessment (see Nervous system)

    c. Evacuation of GI tract to prevent further absorption of protein breakdown products

    d. NG suction to remove stomach contents, followed by laxative to further reduce absorption of protein breakdown products, which are highly toxic to CNS

    e. Nonabsorbable antibiotics to decrease ammonia production by depleting bacteria that act on intestinal contents

    f. Severe protein curtailment — TPN with only essential amino acids, with primarily glucose caloric supplement

    g. Vitamin K in large amounts

    h. Steroid therapy remains controversial

    i. Diuretics must be used with caution (coma may actually be precipitated by electrolyte imbalance secondary to injudicious use of diuretics)

    j. O_2 therapy — assisted ventilation may require use of endotracheal tube (see Pulmonary System for management of patient on ventilator)

    k. Side-rails must be up and padded to prevent injury

    l. Meticulous skin care

    m. Special eye care if corneal reflex is absent

    n. Maintain frequent interaction and support of family

ACUTE PANCREATITIS

1. **Pathophysiology**
   a. Probably due to autodigestion of pancreas by its enzymes
      i. Possibly is result of obstruction of pancreatic duct, which predisposes escape of enzymes from acinar cells
      ii. Increased pressure in ducts and continued secretion of pancreatic juice causes ducts to rupture
      iii. Trypsin enters pancreatic ducts and causes edema, liquefaction, necrosis, and hemorrhage; may activate other pancreatic enzymes — elastase, phospholipase A, and kallikrein
         (a) Hemorrhage in gland may be attributed to action of elastase on walls of small blood vessels
         (b) Phospholipase A probably causes coagulation, fat necrosis, and damage to acinar cell membrane
         (c) Kallikrein probably causes edema, vasomotor changes, increased vascular permeability, and pain

2. **Etiology or precipitating factors**
   a. Exact etiology is unknown
   b. History of biliary tract disease
      i. Common channel theory involving biliary tract and pancreatic duct
      ii. Spasm of ampulla of Vater

      iii.   Reflux of duodenal contents into pancreatic duct

      iv.   Gallstone blocking lower end of common bile duct

  c. Alcoholism theories

      i.   Stimulates pancreatic secretion

      ii.   Precipitates spasm of sphincter of Oddi

      iii.   May impair pancreatic function

      iv.   Causes inflammation of duodenal wall

  d. Trauma, surgery, or an external blow

  e. Drugs

      i.   Thiazides

      ii.   Salicylazosulfapyridine

      iii   Steroids

      iv.   Isoniazid

  f. Infectious processes

      i.   Mumps

      ii.   Scarlet fever

      iii.   Staphylococcic food poisoning

  g. Hyperparathyroidism

  h. Hyperlipidemia

  i. Hereditary factors

3. **Clinical presentation**

  a. Epigastric pain radiating to back

      i.   Peak intensity at time of onset

      ii.   Severe and unrelenting in character

  b. Shocklike symptoms due to large loss of plasma into tissue of pancreas and surrounding tissues

  c. Fever

  d. Dyspnea due to diaphragmatic irritability

  e. Nausea and profuse vomiting due to reflux irritation from inflamed pancreas

  f. Slight jaundice

4. **Diagnostic findings**

  a. History — see Clinical presentation

      i.   Overindulgence in alcohol or fatty foods

      ii.   Steatorrhea; foul-smelling, grayish-colored stool

      iii.   Weight loss

      iv.   Abdominal distention

  b. Physical examination

      i.   Extreme restlessness; agonizing pain causes patient to seek more comfortable position, e.g., fetal or knee chest

      ii.   Mottled skin; extremities cold and sweaty

      iii.   Tender epigastrium, with or without rigidity

      iv.   Ecchymoses in groin and thigh (Grey Turner's sign)

      v.   Ecchymoses around umbilicus (Cullen's sign)

      vi.   Positive Chvostek's and Trousseau's signs; reflects decrease in ionized serum calcium level

      vii. Jaundice from obstruction due to edema of pancreas

     viii. Epigastric mass may be palpable

      ix. Ascites may be present

       x. Diminished or absent bowel sounds

      xi. Rales may be heard at base of lungs

c. Diagnostic studies

    i. Laboratory

      (a) Leukocytosis with increase of neutrophils

      (b) HCT elevated initially because of hemoconcentration due to plasma loss

      (c) HCT will be decreased if hemorrhage is a marked feature of the pathophysiologic process

      (d) Elevated serum amylase — rises sharply during first 24–48 hours

      (e) Elevated lipase

      (f) Hyperglycemia may be attributed to adrenal response to stress or islet damage

      (g) Decreased serum and urine calcium levels

      (h) Increased direct bilirubin

      (i) Increased alkaline phosphatase

      (j) Hypokalemia due to severe tissue destruction

      (k) Decreased serum albumin

      (l) Decreased total protein

      (m) Decreased arterial blood pH indicates metabolic acidosis

      (n) Stool positive for fat and protein

      (o) Increased urine amylase — may remain elevated for up to 7 days

      (p) Increased triglyceride levels — probably present prior to onset of disease

      (q) ECG may suggest myocardial infarction

         (1) Transient S-T segment depression

         (2) T-wave changes

    ii. Radiologic

      (a) Chest film

         (1) Diaphragmatic elevation due to collection of fluid

         (2) Atelectasis, especially in left base

         (3) Left pleural effusion

      (b) Abdominal film

         (1) May diagnose perforated hollow viscus if presence of air under diaphragm is demonstrated

         (2) Presence of pancreatic calcification

         (3) May indicate ileus or intestinal obstruction

      (c) Upper GI series demonstrates delayed gastric emptying and enlargement of duodenum due to edema of head of pancreas

(d) IV cholangiography — ineffective visualization occurs with pancreatitis; reason is unknown

5. **Complications**
   a. Vascular collapse and shock
   b. Myocardial infarction; myocardial depressant factor may be released from acutely inflamed pancreas
   c. Abscess formation resulting from extensive necrosis
   d. Renal failure secondary to hypovolemia
   e. Pseudocysts — result of autodigestion of tissues by proteolytic enzymes, producing a cavity not lined with epithelial cells; may disappear spontaneously over weeks or months
   f. Sepsis
   g. Tetany due to severe hypocalcemia
   h. Pancreatic fistulas as result of operative injury to pancreas

6. **Specific patient care**
   a. See General Patient Care Management, with special emphasis on the following
      i. Establish and maintain adequate blood volume
      ii. Maintain fluid and electrolyte balance
      iii. Prevent secondary infections
      iv. Maintain adequate nutritional intake
   b. Suppress and neutralize pancreatic secretions
      i. NPO
      ii. NG intubation — prevent gastric stimulation of pancreatic secretions and control nausea and vomiting
      iii. Anticholinergic drugs
      iv. Antacids — avoid those flavored with wintergreen, as they increase gastric emptying time
      v. Avoid alcoholic beverages, high coffee intake, and food high in fat
   c. Alleviate pain — prevent vasoconstriction and additional pancreatic damage
      i. Avoid use of morphine and codeine, which produce spasm of biliary and pancreatic ducts and sphincter of Oddi, and may also increase serum amylase levels
      ii. Demerol, even though it has similar spasm-producing effects of a lesser degree, is medication of choice
      iii. Administer papaverine, barbiturates, anticholinergics to promote smooth muscle relaxation
      iv. Institute paravertebral blocks or IV infusion of procaine or lidocaine
   d. Surgical intervention remains controversial. Appropriate intervention is dependent on etiology of disease process

REFERENCES

Baranowski, K., et al.: Viral hepatitis. Nursing 76, 6: 31–38, 1976.

Bates, B.: A Guide to Physical Examination. J. B. Lippincott Co., Philadelphia, 1979.

Boyer, C., et al.: Diseases of the liver. Nurs. Clin. North Am. 12: 257–258, 1977.

Brooks, F.: Gastrointestinal Pathophysiology. Oxford University Press, New York, 1974.

Burke, W.S.: What you should know about Tagamet: new drug therapy for peptic ulcers. Nursing 80, 10:86–87, 1980.

Bynum, T. E.: Axioms on gastrointestinal bleeding. Hosp. Med. 13: 52–56, 1977.

Cohen, A., et al.: Medical Emergencies. Little, Brown & Co. Boston, 1975.

Eshchar, J.: The case for intensive care in hepatic coma. Heart Lung 4: 775–782, 1975.

Given, B. A., and Simmons, S. J.: Nursing Care of the Patient with Gastrointestinal Disorders. C. V. Mosby Co., St. Louis, 1979.

Given, B. A., et al.: Gastroenterology in Clinical Nursing, 2nd ed. C. V. Mosby Co., St. Louis, 1979.

Go, V. L.: Gastrointestinal hormones: diagnostic and therapeutic advances in gastroenterology. Mayo Clin. Symp., March 29–31, 1978.

Greenberger, N., et al.: Gastrointestinal Disorder: A Pathophysiologic Approach. Year Book Medical Publishers, Chicago, 1976.

Guyton, A: Textbook of Medical Physiology, 5th ed. W. B. Saunders Co., Philadelphia, 1976.

Hauge, K., et al.: Hepatic crisis, nursing grand rounds. Nursing 74:15–19, 1974.

Klebanoff, G., et al.: Resuscitation of a patient in state IV hepatic coma using total body washout. J. Surg. Res. 13: 159, 1972.

Long, G. D.: G.I. bleeding: what to do and when. Nursing 78, 8:44–50, 1978.

Martin, F. L.: Nursing decisions. How to salvage a bleeding cirrhosis patient. Part 21. RN 43: 59–65, 1980.

Mitchell, H. S., et al.: Nutrition in Health and Disease. J. B. Lippincott Co., Philadelphia, 1976.

Myers, R. T.: Esophageal bleeding. Hosp. Med. 14: 80, 1978.

Penn, I.: Management of the perforated duodenal ulcer. Heart Lung 7: 111–117, 1978.

Price, S. A., and Wilson, L. M.: Pathophysiology: Clinical Concepts of Disease Processes. McGraw-Hill Book Co., New York, 1978.

Sause, R. B.: Antacid therapy. J. Nurs. Care 12: 8–12, 1979.

Sleisenger, M. H., and Fordtran, L. S.: Gastrointestinal Disease, 2nd ed. W. B. Saunders Co., Philadelphia, 1978.

Sodeman, W. A., Jr., and Sodeman, W. A.: Pathologic Physiology: Mechanisms of Disease, 6th ed. W. B. Saunders Co., Philadelphia, 1979.

Strauss, E.: Explosion of G. I. hormones. Med. Clin. North Am. 62:21–37, 1978.

Vander, A. J., Sherman, J. H., and Luciano, D. S.: Human Physiology: The Mechanisms of Body Function. McGraw-Hill Book Co., New York, 1978.

PSYCHOSOCIAL IMPLICATIONS

prepared by

JOHN L. CARTY, R.N., M.S.N. and
NANCY PIERCE-ERCK, R.N., M.S.N.

BEHAVIORAL OBJECTIVES

1. Define and discuss psychosocial concepts that affect the critically ill person, e.g., self-concept, self-esteem, stress, body image, and pain.

2. Describe the psychosocial impact of the critical care environment on patients, family members, and staff.

3. Given a critically ill person, identify reciprocal conceptual relationships operating in selected phenomena, e.g., crisis, loneliness, powerlessness, fear/anxiety, and the dying process.

4. Utilize the general tool for assessing the psychosocial status of an individual as a guide in preparing an effective nursing plan of care.

PSYCHOSOCIAL IMPLICATIONS

INTRODUCTION

In nursing, human beings are viewed as whole entities consisting of interacting physiologic, psychologic, social, and spiritual dimensions. Interactions between the psychologic and social dimensions are emphasized in the *Core*, but it is recognized that each dimension of man impinges upon every other dimension in many powerful, reciprocal ways. Such interactions expand the experience of the self and form an ongoing, dynamic, psychosocial process throughout the life cycle. One's physiologic state may be expressed in biologic as well as psychosocial ways, which ultimately affect the manner in which one views the world and oneself within it.

The physiologic dimension is almost completed at birth, but the psychologic dimension is only a potential at that time. Each human develops the psychosocial aspects of self over time, in interaction with others and with nonhuman elements in the environment. It is important to note that some universal experiences are common to all humans in their psychosocial development.

It is intended to present basic concepts of psychosocial development that describe how humans encounter, create, and incorporate their reality in wellness and in illness, so that critical care nurses may better understand the experiences of those threatened by serious illness. In other words, a phenomenologic approach has been selected in presenting the following material.

Situations resulting from the interaction of basic concepts with other variables will also be discussed.

This knowledge should be helpful to the nurse in accurately assessing needs, effectively planning and implementing nursing strategies, and evaluating expected patient outcomes in the process of providing holistic, ongoing care to critically ill patients and their families.

CONCEPTUAL FOUNDATIONS OF HUMAN BEHAVIOR

PERCEPTION

1. **Definition:** perception is the experience of sensory input, i.e., all stimuli experienced through sight, hearing , touch, taste, and smell

2. **Discussion**
   a. Perceptions are regulated by invisible filters that allow some perceptions to make an impression upon a person, and others to be kept out of a person's awareness
   b. The filters that regulate the degree of impact individuals experience depend on
      i. The meaning the stimuli have for them at a given moment
      ii. How they feel about themselves at a given moment, e.g., weak or strong, overwhelmed or in control, peaceful or agitated
      iii. The unfulfilled needs operating in them when they experience the stimuli
   c. Perceptions lead to thoughts and often to feelings. Individuals' thoughts and feelings influence the way in which they receive the next perception
   d. Therefore, two people experiencing the same event may perceive it very differently, and may have different thoughts and feelings about the shared experience. Perceptions are unique to each individual

3. **Example**
   A nurse meeting a stranger in a social context may meet the stranger's gaze while being introduced. Little attention may actually be paid to the person's eyes
   When the same nurse meets the gaze of a patient in a critical care unit, the nurse may note pupil reactivity when looking at the patient's eyes
   The nurse's perceptual filters allow the nurse to screen out certain information about eyes in the first instance, and accept the information in the second instance because of the particular meaning the nurse gives to the information in the professional setting

SELF-CONCEPT

1. **Definition**
   a. Self-concept is all that one can identify as being characteristic of oneself
   b. The components of self-concept are those things one believes about oneself based on
      i. Past experiences
      ii. Present experiences currently being confronted

2. **Discussion**
   a. Self-concept is formed over time in the context of others and in the presence of the beliefs, values, and norms of the culture/ society. It consists of what one *believes* others think of one (not

to be confused with what others may *actually* think of one) in light of one's own beliefs and value system

b. Self-concept is always seeking consistency; i.e., one is continually attempting to find information to reinforce one's beliefs about oneself, even if those beliefs are negative or incorrect.

c. When one's self-concept is threatened, one will fight to hold on to one's beliefs about oneself

d. One behaves in a manner that is consistent with one's self-concept, i.e., in a way that demonstrates one's beliefs about oneself

e. The state of one's self-concept is one of the most important influences on behavior

f. The more positive one feels about oneself, the more comfortable one will feel, and the more open one will be to new perceptions and new information

SELF-ESTEEM

1. **Definition**: self-esteem refers to the feelings one has about oneself — one's perceived self-worth. As such, it is a part of self-concept

2. **Discussion**
   a. Self-esteem is based on one's personal goals, measured against one's perceived successes, in interaction with the beliefs and values of the culture/society
   b. In other words, self-esteem is derived from a comparison between the strengths one believes one possesses and the limitations one believes one possesses
   c. The amount of self-esteem one enjoys influences the manner in which one behaves. The impact is seen through demonstrations of self-confidence and the level of comfort with self
   d. When one's self-concept is raised, one's self-esteem is enhanced, and a greater degree of comfort is experienced

3. **Examples**
   a. A 40 year old woman with a healthy self-concept and a high level of self-esteem has a total mastectomy because of malignancy. She is seen reacting with spontaneous signs of grief, but does not report feelings of helplessness or devastation. She appears to be able to maintain herself, and to find sufficient strength to cope with the situation, much as she remembers having done with previous painful situations. She is overheard remarking to a doctor in the ICU: "I'm what you call a survivor. I've gotten through some pretty difficult times in my life, and I guess I've got what it takes to deal with this one too, but I'm scared about how long it will take for me to feel well enough to take care of my teenagers again"

    b. A 15 year old boy steals a car and subsequently is involved in a two-car collision. Because of his multiple injuries, he is admitted to an ICU for observation. While in the unit, he constantly complains about his care, the poor quality of food, and the fact that he is "with all these sickees." He repeatedly states his beliefs that "the nurses are mean" and "my parents don't like me anyway." He refuses to cooperate in having vital signs taken, and yells out rather than use his call light. The night he spends in the unit is obviously difficult for him and he is unable to sleep. A night nurse spends some time with him and begins to explore his behavior to try to find out what he is feeling and to see if she can be of assistance. She finds that the boy feels ashamed because he has "caused trouble" for his family twice during the past year. He views himself as "a rotten kid — just like my father said I was." The boy acts the role of a rotten kid

NEEDS

1. **Definition**: human needs are an individual's perceived physical and psychosocial requirements for developing, maintaining, and enhancing self

2. **Discussion**
   a. Maslow has categorized human needs according to the following levels (the first level being the most basic)
      i. Physiologic
      ii. Safety and security
      iii. Love and belonging
      iv. Self-esteem
      v. Self-actualization
   b. Need satisfaction progresses from basic needs to higher level needs; i.e., one does not become preoccupied with meeting higher level needs until basic needs are satisfied
   c. Unfulfilled needs are constantly operating in humans, influencing their behavior. A person consistently strives to fulfill perceived needs in an ongoing dynamic process throughout the life cycle. The influence of needs on behavior is sometimes a conscious process, and at other times unconscious. In other words, one is sometimes aware of one's unfulfilled needs, and at other times unaware of them. Even when one does not recognize one's unfulfilled needs, those needs continue to influence one's behavior
   d. The greatest human need is to perceive the self as an adequate person
   e. Major life changes (e.g., illness) may necessitate a refocusing of energies to meet a more basic need

3. **Example**

A young man purchases a motor cycle to help him act out his wish to be daring

Analyzing his conversation concerning how he thought he would look to his girlfriend when he picked her up on his cycle, one could hypothesize that he was attempting to meet his need for belonging and for self-esteem at the time of his purchase

Within three weeks he suffers an accident in which he sustains a crushed chest, internal bleeding, and a concussion. In the ICU his energies become intensely focused on all the apparatus to which he is attached for survival and treatment. His need level has apparently reverted to physiologic and safety requirements

STRENGTHS, POTENTIALS, LIMITATIONS

1. **Definitions**
    a. Strengths are perceived as positive attributes believed to be characteristic of self or others
    b. Potentials are perceived as latent strengths believed to be characteristic of self or others
    c. Limitations are perceived inadequacies or shortcomings believed to be characteristic of self or others

2. **Discussion**
    a. Generally, people are more aware of their perceived limitations than of their perceived strengths
    b. Often, one desperately attempts to hide the limitations one believes one possesses in an effort to protect one's self-concept and self-esteem
    c. Humans consciously and unconsciously *choose* the boundaries of their lives through
        i.   The strengths they choose to maintain
        ii. The potentials they choose to develop, as well as those they choose not to develop
        iii. The limitations they choose to maintain
    d. Since all humans struggle to maintain the "self" as adequate, focusing on their strengths and potentials (instead of their shortcomings) enables them to feel more competent and to deal more effectively with perceived or actual limitations. Learning and growth also are greatly facilitated by recognizing strengths in oneself and in others
    e. A poor self-concept and self-esteem are facilitated by focusing only on one's limitations

3. **Example**

A nurse working in a critical care nursery observes a mother anxiously attempting to feed her four week old infant who has just been removed from the incubator. The mother's efforts look awkward and the baby is crying loudly

The mother says to the nurse: "I feel like a klutz when she cries like this. I want to give her all the love I feel for her, but I'm so uncoordinated!"

The nurse responds: "Jenny is awfully lucky to have such a caring mother. I wonder if she would feed more easily if you held her head a little higher. That way, she might stop crying and you might better enjoy feeding her"

The nurse realistically focuses on the mother's strengths, and attempts to assist her in developing potential as a competent caregiver. The interaction helps to increase the mother's self-concept, facilitates her feelings of adequacy, and enables her to perform in a manner that makes her feel more comfortable

GROWTH AND DEVELOPMENT PATTERNS

1. **Definition:** growth and development patterns are those repeated cumulative behaviors frequently exhibited by individuals as they confront and deal with issues that typically arise during life stages

2. **Discussion**
    a. Some types of growth seem to occur automatically, whereas others take place through focused effort
    b. Because growth and development processes are constantly operating within an individual, they have an influence on behavior
    c. In the ongoing process of evaluating self to see if one is adequate, a measuring stick frequently used is one's success in mastering developmental tasks. For example, during adolescence, many people measure their adequacy in part by evaluating their success in forming relationships with members of the opposite sex
    d. If one does not master the developmental tasks of a particular life stage, one will have increased difficulty in mastering the developmental tasks of future stages

3. **Example**

During a spring break vacation in Florida, a 19 year old man is involved in a diving accident and is left hemiplegic. While in the ICU, he constantly struggles with being dependent on the nursing staff for many basic needs

He had recently begun to enjoy a great deal of independence while away at college, and finds his dependent position in the hospital almost unbearable

The struggle makes him reluctant to ask nurses to assist him when he needs help, and he becomes increasingly irritable, frustrated, demanding, and depressed

STRESS

1. **Definition**
    a.   Stress is the condition that exists in an organism when it meets with stimuli
    b.   Selye has identified two types of stress
        i.   Distress — the condition that exists in an organism when it meets with *noxious* stimuli; i.e., when an individual encounters threatening stimuli
        ii. Eustress — the condition that exists in an organism when it meets with *nonthreatening* stimuli

2. **Discussion**
    a.   Individuals may experience the same stressors differently. Stressors that may cause distress in one person may evoke eustress in another
    b.   Individuals respond to stressors differently because their perceptions of the stressful event may be different, and they may possess different coping abilities
    c.   A person experiencing distress feels uncomfortable. The discomfort provides the motivation to find a way to deal effectively with the stressor, so that the discomfort will be decreased
    d.   If one perceives oneself as adequate in the face of stressors, self-concept is maintained and may even be enhanced; growth is experienced and self-esteem is heightened. One functions out of strength
    e.   On the other hand, if one perceives oneself as inadequate in the face of stressors, one may use defense mechanisms (e.g., denial, projection) to mask the fact that one views one's handling of the stressor as inadequate; however, one will feel overwhelmed and helpless. One functions out of a sense of frustration and helplessness
    f.   If one continues to experience oneself as inadequate in the face of stressors for a prolonged period, crisis will result

3. **Example**
    Two critical care nurses begin orientation to a new hospital on the same day. Three weeks after completing orientation, one

nurse begins to relax and talk about feeling more comfortable on the unit, and about how much she is learning. This nurse has worked in an ICU in the past, knows generally what to expect, and has learned to deal effectively with occupational stressors. She generally finds ways to take allotted breaks with other staff members, and to discuss any difficulties she is having in adjusting to the unit. She feels comfortable enough to seek the advice of a clinical specialist in planning care for a very involved patient

The second nurse begins to report feeling nervous, fatigued, overwhelmed, and constantly on the verge of tears or a "blow-up" whenever a patient or colleague asks her to do anything she has not anticipated. This nurse has no previous experience in critical care nursing, and has not yet found ways to deal effectively with the stressful stimuli with which she was constantly being bombarded. The life/death atmosphere of urgency within the unit is a constant source of stress

PAIN

1. **Definition:** pain is a concept denoting the experience of multiple stimuli, all perceived as unpleasant by the individual involved. It is a multidimensional perception that has an influence upon all aspects of one's life

2. **Discussion**
   a. Pain is an individual and personal experience. Behavioral expressions of pain are socially and culturally determined. Because of the complexity of pain phenomena, there is no one theory that takes into account all the ramifications. Scientists and clinicians view pain from as many perspectives as there are clinical specialties. However, there appear to be three elements common to most definitions of pain
      i. There is a break in the protective barrier of the individual
      ii. It is perceived as a danger signal
      iii. It is an expression of all previous pain experiences
   b. Painful stimuli and their associated responses are composed of both physiologic and psychosocial elements. Human beings almost always are born with the physiologic ability to experience pain
   c. It is within the psychosocial realm that one develops behavioral responses to pain. Humans are both blessed and cursed by the fact that they can experience pain, and remember it. The moment one experiences an unpleasant (painful) stimulus, it is integrated with memories of previous painful experiences, and a response occurs. One responds not only to the immediate painful stimulus, but also to the memories of other experiences.

In fact, the ability to think and remember allows one to feel discomfort without presently experiencing a physiologically unpleasant stimulus

d. The meaning one places upon an unpleasant sensation is determined by one's beliefs and values within the context of societal beliefs, values, and norms

e. Pain, like beauty, is in the eye of the beholder. It is whatever the individual experiencing it says it is, whenever it is being experienced

3. **Example**

A 48 year old male has been admitted for the fourth time to the ICU with chest pain and shortness of breath. Four months ago, he experienced a myocardial infarction with residual heart damage. The patient describes events prior to admission as follows: "I started to breathe more rapidly, felt dizzy, light-headed, and faint with increasing chest pain. I felt like this while I was driving to a job interview"

While the nurse is talking to the patient he reports that he is becoming more nervous and anxious. His breathing becomes more rapid, and he mentions that his dizziness is more pronounced

The following diagnosis is made

i. Angina (normal for this individual)

ii. Hyperventilation secondary to anxiety

The patient's past memories of the heart attack and feelings of anxiety about the job interview are expressed behaviorally in terms of hyperventilation and its sequelae. He perceives his symptoms of hyperventilation as chest *pain,* and associates it with a heart attack

INTERPERSONAL COMMUNICATION

1. **Definition**: interpersonal communication is a dynamic process involving verbal and nonverbal means of conveying and receiving information

2. **Discussion**

a. One of the most important aspects of interpersonal communication is that one *cannot not* communicate. Interpersonal interactions means that every word (spoken or written), movement, facial expression, and body posture conveys information. This begins the circular process of communication

b. The receiver accepts information conveyed through the words, gestures, facial expressions, and postures of the sender, and assigns meaning to that information. The meaning assigned is understood in context of the situation and in light of the beliefs, values, knowledge, and self-concepts of both sender and receiver. The meaning and significance of the information influences how the receiver responds. The response is based on the meaning the receiver has given the information. The sender then receives the response

c. The response may not be what the sender desired to know, and a breakdown in communication could result. This can be forestalled by verification, i.e., verifying the information received and its meaning with the sender. Verification can be accomplished in a variety of ways, e.g., directly questioning, restating, and reflecting the information received. Through verification, the receiver and sender both achieve a clearer understanding of the information conveyed. In order to accomplish effective communication, it is not necessary to agree with what another says — only that both parties understand that which is communicated

3. **Example**

A 26 year old man is admitted to the ICU after an auto accident. His medical diagnoses are

Three fractured fingers of the right hand

No internal abdominal injuries

No closed head injury

Trauma to the throat requiring a tracheostomy

The patient, a pianist by profession, is oriented and alert

The nurse says: "How are you?

The patient stares at his right hand, which is wrapped in bandages and elevated

The nurse observes the patient's staring, shares with him the meaning she assigned to his behavior, and attempts to verify it by saying: "Does this mean that you are having pain in your hand?"

The patient clarifies his meaning by shaking his head to signify "no," and points to his right hand with his left hand. He opens and closes his left hand

The nurse now shares her perception and thoughts about the patient's new behavior by asking: "Are you saying that you have no pain, but you want to know about being able to move your right hand?"

The patient verifies for the nurse by nodding his head to signify "yes"

BODY IMAGE

1. **Definition**: body image is the concept of one's own body. It is formed through an accumulation of all perceptions, information, and feelings incorporated about one's body as different and apart from all others

2. **Discussion**
   a. One is not born with a body image. The concept of body is built slowly over a period of time as an integral part of one's growth and development. Body image is an essential component of the self-concept, and as such is grounded in interactions occurring between individuals and their environment
   b. Like self-concept, body image reflects sociocultural beliefs and values. Body image evolves in a dynamic, ever-changing process that incorporates not only one's body, but also devices attached to it, e.g., clothes, rings, watches, dialysis machine, pacemaker. It is more than a portrait in the mind: it is the *significance* attached to the structures and functions of the body that are truly significant
   c. Body image is social in nature, yet is individually experienced. If an individual experiences a positive body image, then self-concept and self esteem are likely to be influenced favorably. Conversely, a negative body image could lead to a less than favorable self-concept and self-esteem. Changes in body image influence an individual's perception of consequential events

3. **Example**
   A 33 year old woman with a postbilateral mastectomy has experienced an altered body image. She perceives herself as less than whole and less feminine
   Her changed body image has affected her self-concept
   She complains that, when she is alone with her husband, he seems nervous and afraid to touch her. Her perception is that he no longer "cares for me or finds me desirable." She feels repulsive
   The woman's altered body image influences her perception of her husband's attitude toward her

HUMAN SEXUALITY

1. **Definition**: human sexuality is a developmental process encompassing a blend of the physiologic aspects of genetic sex and the psychosocial aspects, which include gender identity, sexual behavior, and sexual attitudes or values. Sexuality is part of one's self-concept

2. **Discussion**
   a. The interaction between the psyche and the soma is nowhere more evident than in the area of sexuality where perception, self-concept, self-esteem, body image, and personal values clearly combine with basic mechanisms of physiologic functioning in a complex system. Although the genetic sex of an infant is determined by chromosomal factors before birth, the psychosocial impact on gender identity becomes predominant after

birth. The concept of sexuality, or more specifically the psychosocial aspect of sexuality, primarily involves the quality of an individual's interactions with significant others throughout the life cycle. One's gender identity, sexual behaviors, and sexual attitudes and values are integrated into the fabric of one's self-concept. Sexuality is so closely interwoven with the self-concept that a perceived threat can have an impact upon one's sexuality, which is expressed in both physiologic and psychosocial realms

b. For different reasons, sexuality is as important to a 70 year old person as it is to a 20 year old. Younger individuals often are concerned about their sexual attractiveness as well as their ability to reproduce. Older people usually are concerned with feeling like a sexual being and being perceived by others as such

c. A perceived threat to the self within a critical care environment has an effect upon sexuality. The effects can be expressed in a variety of symptomatic behaviors, e.g., depression or anger, a sense of loss, sexual aggressiveness, noncompliance, or demands upon others. Such behaviors can result in decreased self-esteem, influencing the individual's perception of events occurring in the environment

3. **Example**

A 37 year old male is admitted to the hospital with chest pain and shortness of breath. Lab studies confirm that he has suffered a myocardial infarction. The patient married for the second time 18 months ago. His wife is 27 years old, and they have two children from her previous marriage. The patient appears to be apprehensive, restless, and withdrawn, and these symptoms seem to increase after his wife's visit. He discusses his apprehensiveness with a nurse after his wife's visit

The patient says: "Things won't be like they have been. I won't be able to support my family now." He then grimaces and quickly looks away

The nurse says: "Is there something wrong right now?"

The patient replies: "I'm just thinking about my wife. Because of my heart attack, I won't be able to be the husband she's known. She's younger than me and can have almost any guy she wants"

The myocardial infarction is a threat to the patient's self-concept, self-esteem, body image, and sexual identity

FAMILY

1. **Definition**: the family is a social group with culturally determined characteristics, which include economic cooperation, reproduction, and the rearing and socialization of children. It is an interacting and transacting group in relation to the larger society

2. Discussion
   a. The family is the conveyor of the beliefs, values, norms, and roles of society. The entire family participates in the socialization process of its members. A child must acquire an immense amount of traditional knowledge and skill, and must learn to subject some natural inborn impulses to the discipline prescribed by society, before being accepted as an adult member. One of the immutable facts about the family is that it is a primary building block of all societies
   b. Within the family, norms are found, usually modeled after those of the larger society, which prescribes role-appropriate behaviors for family members — each member has a role. The family usually acts to support and protect its members, both collectively and individually
   c. Like individuals, families attempt to maintain a steady state. Any perceived threat to the family's function or structure causes it to feel anxious and to close ranks
   d. If one family member is in an ICU, other members attempt to assume the role-behaviors of the absent member. If a family feels the threat of losing one of its members, it mobilizes to defend against the loss
   e. A patient in an ICU may experience a biologic crisis, and at the same time his family may undergo a psychologic crisis. The provision of effective care for an individual necessarily involves extending care to available family members

3. Example
   Mr. B. is a 36 year old married man with three children: two boys, ages 9 and 12, and a 10 year old girl. He is admitted to the ICU with renal and liver impairment secondary to cancer
   During the first week of hospitalization, Mrs. B. is present nearly all day every day. She looks tired, and behaves as if she were quite anxious
   During the second week of hospitalization, Mrs. B. visits less frequently and has dark circles under her eyes. Her behavior appears increasingly agitated, except when with her husband: when talking to him and holding his hand, she seems to relax considerably. While talking to a nurse, Mrs. B. starts to cry and tremble, saying: "We try to carry on, but it's so hard. My oldest son tries to be the father for the other children, and when I am not home my daughter cooks. But it is so hard"

PSYCHOSOCIAL IMPACT OF THE CRITICAL CARE ENVIRONMENT

1. **Definition:** the critical care environment is defined as the sum of interactions among all people, objects, and circumstances that affect the well-being of individuals present in an ICU

2. **Discussion**

   a. Stressors within the critical care environment that have an impact upon individuals include: machines, the noise level, spatial structures, individuals' preconceived ideas, human interactions, thwarted needs and desires, and volumes of decisions. Interactions that occur within this environment are significant in that they regulate the amount of distress as well as the amount of support experienced by individuals, in addition to the amount of control each has over the environment

   b. In order to deal with the ever-changing demands of the environment, those present utilize a variety of coping mechanisms to assist them with their struggles to feel adequate. If an individual's coping mechanisms fail to provide sufficient protection, the environment is usually perceived as overwhelming, and dysfunctional behavior can result

   c. Dysfunctional behavior is commonly seen in the following ways
      i. Among patients — by demanding and acutely aggressive behaviors as well as by withdrawn behaviors
      ii. Among family members — by repetition of questions or statements, putting blame upon nurses, and making unrealistic demands upon staff as well as by withdrawn behaviors
      iii. Among staff — by rashes of errors, avoiding patients, other staff members, or family members; increased feelings of competitiveness; and emotional lability "for no apparent reason"

3. **Example**

   A 37 year old man is admitted to the CCU with diagnosis of myocardial infarction. He has chest pain and shortness of breath. On the third day after admission, the patient appears apprehensive and restless, jumping at all noises and whenever he is touched. He continuously handles his monitor leads and is unable to sleep for more than two hours at a time. When an alarm goes off anywhere on the unit he becomes ashen, and he pushes the call button every couple of minutes. He repeatedly asks the nurses for reassurance that he will not die, and nothing the nurses do satisfies him

   The nurses' reactions become characterized by irritation, as they grow weary of his demands for their time and attention. As the days wear on the staff increasingly avoid the patient who becomes increasingly symptomatic

_____ PSYCHOSOCIAL PHENOMENA ENCOUNTERED _____

CRISIS: In order that the reader may better understand the phenomenon of crisis, it is recommended that appropriate concepts on the preceding pages be reviewed.

1. **Definition:** crisis is the state of feeling overwhelmed by stressors and struggling unsuccessfully to cope with the situation. It involves an attempt to regain equilibrium. Crisis is not an illness; it is an opportunity for growth

2. **Discussion**
   a. Like stress, crisis is a matter of perception. Events that trigger crisis in one person may not do so in another
   b. Crisis usually lasts from four to six weeks and is characteristically self-limiting. The reason for this is related to the fact that humans become depleted of energy after enduring significant distress over a prolonged period. They then begin to adapt to the crisis in order to recoup their energies
   c. There are two identified types of crisis commonly experienced
      i. Situational — derived from a particular set of circumstances that occasion major changes in a person's life, e.g., role change, illness, divorce, death
      ii. Maturational — derived from difficulties in mastering developmental tasks associated with life stages, e.g., going to school, puberty, middle age, involutional changes
   d. It is important to remember that crisis is part of normal growth and development
   e. Whether the crisis is experienced by critical care nurses, their patients, or the patients' families, four observable phases can be distinguished. Fink has identified these as follows
      i. Shock — one perceives a threat to existing familiar structures, views reality as overwhelming, and experiences anxiety, helplessness, and thought disorganization
      ii. Defensive retreat — one attempts to maintain one's usual structures; tries to avoid reality by wishful thinking, denial, or repression; and experiences indifference or euphoria, *except* when challenged. Challenge makes one angry and resistant to change because one is defensively reorganizing one's thoughts
      iii. Acknowledgment — one gives up the existing, familiar structures; faces reality; and feels depressed. One may

experience apathy, agitation, bitterness, mourning, high
anxiety, or suicidal thoughts if the stressor is too overwhelming. The thought process is disorganized owing to
a reorganization in light of altered perceptions of reality.

    iv.   Adaptation and change — one establishes a new structure,
feels a renewed sense of self-worth, engages in new reality
testing, and experiences a gradual increase in satisfaction.
The thought process is reorganized in light of present
resources and abilities

  f. The outcomes of crisis fall into three categories

    i.   Some individuals break down under the stress and never
learn to cope with the traumatic change

    ii. Others experience the crisis and emerge from it about the
same as they were before

    iii. Others learn about themselves and their ability to handle
new situations, and emerge feeling stronger and with
increased self-esteem

  g. People in crisis are more open than usual to help

CRISIS INTERVENTION

1. **Minimal goal**: to assist persons in crisis with the psychologic
resolution of the immediate crisis, and to help restore their level of
functioning to at least that which existed before the crisis

2. **Maximal goal**: to assist persons in crisis to improve their level of
functioning beyond the pre-crisis level

3. **Factors that influence the outcome**

  a. How serious and how unexpected was the crisis?

  b. What is the individual's perception of the stressful event precipitating the crisis? Is the perception realistic?

  c. What strengths do persons in crisis possess to help them
through it?

  d. What coping skills have they used successfully in the past?

  e. What is their physical condition and energy level?

  f. What sociocultural supports are available to them (e.g., religion,
social agencies)

  g. Is there anyone willing to assist them?

4. **Steps involved**

  a. Begin the interaction by sharing with people in crisis your own
perception, thought, or feeling that is causing you to initiate the
interaction. *Validate* with them to find out if what you think is
happening is actually happening to them

  b. Help them to identify the problem in reality; help to correct
apparent distortions

   c. Help them to identify coping mechanisms that might be of assistance, and support them while they use the mechanisms. It might be beneficial to say something such as: "What have you done to help yourself endure other very difficult times?"

   d. Help them to identify and contact people-supports who might assist them. If no such people are available, *you* become the temporary support. You might say something such as "Who would you like to have with you during this difficult time?"

   e. Help them to plan realistically for only the next step or two (help them to know what to expect next)

   f. The process for intervening is the same for patients, family members, and nurses

   g. Some final tips

      i. Short, simple interactions are the most helpful

      ii. Help people in crisis face issues they are able to acknowledge, and facilitate their expression of feelings

      iii. Support them in confronting a doubtful outcome. One cannot control the outcome, but one can provide needed support and facilitate a discussion of what is happening

      iv. At times it is helpful for people in crisis to perform an actual constructive task

      v. It is important that people in crisis are not overmedicated, so that resolution and growth can occur and self-esteem can increase

FEAR/ANXIETY

1. **Definition**: fear and anxiety are unpleasant feeling states, precipitated by perceived threats to the self and manifested by psychophysiologic symptoms

2. **Discussion**

   a. The psychophysiologic symptoms of fear and of anxiety are indistinguishable from each other. Commonly identified symptoms are: increased heart rate, increased muscular tension, trembling, increased startle response, perspiration, sinking feeling in stomach, dry mouth and throat, frequent urge to urinate, irritability, aggressiveness, urge to cry or run and hide, confusion, feelings of unreality, feelings of faintness, nausea, fatigue, restlessness, appetite changes, insomnia or increased sleep, nightmares, speech pattern changes, and meaningless gestures. Each of these symptoms can be experienced as normal, everyday feelings at a low intensity level. Some are adaptive in nature, such as

      i. Increased heart rate and respiratory exchange, which results in increased oxygen and blood supply to muscles

      ii. Increased oxygen supply, which enhances mental alertness

b. Adaptive functions enable the individual to be in peak condition to respond more effectively to stress

c. When the symptoms of fear and anxiety reach a certain level of intensity, they cease being adaptive and become maladaptive for the individual. When one perceives that one's symptoms are becoming harmful, one begins to channel energies toward achievement of a steady state. This process decreases the amount of energy available to cope with incoming stimuli, and increased anxiety and fear may result. One feels vulnerable and cannot experience oneself as safe

d. Critical care nurses often encounter patients who are unable to sleep because of fear related to illness or to the unfamiliarity of their surroundings. The longer patients are unable to sleep, the greater the fear and anxiety become. When fear and anxiety increase, other symptoms are demonstrated, e.g., confusion, restlessness, irritability, and signs of aggression. Patients experience themselves as threatened, and may behave in noncompliant ways. They may even hallucinate or speak from a delusional frame of reference

e. When assessing patients who are experiencing high levels of fear and anxiety, the nurse will want to ascertain

   i. What they are experiencing, and what is the perceived threat

   ii. What in the environment can be modified to decrease the sense of threat

   iii. What support resources (from within patients as well as externally) are available to help decrease their fear and anxiety

   iv. What identified needs for help can be met by the nursing staff

f. The goal of intervention with those who are highly anxious and fearful is not to try to remove all fear and anxiety (this is impossible), but rather to help reach a level with which they can cope. The hope is that they will find ways of adapting to their situation through the help of internal and external supports

g. The following are suggestions for intervening with persons who are experiencing high levels of fear and anxiety

   i. Through interactions, assist them to clarify the perceived threat, and to dispel misconceptions

   ii. Reinforce their self-esteem by emphasizing identified strengths that you observe them using to cope with the situation

   iii. Help them to control pain by eliciting information about its source and the reason for it; by discussing with patients the meaning of the pain for them; and by administering medication appropriately

  iv. Utilize safety, security, and comfort measures, as
       appropriate
  v.   Involve patients and significant others in the care process, as
       appropriate
  vi. Communicate your concern and care for patients through
       verbal and nonverbal means

LONELINESS

1. **Definition**: loneliness denotes uncomfortable feelings of alienation
    caused by separation from significant relationships, events, and
    objects — painful aloneness

2. **Discussion**
    a. Loneliness often accompanies major life changes in which some
        familiar structures are lost. Illness and hospitalization are
        prime precipitators of feelings of loneliness
    b. Everyone experiences loneliness at times, but for some it is a
        characteristic way of life
    c. When attempting to assist someone who is lonely, the goal is to
        facilitate the individual's sense of relatedness to
        i.   His body
        ii.   His psyche
        iii. Significant others
        iv.   Familiar events
        v.   Yourself, the nurse
    d. This goal can be accomplished through interventions such as
        i.   Encouraging patients and family members to participate in
              their care, when appropriate, and to ask questions
        ii.   Initiating and facilitating discussion about patients' pain/
              surgery/illness, feelings about self/visitors/environment/
              cherished possessions, and other topics of importance to
              them
        iii. Allowing patients to get to know you, insofar as it seems
              helpful in enabling them to relate to the caregivers on whom
              they are dependent
        iv.   Relating on a person-to-person basis, which fosters
              personalized care
    e. Promoting relationships, providing familiar activities, and
        permitting patients to have objects that hold positive meaning
        for them are the focus of interventions
    f. It is important to remember, however, that the nurse can only be
        a facilitator when working with those who feel lonely. If, during
        your intervention, patients refuse to relate to others, or feel too
        angry or depressed to focus on familiar (usually comforting),
        activities, they must make their own choice as to what to do to
        help themselves feel more comfortable

g. Patients will make choices based on their self-concept, self-esteem, and need levels at the time. It is not helpful for the nurse to attempt to coerce them into feigning interest when they clearly are not interested: coercion makes them feel more alienated, and thus more lonely

POWERLESSNESS

1. **Definition**: powerlessness is a perceived lack of control over the outcome of a specific situation

2. **Discussion**
    a. Powerlessness derives from the belief that, no matter how one behaves, one is unable to influence the outcome of a situation
    b. In the process of concluding that one is incapable of effecting a desired change, one attempts to problem-solve in as many ways as one can. However, one consistently runs up against obstacles, and all efforts to bring about a desired outcome are ineffective
    c. As this process is repeated, one begins to feel frustrated, inadequate, hopeless, angry, and depressed
    d. In the critical care environment, all parties are capable of experiencing themselves as powerless — patients, family members, and staff
    e. In order to counteract the powerlessness phenomenon, one must believe that one is able to behave in ways that will make a difference in the resulting outcomes
    f. In an effort to help those who feel powerless, a nurse might consider the following interventions
        i. Assist them to redefine goals that they are unable to accomplish, in the hope that they will consider shorter, more attainable goals
        ii. Assist them to identify ways in which they can be effective in given situations; i.e., help them to focus on ways in which they can be powerful, if they choose
        iii. Help them by giving information they need in order to be effective in given situations
        iv. Support them by attempting to understand their feelings of impotence when they express them
    g. It is helpful to remember that the nurse cannot take away another's feelings of powerlessness, since they grow out of an individual's life situation, and one cannot change another person's life. However, patients themselves can work with inner strengths to discover new meaning in life and to problem-solve by determining ways in which they can be effective in influencing desired changes
    h. A nurse can be helpful by displaying a caring presence, by actively listening, and by using empathy. The nurse can provide feedback in relation to knowledge gaps, strengths, or confusions

that are expressed by patients, and can let them know that their emotional pain is recognized

    i.   It does no good to tell patients how to solve their problems: this only reinforces their view of themselves as inadequate and adds to their feelings of powerlessness

SENSORY OVERLOAD

1. **Definition**: sensory overload indicates repeated multisensory experiences that occur with greater intensity than is normally experienced by an individual. Often, the excessive stimuli are experienced suddenly. Sometimes, they are not understood by the individual, but rather are perceived simply as bothersome, meaningless experiences. In general, excessive sensory stimuli are caused by an onslaught of unfamiliar, uncomfortable, unexpected stimulation

2. **Discussion**
   a. Sensory stimuli are stressors. Since ICUs are areas of excessive sensory stimuli for patients, family members, and staff, stress levels are excessively high. Individuals frequently tend to act out high stress levels by creating a noisy environment, which perhaps relieves some of the tension for those creating the noise!
   b. However, the increased noise level creates new stressors for all in the environment, adding to the sensory stimuli
   c. Along with auditory stimuli, the ICU hosts a myriad of visual, tactile, olfactory, and gustatory stimuli 24 hours a day, which are absorbed by those in the environment. Family members and staff are able to change the types and patterns of stimuli to which they are exposed by routinely leaving the critical care area. Patients, of course, are continually subjected to high levels of stimulation for as long as they are housed on the unit. *All* who encounter this environment are prone to experience sensory overload
   d. Some common symptoms of sensory overload include: confusion, restlessness to the point of agitation, anger, and sometimes hallucinations
   e. In attempting to prevent or minimize sensory overload, the nurse could
      i. Assess the noise level on the unit, particularly at the bedside of patients, since it is here that many noise-producing mechanical devices are located, e.g., the bellows of ventilators and the alarm mechanism of cardiac monitors
      ii. Assess the visual intensity generated by the unit lighting
      iii. Assess the environment for malodorous stimuli
      iv. Assess each patient's level and type of gustatory stimuli
      v. Assess how staff and family members touch individual patients, and the amount of pain experienced by each patient

vi. Implement modifications that seem appropriate regarding
   (a) Noise levels — attending particularly to the intensity of conversational tones used by staff members; the positioning of noisy machinery in relation to the head of each patient; and loud, banging noises caused by dropped equipment, bedpan hoppers in need of repair, mishandled food trays, and messengers delivering supplies
   (b) Visual intensity — monitoring the light intensity on the unit to ensure that the environment is as safe and comfortable as possible, and attempting to simulate natural light cycles from morning to night
   (c) Environmental odors — using air deodorizers and disposing of malodorous substances appropriately
   (d) Gustatory stimuli — assisting patients with mouth care when needed, and offering palatable fluids and foods as appropriate
   (e) Tactile communication — each time the nurse makes physical contact with patients she should be aware of the message one may convey through touching. This can be accomplished by appropriate gentleness as a nurse turns patients, changes dressings, administers injections, gives baths and back rubs, and provides hair care. When a nurse becomes aware of the amount of invasive tactile stimulation experienced by patients, the method of evaluating their need for pain medication may change. Administering pain medication effectively greatly helps to decrease tactile overload

SENSORY DEPRIVATION

1. **Definition**: sensory deprivation denotes a lack of sensory input or a lack of variety, intensity, or perceived meaning of sensory stimulation

2. **Discussion**
   a. Since most critical care patients are immobile, they are generally confined to a limited space in a machine-oriented, totally unfamiliar environment. They often experience consciousness-altering drugs that numb sensory receptors. Sometimes, the nature of their illness reduces sensitivity to stimuli. At other times, technical assists are so complex as to require much time and attention from caregivers, perhaps more than are focused on the patient. All these factors predispose critical care patients to sensory deprivation
   b. The goal of nursing interventions aimed toward preventing or eliminating sensory deprivation is to provide sensory stimuli that patients can experience and find meaningful, in order to facili-

tate their relatedness to themselves and the unfamiliar world in which they find themselves

c. Communicating through meaningful touch and conversation is one way in which a nurse can assist patients to increase their ability to relate, thereby decreasing sensory deprivation. Encouraging family members to provide familiar personal items, when possible is also helpful as is the presence of loved ones.

d. Usual symptoms of sensory deprivation can mimic symptoms of sensory overload, including lethargy

e. To distinguish between sensory hunger and sensory overload, the nurse must carefully assess the types and amounts of sensory stimuli experienced by individual patients, and make judgments based on the data collected

f. In general, sensory alterations are caused by a variety of factors found within the ICU. Some common factors include

  i. Abnormal physiologic conditions

  ii. Ingestion of drugs

  iii. Prolonged experience of pain

  iv. Lack of familiar persons and objects

  v. Fear

  vi. Lack of understanding about one's condition

  vii. Sleep deprivation caused by interrupted sleep cycles that deny a person opportunity to adequately restore depleted energy supplies

g. Effective nursing interventions involving sensory deprivation and overload are crucial for the protection of patients' compromised health states

ADDICTIONS

1. **Definition**: addiction is a phenomenon that refers to dependence on a chemical substance outside the self that is perceived by the individual as being necessary for self-maintenance and for the self to feel complete, i.e., adequate

2. **Discussion**

a. The addiction phenomenon is a maladaptive effort to help the self feel adequate. The process is considered maladaptive because the end result involves the individual in spending time and energy numbing the self, so that spontaneous, growth-producing doubts, fears, and stressors are not experienced or dealt with constructively. Growth does not take place, and the individual stagnates

b. When a nurse encounters addicts in the ICU it is important to remember the following

  i. If individuals are still under the influence of the addictive substance, their perceptions of reality will be altered

      ii.   Patients' self-concept and self-esteem will be threatened because they do not have access to that which they believe will make them complete; they probably feel incomplete, and desperate for the substance

     iii.   There is usually some concern on the part of addicts regarding how others will view them, so that self-concept and self-esteem are again threatened

     iv.   While withdrawing from the substance, patients will be acutely reactive to physical and emotional stimuli

c. In attempting to deal effectively with addicts, the nurse should remember that they may feel threatened. Their behavior, therefore, may reflect a strong need to defend themselves by keeping people at a comfortable distance

d. Distancing maneuvers include withdrawal behaviors as well as those that tend to push others away by evoking feelings of anger, frustration, repulsion, or fear

e. The nurse will not want to make addicted patients feel even more threatened (which would occasion further acting-out behaviors), and so might consider the following

     i.   Attempting to understand their suffering and concerns

     ii.   Communicating in a straightforward manner; i.e., if patients' behavior is disruptive to the nurse or to the unit, telling them so and requesting that they behave in a specifically different manner

     iii.   Assisting patients to feel secure on the unit by providing simple, clear explanations regarding what is happening to them

     iv.   Avoiding power struggles and arguments by approaching conflicts from the perspective of understanding patients' feelings about the issues, and making clear statements about how the nurse views the situation

f. In general, communicating that the nurse cares about addicted patients and wants to be of help during this difficult time is an important factor in establishing a helping relationship. At times, attempts to help will include insisting that patients do things they may not want to do

SUICIDAL PHENOMENON

1. **Definition:** suicide is an active or passive self-destructive act by an individual that results from a perceived, overwhelming threat to the self

2. **Discussion**

    a. Everyone at one time or another has suicidal thoughts. These can be as casual as a morning wish to cancel the day owing to lack of interest, which one generally would not act upon because less drastic coping mechanisms can effectively handle the situation

b.   Every case of self-destructive behavior involves the pressure of a phenomenologically unbearable threat to self. Other less drastic and less destructive coping mechanisms no longer are experienced as effective in handling the perceived overwhelming threat. Suicide, therefore, as the ultimate attempt to deal with threat, is considered and sometimes acted upon. In a sense, suicidal behavior is seen as an escape from, rather than a movement toward, something

c.   A suicidal individual experiences many emotions, e.g., despair, guilt, shame, dependency, hopelessness, weariness, boredom, depression. There is a point at which despair becomes overwhelming and unbearable. For some, there is a sense that life is just not worth living anymore — it no longer has meaning. Others feel that someone does not want them around, or that their individual problems can never be resolved

d.   In providing nursing services to patients who have attempted suicide, nurses should be aware of the following common characteristics of the suicidal phenomenon
   i.   The acute crisis period or high lethality time is of short duration — it can be counted in hours or days
   ii.   Suicidal individuals are usually ambivalent about dying. At the same time at which they plan suicide, they have fantasies of rescue
   iii. People who talk about it commit suicide as well as those who do not talk about it
   iv.   Suicidal individuals usually give clues about their intentions
   v.   Suicidal behavior has no racial, social, religious, cultural, or economic boundaries
   vi.   Suicide has no characteristic genetic qualities; however, its incidence is greater in families in which there have been previous suicides
   vii. Suicidal behavior does not necessarily mean that the individual is mentally ill; in some cases, suicide is viewed as a logical last step by one who is overwhelmed with stress
   viii. Most important, directly asking an individual about suicidal intent will *not* cause suicide

e.   In addition to *knowing* about suicide, one must also be aware of one's own *feelings* about it. Dealing with suicidal individuals can raise fears and reactions within caregivers, e.g., anger, anxiety about one's own suicidal thoughts, dislike/resentment toward those who have attempted suicide, a wish to avoid the suicidal person in favor of other patients whose conditions do not appear to be self-inflicted, and doubts about one's ability to care for them. It is easier to care for suicidal patients if one is able to understand why they attempted suicide

    f. Nursing interventions must take into consideration that which is real for suicidal patients — those things that they perceive to be an overwhelming threat.

    g. The following are suggestions for intervening with patients who have attempted suicide

        i. Accept the suicidal behavior as logical from the patients' point of view

        ii. Utilize all communication modes (verbal and nonverbal) in an attempt to understand how they perceive their world, and themselves in that world

        iii. Reinforce positive aspects of their self-concept, if any are expressed

        iv. Reinforce self-esteem by interacting with them in a manner that accords them dignity

        v. Recognize that which they perceive to be real

        vi. Avoid participation in power struggles with those who behave in a belligerent and noncompliant manner

        vii. Assist them to re-establish supportive relationships with those whom they choose

        viii. Support the patient's significant others, so that they in turn can support the patient

        ix. Provide an environment that is as safe and secure as possible (this includes a nonthreatening emotional climate).

        x. Be aware of and attempt to deal with your own fears, feelings, and conflicts. Reciprocal staff support is essential

THE DYING PROCESS AND DEATH

1. **Definition**
   a. Dying is a psychophysiologic process that evokes many stresses and crises, and that ultimately terminates in death for the dying and in suffering for significant survivors
   b. Death is the antithesis of life

2. **Discussion**
   a. Death is not amenable to change or intervention. It incorporates the greatest loss
   b. The dying process is part of the life cycle. When one is conscious of this process, the threat of death unleashes the primordial feelings of hopelessness, helplessness, and abandonment. The fear of the unknown in death evokes fears of the unknown of annihilation of self, of being, and of identity
   c. The dying process imposes a twofold burden
      i. Intrapsychic stress — preparing oneself for death
      ii. Interpersonal stress — preparing oneself for death in relation to significant others, while simultaneously preparing those others to be survivors

d. This twofold task evokes a pervasive state of grief about the impending death, and anger about one's impotence. The anger can be directed toward God, loved ones, or caregivers. In addition, dying individuals may experience anxiety related to fear of pain, loss of identity, loneliness and abandonment, powerlessness, fear of the unknown, and fear of annihilation

e. Elizabeth Kubler-Ross has described five psychologic stages of the dying process
   i.   Denial or isolation — "no, not me"
   ii. Anger, rage, envy, resentment — "why me?"
   iii. Bargaining — "if you will. . . .then I will"
   iv. Depression — "what's the use?"
   v.   Acceptance — the final resting stage before the long journey

f. Some who are inexperienced in working with the dying may expect individuals to follow the exact sequence described above. In reality, the dying process may include all the stages (although some never get beyond the denial stage), but the stages shift, depending on what the individual experiences. A person may fluctuate from depression to anger, or may revert to the denial stage once again

g. Providing care for the dying may evoke strong emotions in caregivers — anger, frustration, or dislike. These reactions may result in a desire to avoid dying patients or their families. Like-wise, being with a dying loved one may evoke strong emotions in family members, and may cause them to be less and less available as the process continues. The dying process predisposes individuals to a sense of abandonment

h. Because psychologic states are complicated clusters of intellectual and affective factors that occur in the context of individuals' perception of their world and of themselves in that world, it is important to remember two principles: denial and hope
   i.   *Denial can be an important coping mechanism for enabling individuals to maintain some control over the most threatening of situations.* Denial can make it possible for them to block out information with which they cannot successfully cope, and to begin to deal with reality in smaller, more manageable segments
      (a) Because denial operates protectively in persons on the verge of crises, it is important for the nurse to respond to dying patients by
         (1) Listening to find out their perception of their situation
         (2) Showing acceptance whenever they are found to be in the dying process
         (3) Not encouraging false beliefs
         (4) Attempting to understand why they are behaving as they are

(b) Examples
   (1) A man who suffered a life-threatening myo-
       cardial infarction two days ago says: "I
       think I'm well enough to go home now." The
       nurse responds: "I'm trying to appreciate
       how badly you want to go home, but it
       wouldn't be beneficial for you now because
       of your illness"
   (2) A 64 year old, recently retired woman
       has been diagnosed as having cancer, and
       told that she will probably live another six
       months. She tells a nurse that she plans to
       buy a new Mercedes, "even though it will
       probably take me three years to pay for it."
       The nurse responds: "I can hear how much
       you want to own that car. I hope you might
       be able to do it"
ii. *Hope is usually present throughout the dying process in
    some degree.* Hope, a belief in the desirability of
    survival, is usually found in persons demonstrating a
    healthy self-concept and self-esteem, but can be lost
    when individuals are unable to act on their own behalf
    and must submit to the influence of others
    (a) To a large extent, denial and hope are necessary
        for an individual to experience the dying process
        with some control. Denial provides a sorely
        needed locus of control over the primordial
        feelings unleashed during that process. Hope is
        the core of strength needed to withstand the pain,
        suffering, fears, and conflicts encountered
        throughout
i. In order to provide quality care to dying patients, it is helpful
   for nurses to be aware of the following
   i. Through caring for the dying, the nurse is often made aware
      of the fact that nurses also must one day face death, and
      perhaps the dying process. All the fears, feelings, and con-
      flicts demonstrated in dying patients are also evoked in the
      nurse, which in turn evokes the nurse's coping mechanisms.
      It is essential that nurses be aware of and accept their own
      fears about dying
   ii. Like all other kinds of nursing assessments, the assessment
       of dying patients is aimed at achieving an understanding of
       the needs of the individual and of family members. This can
       be accomplished by ascertaining the following
       (a) How do dying patients perceive their situation? What
           feelings are being expressed?
       (b) How does the family perceive the situation? What
           feelings are they expressing?

(c) What strengths and supports are the patient and family members utilizing to help them cope with the stress?

(d) What needs does the patient wish to have met? Who are the most appropriate people to meet those needs?

(e) Are body image and sexual identity significantly affected? Can interventions be designed to reaffirm these?

(f) Are loneliness and powerlessness causing the dying process to be more painful than is necessary? Can these factors be altered through interventions?

j. The goal of intervention is to respond effectively to the patient's identified needs for help. Because dying is an individual experience, the nurse will want to respond to the needs identified at a given point in time. The following are suggested interventions for the feeling stages identified by Kubler-Ross

   i. During the denial stage

     (a) Attempt to have someone stay with dying patients for a time

     (b) Take cues for conversation from the patients

     (c) Listen (one need not attempt to provide solutions to the questions raised, unless specifically requested to do so)

     (d) Respond to patients by sharing your reactions, when you think it might be helpful to them or their families

     (e) Provide opportunities for continued communication

   ii. During the anger stage

     (a) Allow patients to express their feelings to you and to ask: "Why me?"

     (b) Remember that you need not attempt to answer that unanswerable question

     (c) Try to remember that the anger patients are expressing is not directed at you, personally, but rather toward that which you represent (continued life) and toward their own painful situation ·

   iii. During the bargaining stage

     (a) Find out what kind of help patients need to complete their unfinished business.

     (b) Try to make time just to be with dying persons and to listen

   iv. During the depression stage, patients mourn all that they are losing. One can help by

     (a) Not interrupting the grieving process

     (b) Supporting patients in their grief

     (c) Sharing your feelings of sadness appropriately, if you feel sad

   v. During the acceptance stage, the issue of letting go of dying persons arises. One can be helpful by

     (a) Not deserting them

(b)   Respecting their acceptance of death

(c)   Assisting the family with their letting go of someone whom they love by listening, and by intervening in areas in which the family feels that it needs help

k.   Providing comfort measures for dying patients is reported to be a most important nursing intervention, for the sake of both the patient and the family. Effective verbal and nonverbal communication is essential to evaluate the need for the following

i.   Adequate medication for control of pain

ii.   Frequent mouth care

iii.   Positioning for comfort

iv.   Allowing family members to visit more frequently when the patient desires closer contact with loved ones

v.   Supporting the family's involvement in providing comfort measures for the dying person

l.   Providing nursing care for dying patients can be one of the most rewarding experiences, if critical care nurses are knowledgeable about and prepared to confront the dying process and themselves. Knowing that one may experience the ups and downs of the grieving cycle along with a few dying patients helps to diminish the fear of getting involved. Recognizing personal strengths and limitations helps to prevent burnout. Realizing that one will ultimately learn more about life and about oneself while working with dying patients helps one to take advantage of opportunities for growth

COPING WITH CRITICAL CARE

a.   Since nurses who work in critical care environments are exposed to the same environmental stressors as are patients and family members, one can expect similar emotional reactions to occur in staff over a prolonged period. Nurses are subject to additional stresses: responsibility for knowing how to respond appropriately to patients' medical and emotional crises, and desiring to be viewed by peers as competent practitioners. The nurse's position in the administrative structure is sometimes a source of further distress. All of this can lead to exhaustion if the nurse is not able to build in effective ways to deal with the distress

b.   It is helpful for nurses to remember that they are effective in the work setting to the degree that their own needs are met, and in accordance with the level of self-esteem experienced at a given moment

c.   To help promote self-esteem and to provide mechanisms for discharging distress, nurses may find it useful to

i.   Identify their reasons for choosing the critical care setting for practice

  ii. Identify their strengths as critical care nurses

  iii. Identify their own individual professional potentials (goals)

  iv. Identify their limitations as critical care nurses

  v. Routinely identify the effect critical care nursing is perceived to have on them individually

  vi. Develop peer relationships that allow them to feel safe enough to be comfortable in the critical care setting

  vii. Develop peer relationships that promote open communication (exchanging ideas, complaining, sharing difficult and positive experiences, resolving conflicts)

  viii. Utilize formal and informal multidiscipline clinical care conferences

  ix. Utilize staff groups facilitated by a mental health resource person

  x. Devise work plans that allow for sharing responsibilities, as needed

  xi. Utilize break and meal times to replenish energy levels constructively

  xii. Utilize moments alone when feeling overwhelmed by excessive stimuli

  xiii. Develop a relationship with supervisors that promotes open communication

  xiv. Utilize people-supports available outside the critical care unit (e.g., clinical nurse experts, in-service personnel, staff clergy)

  xv. Routinely schedule participation in continuing education events

  xvi. Develop sources of support and areas of enrichment outside their professional lives

d. It is suggested that nurses utilize the critical care environment in such a way that an area be established for staff use only, out of the view of patients and family members

e. Virginia Satir relates a story from her childhood that seems appropriate for critical care nurses. When she was growing up on a farm, the family water supply was located outside in the yard. Every time the water bucket was empty, someone had to go to the well to refill it. So, too, nurses working in high stress areas must go out and "refill" themselves when they feel empty and unable to give anymore. We hope you may always be "refilled"!

ASSESSMENT TOOL

Item to be assessed	Suggestion(s)
1. PERCEPTION – How do individuals view their situation, or particular issues in their situation?	1, 2. *Ask:* "What is it like for you right now . . . (having this illness, having had this surgery, being in these surroundings, having your wife in the hospital)?"
2. SELF-ESTEEM – Do individuals view themselves as adequate or inadequate in the present situation?	*Listen* for remarks disclosing self-perception, and
	Clarify the remarks if you see the need
	Say something like: "I think that if I were in your shoes, I might feel a little_____ (unsure, helpless, sorry, worried) about myself right now. I wonder if you might be having any of these feelings"
3. NEEDS/STRESS LEVELS AND PERCEIVED LIMITATIONS – What do individuals think their greatest need is right now?	3. *Listen* for requests to have needs met and for stressors that individuals talk about most frequently.
	Ask: "What is the most difficult thing for you right now that I may be able to help you with?"
4. STRENGTHS AND POTENTIALS – What positive attributes or resources can individuals identify as being of possible help in their situation?	4. *Observe* the coping mechanisms that patients are using successfully.
	Support them in their use of such successful mechanisms
	Ask: "Can you think of anything that could help you through this time?" and "How have you handled previous difficult situations that might be helpful to you now?"

ASSESSMENT TOOL *(Continued)*

Item to be assessed	Suggestion(s)
5. PAIN	5. *Observe* patients' verbal and nonverbal indications of pain, fear, and anxiety
	Ask them to describe the location, intensity, and frequency of pain
	Say: "On a scale of 1 to 10 (with 10 indicating the most severe), where would you place your pain at the moment?"
6. BODY IMAGE	6. *Listen* to the words patients use to describe themselves and to describe equipment to which they are attached
	Observe the body parts on which individuals focus their attention
7. SLEEP PATTERNS	7. *Observe* the length of time individuals appear to sleep
	Ask them if they think they are able to get sufficient sleep
8. COMMUNICATION PATTERNS	8. *Observe* the mode of communication used most expressively, verbal or nonverbal
	Observe those with whom patients initiate interactions
	Listen for questions and phrases repeated frequently

ASSESSMENT TOOL *(Continued)*

Item to be assessed	Suggestion(s)
9. GENERAL RESPONSE TO THE CRITICAL CARE ENVIRONMENT	9. *Observe* patients' level of irritability, startle response, and type of communication with staff and loved ones
	Ask them how they would like their immediate territory arranged regarding: light, the door (open or closed), placement of personal items, accessibility of food and beverage containers, positioning of necessary equipment, etc.
	Ask them if they have questions regarding the routine of the unit, their own care, or the use of equipment in their territory

Note: Since a direct psychosocial assessment of comatose patients is impossible, one can refer to the chart and talk with their families to ascertain the following information about them: location of residence; marital status; occupation; interests and activities; social supports.

When approaching comatose patients, it is suggested that the nurse use a consistent format, e.g., *call* them by name; *tell* them your name and that you are a nurse, and attempt to orient them to place, day, and time; *say:* "I know you are unable to talk to me right now, and I don't know if you can hear me, but I'm going to explain to you what I will be doing for you before I do it."

While administering care, consider talking briefly to patients about such things as the weather, where they live, their interests, etc.

REFERENCES

Aquilera, D. C., and Messick, J.: Crisis intervention: Theory and Methodology. C. V. Mosby Co., St. Louis, 1980.

Bandman, E. L.: The dilemma of life and death: should we let them die? Nurs. Forum *17*: 118–132, 1978.

Bechervaise, M. D.: The riddle of communication—1. Nurs. Times *75:*1434–1436, 1979.

Benoliel, J. Q., and Crowley, D. M.: The patient in pain: new concepts. American Cancer Society Professional Education Publication, 1974, pp. 1–9.

Benson, H.: The relaxation response. Psychiatry *37*: 37–46, 1974.

Berni, R., and Fordyce, W. E.: Behavior Modification and the Nursing Process. C. V. Mosby Co., St. Louis, 1973.

Billie, D. A.: The role of body image in patient compliance and education. Heart Lung 143–148, 1977.

Bolin, R. H.: Sensory deprivation, an overview. Nurs. Forum *13:* 240–258, 1974.

Breu, C., and Dracup, K.: Helping the spouses of critically ill patients. Am. J. Nurs. *78:* 50–53, 1978.

Briggs, D.: Your Child's Self-Esteem. Doubleday, New York, 1975.

Brissett, D.: Toward a clarification of self esteem. Psychiatry *35:*255–263, 1972.

Bugental, J.: The listening eye. J. Hum. Psychol. *16:*55–65, 1976.

Cabanac, M.: Physiological role of pleasure. Science *173:*1103–1107, 1971.

Calhoun, G., and Perrin, M.: Management, motivation and conflict. Top. Clin. Nurs. *1:* 71-80, 1979.

Cassem, N. H.: Treating the person confronting death. *In* Nicholi, A. M. (ed.): The Harvard Guide to Modern Psychiatry. Harvard University Press, Cambridge, 1978.

Cassem, N. H., and Hackett, T. P.: Stress on the nurse and therapist in the intensive care unit and the coronary care unit. Heart Lung *4:*252–258, 1975.

Chapman, R.C.: Role of anxiety in acute pain. Pain Overview pp. 6–13, 1980.

Chatham, M. A.: The effect of family involvement on patients' manifestations of postcardiotomy psychosis. Heart Lung *7:*995–999, 1978.

Chodil, J.: The concept of sensory deprivation. Nurs. Clin. North Am. *5:*252–255, 1970.

Cohe, C., Levin, E., Whitly, J., and Young, S.: Brief sexual counseling during cardiac rehabilitation. Heart Lung *8:* 124–129, 1979.

Collins, V. J.: Ethical considerations in therapy for the comatose and dying patient. Heart Lung *8:*1084–1088, 1979.

Combs, A., Richards, A. C., and Richards, F.: Perceptual Psychology: A Humanistic Approach to the Study of Persons. Harper and Row, New York, 1976.

Cooley, G. H.: The Social Self. *In* Farrell R., and Swigert, V. (eds.): Social Deviance. J. B. Lippincott Co., New York, 1975.

Coopersmith, S.: The Antecedents of Self-Esteem. W. H. Freeman Co., San Francisco, 1960.

Corbeil, M.: Nursing process for a patient with a body image disturbance. Nurs. Clin. North Am. *6:*155–163, 1971.

Cornish, R. D., and Miller, M. V.: Attitudes of registered nurses toward the alcoholic. J. Psychiatr. Nurs. *14:*19-22, 1976.

Costello, A. M.: Supporting the patient with problems related to body image. American Cancer Society Professional Education Publication, 1975, pp. 1–5.

Difabio, S.: Crisis: a complex process. Nurs. Clin. North Am. 9:47–56, 1974.

Dossett, S. M.: Nursing staff in high dependency areas. Nurs. Times *74:*888–891, 1978.

Downs, F.: Bedrest and sensory disturbances. Am. J. Nurs. *74:*434–438, 1974.

Drakontides, A. B.: Drugs to treat pain. Am. J. Nurs. *74:*508–513, 1974.

Eisendrath, S. J., and Dunkel, J.: Psychological issues in intensive care unit staff. Heart Lung *8:*751–758, 1979.

Erikson, E.: Identity and the Life Cycle: Selected Papers. International Universities Press, New York, 1959, Chap. 2.

Erikson, E.: Childhood and Society, 2nd ed. W. W. Norton and Co. New York, 1963, Chap. 7.

Erikson, E.: Identity, Youth and Crisis. W. W. Norton Co., New York, 1968, Chaps. 3 and 4.

Farberow, N. L., and Shneidman, E. S.: The Cry for Help. McGraw-Hill Book Co., New York, 1961.

Fink, S. L.: Crisis and motivation: a theoretical model. Arch. Phys. Med. Rehabil. *48:*592–597, 1967.

Fisher, S., and Cleveland, S.: Personality, body perception, and body image boundary. *In* Wapner, S., and Werner, H. (eds.): The Body Percept. Random House, New York, 1965.

Fitts, W.: Interpersonal Competence: The Wheel Model. Counselor Recordings and Tests, Nashville, 1970.

Fleming, M. L.: The nurse, the family system, and the client. Top. Clin. Nurs. *1:*1003, 1979.

Gardner, D., and Stewart, N.: Staff involvement with families of patients in critical care units. Heart Lung *7:*105–110, 1978.

Garfield, C. A.: Stress and Survival: The Emotional Realities of Life-Threatening Illness. C. V. Mosby Co., St. Louis, 1979.

Garfield, C. A.: Psychosocial care of the dying patient. *In* Patterson, M. E. (ed.): The Living-Dying Process. McGraw-Hill Book Co., New York, 1978.

Gick, R., and Whipple, B.: A holistic view of sexuality—education for the health professional. Top. Clin. Nurs. *1:*91–98, 1980.

Gowan, N. J.: The perceptual world of the intensive care unit: an overview of some environmental considerations in the helping relationship. Heart Lung *8:*340–344, 1979.

Graven, R. F., and Sharp, B. H.: The effects of illness on family functions. Nurs. Forum *11:*186–193, 1972.

Grollman, E. A.: Suicide. Beacon Press, Boston, 1971.

Guzetta, C. E.: Relationship between stress and learning. Adv. Nurs. Sci. *1:*35–49, 1979.

Hamachek, D. E.: Encounters with the Self. Holt, Rinehart and Winston, New York, 1971.

Hampe, S. O.: Needs of the grieving spouse in a hospital setting. Nurs. Res. *24:*113–120, 1975.

Hartl, D. E.: Stress management and the nurse. Adv. Nurs. Sci. *1:*91–100, 1979.

Hatten, C., Loing, V., McBride, S., and Rink, A.: Suicide assessment and Intervention. Appleton-Century-Crofts, New York, 1977.

Hein, E. C.: Communication in Nursing Practice, 2nd ed. Little, Brown & Co. Boston, 1980.

Heinemann, M., and Smith-DiJulio, K.: Learning to understand alcoholism. Nurs. Clin. North Am. *11:*493–505, 1976.

Hoff, L. A.: People in Crisis: Understanding and Helping. Addison-Wesley Publishing Co. Reading, 1978.

Hoffman, M., Donckers, S., and Hauser, M.: The effect of nursing intervention on stress factors perceived by patients in a coronary care unit. Heart Lung *7:*804–809, 1978.

Hoggatt, L., and Spilka, B.: The nurse and the terminally ill patient: some perspectives and projected actions. Omega, J. Death Dying *9:*255–266, 1978–79.

Hott, R.: Sex and the heart patient: a nursing view. Top. Clin. Nurs. *1:*75–84, 1980.

Huckabay, L. M. D., and Jagla, B.: Nurses' stress factors in the intensive care unit. J. Nurs. Admin. *9:* 21–26, 1979.

Jackson, W.: Sensory deprivation as a field of study. Nurs. Res. *20:*46–54, 1971.

Jacox, A.: Pain—A Source Book for Nurses and Other Health Professionals. Little, Brown, & Co., Boston, 1977.

Johnson, M. N.: Anxiety/stress and the effects on disclosure between nurses and patients. Adv. Nurs. Sci. *1:*1–20, 1979.

Jourard, S. M.: Suicide: invitation to die. Am. J. Nurs. *70:*269, 1970.

Kendal, M.: The community health nurse and alcohol-related problems. National Institute on Alcohol Abuse and Alcoholism, June, 1978, pp. 25–44.

Kolodny, R. C., Masters, W. H., Johnson, V. E., Biggs, M. A.: Textbook of Human Sexuality for Nurses. Little, Brown & Co., Boston, 1979. pp. 31–78.

Kubler-Ross, E.: On Death and Dying. Macmillan Co., New York, 1969.

Lazarus, R.: Psychological Stress and the Coping Process. McGraw-Hill Book Co., New York, 1966.

Lewis, G.: Nurse-Patient Communication. W. C. Brown Co., Dubuque, Iowa, 1978.

Lief, H., and Payne, T.: Sexuality, knowledge and attitudes. Am. J. Nurs. *75:*2026–2029, 1975.

Limandri, B. J., and Boyle D. W.: Instilling hope. Am. J. Nurs. *1:*78–80, 1978.

Maconachy, M. M.: The riddle of communication—2. Nurs. Times *75:*1493–1496, 1979.

Maslach, C.: How people cope. Public Welfare Association, Spring, 1978.

Maslow, A. H.: Toward a Psychology of Being. Van Nostrand, Princeton, 1968.

Mastrovizo, R. C.: Psychogenic pain. Am. J. Nurs. *3:*514–519, 1974.

McChoskey, J.C.: How to make the most of body image theory in nursing practice. Nursing *76:*68–72, 1976.

McCullougy, W. B.: The postoperative pain-anxiety circuit: a general surgeon's persepective. Pain Overview 1980, pp. 14–19.

Modlin, H. C.: Crisis intervention. J. Contin. Educ. Psychiatry 42:13–22, 1979.

Molter, N.C.: Needs of relatives of critically ill patients, a descriptive study. Heart Lung 8:332–339, 1979.

Moritz, D. A.: Understanding anger. Am. J. Nurs. 78: 81–83, 1978.

Murphy, G.: Human Potentialities. Basic Books, Inc., New York, 1958.

Nash, M.L.: Dignity of person in final phase of life—an exploratory study. Omega, J. Death Dying 8:71–80, 1977.

Orlando, I. J.: The Dynamic Nurse-Patient Relationship. G. P. Putnam's Sons, New York, 1961.

Oskins, S. L.: Identification of situational stressors and coping methods by intensive care nurses. Heart Lung 8:953–960, 1979.

Otto, H.: The human potentialities of nurses and patients. Nurs. Outlook 13:32-35, 1965.

Otto, H.: New light on human potential. Saturday Review, Dec. 20, 1969, pp. 14–18.

Parad, H. J.: Crisis Intervention: Selected Readings. Family Service Association of America, New York, 1965.

Pluckhan, M. L.: Human Communication, The Matrix of Nursing. McGraw-Hill Book Co., New York, 1972, Chap. 2.

Puksta, N. S.: All about sex – after a coronary. Am. J. Nurs. 77: 602–605, 1977.

Rahe, R., and Arthur, R.: Life changes and illness studies. J. Hum. Stress 4:3–15, 1978.

Reichman, W.: The alcoholic stigma – in the eye of the beholder. Alcoholism Dig. 6: 5–6, 1977.

Richter, J. M.: Physical symptoms – a signal of distress in the family system. Top. Clin. Nurs. 1:31–40, 1979.

Roberts, S.: Behavioral Concepts and the Critically Ill Patient. Prentice-Hall, Inc. Englewood, 1976.

Robinson, L.: Liaison Nursing: Psychological Approach to Patient Care. F. A. Davis Co., Philadelphia, 1974, pp. 19–27.

Rogers, B. J., and Mengel, A.: Communicating with families of terminal cancer patients. Top. Clin. Nurs. 1: 55–61, 1979.

Rosel, N.: Toward a social theory of dying. Omega, J. Death Dying 9:49–55, 1978–79.

Sanford, S., and Paul, L.: Dying in a hospital intensive care unit: the social significance for the family of the patient. Omega, J. Death Dying 8:29–40, 1977.

Satir, V: Psychology of Self-Esteem. Bantam Books, New York, 1971.

Satir, V.: Peoplemaking. Science and Behavior Books, Inc., Palo Alto, 1972.

Satterfield, S. B., and Stayton, W. R.: Understanding sexual function and dysfunction. Top. Clin. Nurs. 1:21-32, 1980

Scalzi, C., and Dracup, K.: Sexual counseling of coronary patients. Heart Lung 7:840–845, 1978.

Seligman, M. E. P.: Submissive death: giving up on life. Psychol. Today 10:80–85, 1974.

Selye, H.: Stress Without Distress. J. B. Lippincott Co., Philadelphia, 1974.

Selye, H.: The Stress of Life. McGraw-Hill Book Co., New York, 1956.

Shneidman, E. S.: On the Nature of Suicide. Jossey-Bass, San Francisco, 1970.

Shneidman, E. S.: Deaths of man. Penguin Books, Inc. Baltimore, 1973.

Shontz, F.: Body image and its disorders. In Lipowski, Z., Lipsitt, D., and Whybrow, P. P. (eds): Psychosomatic Medicine: Current Trends and Clinical Applications. Oxford University Press, New York, 1977, pp. 150–161.

Shubin, S. Prescription for stress – your stress. Nursing 9:52–55, 1979.

Slater, P.: The Pursuit of Loneliness. Beacon Press, Boston, 1970.

Slocum, J. W., Susman, G. I., and Sheridan, J. E.: An analysis of need satisfaction and job performance among professional and paraprofessional hospital personnel. Nurs. Res. *21*:338–341, 1972.

Smith, M. J. T., and Selye, H.: Reducing the negative effects of stress. Am. J. Nurs. *79*:1953–1955, 1979.

Stevens, B. J.: A phenomenological approach to understanding suicidal behavior. J. Psychiatr. Nurs. *9*:33–35, 1971.

Stewart, J.: Bridges Not Walls. Addison-Wesley, Reading, 1972.

Stone, L. J., and Church, J.: Childhood and Adolescence—a psychology of the Growing Person. Random House, Inc. New York, 1975.

Tierney, E.: Accepting disfigurement when death is the alternative. Am. J. Nurs. *75*:2149–2150, 1975.

Vaillot, C.: Hope: the restoration of being. Am. J. Nurs. *70*:268–273, 1970.

Wepman, B. Pain as an interpersonal device. Psychosomatics *20*:561–562, 1979.

Whitley, M. P., and Willingham, D.: Adding a sexual assessment to the health interview. J. Psychiatr. Nurs. *16*:17–27, 1978.

Wise, T.: Sexual difficulties with concurrent physical problems. Psychosomatics *18*:56–64, 1977.

Yura, H., and Walsh, M. B.: Human Needs and the Nursing Process. Appleton-Century-Crofts, New York, 1978.

INDEX